TEDDY L. LANGFORD

Dean and Professor
School of Nursing
Texas Tech University Health Sciences Center
Lubbock, Texas

MANAGING AND BEING MANAGED

preparation for

REINTEGRATED PROFESSIONAL NURSING PRACTICE

LANDOVER PUBLISHING CO.
Lubbock, TX 79453

Library of Congress Cataloging Data
Langford, Teddy.
   Managing and being managed
   Preparation for reintegrated professional nursing practice
Includes bibliographies and index.
1. Nursing. 2. Nursing service administration.
3. Reintegration

ISBN 0-9626604-1-8

Editorial /production supervision by Mike Overbey
Interior design by Mike Overbey
Cover design by Kathy Hinson, Hinson Graphics
Printing by Evans Press, Ft. Worth, Texas

Printed in the United States of America

Contents

Preface to the first edition

The days when "ward management" meant knowing how to make out time sheets and when to make rounds are gone forever. Management for nursing care must now be sufficiently broad to provide the professional nurse with the skill to manage nursing in a variety of settings and retain nursing as the primary focus. This book begins at the level of the individual and moves to consider others in health care, the setting for care, and the processes and practical activities involved in managing and improving care. In this way, numerous topics of current and continuing interest, including motivation, group conferences, assignments and staffing, staff development, and nursing audit, are presented.

This book is designed for three different course arrangements: the "management strand in several integrated courses" plan, a single nursing management course, and special-focus continuing education courses. For that reason, the arrangement of the book allows its separate parts to be used at different times in a student's program or all at once in a single course. Part One emphasizes persons, places, and relationships in the work setting. Individuals and their motivation and roles, the various settings where health care is delivered, and the relationships between individuals and among groups are each considered as they affect and are affected by the professional nurse. Processes and practical matters are the themes of Part Two. The nursing process, and planning, organizing, implementing, and evaluating as phases of a mangement process in nursing are detailed. Topics include organizational design, staffing, budgeting, supervision, evaluating care, and evaluating personnel. Staff development and planned change are two other important processes that complete this part. The final brief part returns to the individual professional nurse as the element of emphasis by offering help with seeking and choosing the first position of employment. Throughout, the dual roles of the professional nurse as manager and one who is managed are balanced to aid the student in adjusting to the world of work while retaining tthe professional concern with practice based on principle and theory.

If you notice that there are references to the nurse in the female gender, that is simply a reflection of fact (most nurses are female) along with my own concern that he/she or other forms are awkward. It in no way implies a sexist bias on my part.

If you are a student who reads this, I hope that you will question the content critically. Disagree, form new judgments based on your evidence, or move with and beyond the content to new areas. Talk about the material; do not memorize it. This book will only be useful if it serves as a guide for application in practice.

For graduates who read this text for continuing education, I recommend that you read the original sources cited and that you compare this book's content with monthly publications in professional journals. If you are stimulated to apply some of the content in this text, it will have been useful. If it prompts thought and causes you to ask questions, it will have been doubly useful.

Finally, I warn the faculty who use this as a text that this book is not Basic Management 301 translated into nursing. Rather, I have attempted to present a synthesis of principles that are widely applicable in management of nursing, leaving the basic course in theories of management to be taught in a school of business. The choice of content reflects my belief that in nursing we too often only translate from other fields, with no synthesis and, worse yet, no real critical examination.

I have not included behavioral objectives for the chapters because I believe that a particular learning experience, like a textbook, can meet a variety of objectives when combined with other experiences. The objectives met by text experiences alone are much more fundamental than those required for competent practice. (In the accompanying instructor's manual, I have suggested a variety of objectives and related uses of this text.) The best fit between your curriculum and this text will be made when you, rather than I, make the choices about sequence and use of the material here.

I hope that this text will be used in courses with extensive clinical activity and that you will require that the text's information be used as a prerequisite to attending classes that are conducted as debates, discussion, seminars, and simulation, rather than only lectures and note-taking activities.

Writing this book has been a learning experience for me. I hope that using it will be for others.

Acknowledgments

Many individuals have contributed to the preparation of this text in a variety of subtle ways. Others' efforts were more direct, in the form of reading and commenting on the manuscript at the editor's request. The assistance of those reviewers is gratefully acknowledged. They are R. Evelyn Harper, R.N., M.S.N.. Ed.D., Associate Professor, University of Tennessee at Martin; Yvonne M. Abdoo, R. N., M.S.N., Assistant Professor, The University of Michigan School of Nursing; Ruth Beckmann Murray, R.N., M.S.N., Professor, St. Louis University School of Nursing; Dorothy E. Sassenrath, M.S. N., Associate Clinical Professor, St. Louis University School of Nurisng and Educational Specialist, Veterans Administration Regional Medical Education Center, St. Louis, Missouri; Ann McCormack, R.N., R.S.N., M.S., Instructor and Coordinator for Nursing Education, St. Louis University School of Nursing, St. Louis Veterans Administration Medical Center; Professor Judy Sands, School of Nursing, American University, Washington, D.C.; and Carole A. Shea, R.N., M.S., Assistant Professor, College of Nursing, Rutgers, The State University of New Jersey.

Teddy L. Langford

Preface to the second edition

Since the publication of the first edition, in 1981, the world of the professional nurse has changed in many ways. The economic situation in health care has influenced the acuity of patients receiving care in hospitals and nursing homes. They are returning home earlier in their course of illness and the care in homes is no longer only for convalescence or for chronic illness. Acute care has moved into the home and the nursing home as well. A nationwide shortage of nurses has prompted efforts to improve recruitment to the field and to retain those already in practice. Nurse executives are developing methods to cope with the shortage of staff while attempting to provide effective, safe care. Many nursing managers have found opportunity in this adversity. These leaders have used the crisis to gain increased salaries for staff, to explore practice arrangements which are more professionally satisfying to nurses and to impress on their Boards of Trustees and CEOs the value of professional staff in the overall viability of the agency.

But, much remains constant for the beginning professional nurse. This nurse is entering a field where one is both manager and managed in some respects, even in the entry level positions. And while the work of the nurse may demand even greater technological knowledge to deal with medical treatment, the recipient of care is still the same human for whom we have always cared. The work environment may be changed -- more competition between facilities, new equipment, more computers. But the principles of management applied to our work are the same as in 1981, even while new roles for workers in nursing and new patterns of delivery have been developed.

As a result, some of this edition's content has been changed very little from the prior edition. Of course, updating has been accomplished in each chapter. Material on supervision has been expanded, adding the issue of the impaired nurse. Content on conflict has been increased and introduces the topic of the difficult person. The chapter on planning has been reorganized. Peer review is also considered in the section on evaluation and self governance is addressed. Also, new content, on leadership and on the concept of Reintegration, has been added because I am convinced that this provides useful guidance for one's professional career development and planning.

Managing and Being Managed is still directed first to the student of nursing, the developing professional. Its organization retains the characteristics of the earlier edition, making it useful for various curriculum patterns. I have learned that this text is useful for nurses in practice as well, in nursing homes and in hospitals.

The years between the first and second editions have taught me much. Part of what I have learned is that the professional nurse is a precious resource for our nation's health. I hope that those who are becoming that nurse and those who are continuing to develop as that nurse will find this book useful.

Acknowledgements

This edition benefitted from the groups of students and faculty at Texas Tech University Health Sciences Center who used and critiqued the book during the past several years. They were direct and liberal with their input. Many colleagues have encouraged me with their positive comments about my beliefs about management and administration, thus confirming many elements reflected in this book. Mike Overbey and Judy French also deserve special thanks for their work in preparation of this manuscript.

TLL

PART I

Managing Nursing Care: Persons, Places, and Relationships

● The Individuals in the Work Setting

This first section begins with a view of the individuals who work in health care settings. Chapter 1 focuses on basic concepts of motivation and role development as these relate first to you, the reader, the becoming professional, and more broadly then to others at work. Chapter 2 describes some of the other workers in health care facilities.

● The Environment for Work

Another level of concern, in learning to be both manager and managed as a professional nurse, is the setting in which practice is carried out. Chapter 3 describes the different categories of health care facilities and Chapter 4 moves to the specific aspects of agencies that have the greatest effect on the nurse's professional functions.

● Relationships in the Work Setting

Chapters 5 through 9 provide information on important aspects of interaction among those employed in the work setting, information that is basic to understanding the behavior of these individuals at work. This understanding can mark the critical difference between being able to function effectively as a manager of nursing care instead of just applying management methods in "cookbook" fashion.

Chapter 1

You, the professional nurse

"The professional nurse." This phrase seems to imply that there is an identifiable package that comprises the person you are becoming. If this were true, the task of schools of nursing would be relatively simple. They would merely identify the beliefs, values, knowledge, and skills required. They would then choose students who have these basic attributes, polish them with some learning experiences, and turn out the finished product-"the professional nurse." However, in a society where individual differences are recognized and generally are encouraged, it is no surprise to find that the professional nurse is many people. One aspect of becoming the professional nurse is to have a concept of a desirable professional role. Another aspect is to acquire the basic skills for each element of the professional role as you may choose to develop it. This text focuses on presenting one general view of basic elements of the professional role and on developing useful skills for a subrole, manager of nursing care. This chapter presents an overview of the concept of the Reintegrated Professional Nurse role. And it also presents perspectives for understanding yourself as one who will be both a manager and the one who is managed in the work setting. The facts, principles, and theories presented here are intended to serve as a lens for introspection. This approach is based on the premise that an understanding of oneself and of the rights and obligations of one's own roles is a firm basis for working effectively with others.

Reintegrated Professional Nurse Role, An Overview

Simply put, the concept "Reintegrated Professional Nurse Role" states that any professional nursing role should bring together the elements of the profession that were historically integral parts of the role. They include a clinical practice aspect, an educative function, scholarly activity, and community service. The notion is that one's professional role transcends the specific job and that while the job may expect role activities only in some portion of these role areas, the professional should develop her/his role to encompass at least these basic elements.

The process of bringing together parts to form a new whole. Reintegration of the professional nurse role assumes that a professional nursing role always should have at least the following elements regardless of the position or practice site:

- Clinical
- Educative
- Scholarly /Systematic Inquiry
- Community Service

Figure 1.1 Elements of the Reintegrated Professional Nurse Role

---

The larger emphasis of this text, the managerial function, is often an aspect of the position expectation in the clinical aspect of one's professional role. Managerial skills may also benefit functional abilities in the other three basic role areas. Thus, while you are a student. you have not completed your initial development of basic professional role, you are assembling the parts; the concept of the role elements, the skills of subroles. As you complete this text, in the final chapter, you will consider Reintegration further, as you contemplate moving into your first professional position, or if you are now in practice as you begin to redefine yourself as a professional, a Reintegrated Professional Nurse.

The nursing role, over the past several decades has become increasingly divided. As a result of efforts to develop specializations, and to improve the scientific and educational base of the field, division has occurred. Nurses in education have emphasized their role as educators to the exclusion of their clinical function. Nurses in clinical roles have felt estranged from their scholarly roots and have seen researchers who did not participate in clinical practice begin to develop the science of nursing. Individuals often have viewed their jobs as their only necessary contribution to their community. New roles have developed.

Nurse clinicians, clinical specialists, nurse practitioners are descriptions common in literature since the 1960s. Each of these changes has had its positive aspects. Perhaps they were a necessity if nursing were to develop as a professional field. But a negative aspect of this evolution has been a separation of elements of the professional nursing role. In the 1970s, a small number of nurses working in education began to call for "Unification", seeking a union of nursing service and nursing education.[1] That call emphasized creating organizational roles that expected both clinical and educational aspects. The concept of Reintegration goes beyond that emphasis on organizational roles. It focuses on the expectation that the individual professional nurse should enter practice, in whatever setting, with the commitment to creating her/his own personal professional role as one with at least four core elements. Those elements are the clinical, the educative, the scholarly, and the community service aspects. As nurses bring these personal role expectations, they will affect the organizations and the positions that are within them.

Motivation

It is a quite likely that by the time you encounter this book, you will have studied at least a survey of general psychology and perhaps a general course in management. In doing so, you will have gained some information about current theories of human motivation. No theory is yet sufficiently explicit to predict all behavior. However, there are several approaches that can serve as a basis for understanding the differences as well as the similarities among individuals in nursing. A look at some of these theories follows.

Most current ideas on motivation are compatible with the basic model shown in Fig. 1.2. In the diagram is depicted the relationship between the

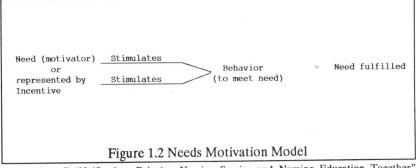

Figure 1.2 Needs Motivation Model

1 Nayer,D."Unification: Bringing Nursing Service and Nursing Education Together" *American Journal of Nursing* 80,6:1110-1114

need (or motive), the behavior, and the goal that represents need fulfill-ment. It is important to note that in this model, motivation comes from within the individual. Choice of behavior as well as choice of goal may be influenced by other persons, but the initial need is within the person. Objects or even activities may represent the fulfillment of a need for a person. For example, if a child needs parental approval and approval has come to mean a bar of candy from the parent, then the candy bar may become an *incentive*. That is, the possibility of receiving it may prompt certain behavior. The motivation is within the child, the child's need for approval. The *incentive* appeals to the child's desire to meet that need. Given the general view of motivation represented by this diagram, the distinction between *motivation* and *incentive* is an important one.

In his text on motivation, Ross Buck provides a very good overview of scientific work on motivation.[2] He uses what he calls "a developmental-interactionist view of motivation and emotion.This view holds that "cogni-tive and physiological factors interact in producing behavior often undergo-ing relatively independent developmental histories."[3] Taking this into ac-count, one must recognize the "need" in the model in Fig. 1.2 can be constituted though a variety of either or both cognitive and physiological bases. The more carefully it is examined, the more complex the relationship of behavior and motivation is found to be.

Theories dealing with human motivation, particularly those focusing on motivation in work settings, can be viewed as being of two sorts: (1) the *universal* type theory is one that purports to explain behavior in absolute terms; that is, "All persons behave in this fashion for the following reasons." (2) The *contingency* theories provide for explanations that are more situa-tion-specific; that is, "Under these circumstances, individuals with these attributes will respond in this fashion." In addition, the nature of a theory may be either *normative*, describing what *should be; predictive,* suggesting what *will be;* or *descriptive*, relating what the theorist believes *is.* The theories that are examined here, related to work behavior, vary also in that some were developed from a general perspective while others focus specif-ically on motivation in the work setting. Abraham Maslow's theory[4] dealing with basic needs as motivators is an example of the general perspective approach while Herzberg, Mausner, and Snyderman considered motivation at work.[5]

[2] Ross Buck,*Human Motivation and Emotion*(New York: John Wiley, 1976).
[3] Ibid., p. 6.
[4] Abraham Maslow, *Motivation and Personality*(New York: Harper & Row, 1954).
[5] Frederick Herzberg, Bernard Mausner, and Barbara Bloch Snyderman, *The Motivation to Work*, 2nd ed. (New York; John Wiley, 1959)

Maslow's Hierarchy of Needs

Maslow proposed a theory of human needs that has been widely discussed. The primary element of this theory is the notion that basic needs motivate all human behavior. Further, the needs of the individual are viewed as being arranged in a hierarchical fashion. This hierarchy is intended to indicate that needs at the lower level serve as motivators until they are met. Once this lower level is met, the needs at the next level are the source of action. According to Maslow, the hierarchy ascends from physiological survival needs to safety, to love, to esteem, to the highest level-the self-actualization need. The physiological level of need is what causes the individual to seek the basic requirements of food, water, shelter, etc. to sustain the body.[6]

Maslow's work implies that in today's United States, the basic needs are seldom the ones that are directly operating in the individual at work since most persons' survival needs are met. Although this may be true in the largest sense, in reference to you as a professional nurse, there is reason to question whether it is true for all the personnel with whom you work. For example, there are many women working as nurse's aids who are the sole support of their children. In order to supply food, shelter, and heat before any other necessities, these women work at jobs that are often difficult. Many of them will tell you that it is precisely the need to provide for themselves and their family that brings them to work.

The safety needs are related to the desire to be free from threats to both physical and psychological security. Following these needs in the hierarchy is the need for love and belonging, that is, the social needs. This level of need is associated with the wish to have close, meaningful interpersonal relationships. The next level is the esteem need or ego need, which develops the individual's desire to gain a feeling of personal worth through feeling competent, knowledgeable, and self-confident. Clearly, much of this estimate of self is derived from the response of others to one's appearance, behavior and communication.

The self-actualization need is at the pinnacle of Maslow's hierarchy. The need is defined as the urge to become the most that one can be. This has been interpreted in a variety of ways. Most interpretations describe the need as one to function in a creative fashion in some aspects of life. The main elements of Maslow's theory are as follows.[7]

1. Human behavior is motivated by unmet needs.

6 Maslow, *Motivation and Personality.*
7 Ibid.

2. Human needs can be viewed as forming a hierarchy, the most basic needs at the base and the self-actualization needs at the pinnacle. This hierarchy is often pictured as a pyramid.
3. An individual can be viewed as behaving in order to meet one level of needs until that level is met or is relatively consistently met. When that occurs, the next higher level of needs becomes the major motivator. Maslow also indicates that an individual can be fixated (permanently stopped in development) at any certain level.

Obviously, statement 3 bears careful consideration. Just because a person consistently has food, water, and shelter, he does not cease to seek them. Rather, the point is that when that need is consistently met, the individual is free to be motivated by the next level of need. This point is basic to making use of the theory in your role as a manager. Identifying the level of need at which an individual is operating may enable you to arrange opportunities for that person to see certain work activities as meeting the particular level of need that is operant.

Another implication is that the individual may move from one level of need to another, perhaps during the period of his employment. For that reason, frequent reassessment of individuals' performances can provide clues to when new needs may be operating or when work activities no longer provide fulfillment of the needs that are primary.

As mentioned before, the ultimate value of the theory is in its ability to provide a framework for analysis of a phenomenon and for prediction in regard to that phenomenon. With these purposes in mind, use Maslow's theory to examine the following situation.

> Alice Ralston, newly licensed as a registered nurse (RN) seven months ago, has been working since graduation ten months ago as a staff nurse in the city health department. She was assigned, until three months ago, to work with an experienced staff nurse. That nurse met with her daily and made several home visits with Alice each week. Alice also assisted the staff nurse in one of the well child clinics. She has learned recently that there is a need for school health visits in a school near her area. She has asked to be given the assignment even though it will mean more work with no increase in pay.

From the description, can you discern what need, according to Maslow's scheme, seems to be the major motivator of Alice's work behavior? If you speculated that the need motivating Alice is self-actualization, this would be consistent with much of what has been derived from Maslow's theory. This assumes, of course, that Alice views the extra activity as a means (instrumental) to become what she is best able to accomplish. However, the motivation may well be need for self-esteem or self-respect. If this is so, then if Alice's manager (supervisor) substituted an additional caseload of families because she could not make arrangements for the school activities, it might serve to meet that need. But the result might be quite different if the self- actualization need were the concern. This is particularly true if the "best school nurse" is what represents self- actualization to Alice. The addition of families and subsequent recognition through supervisory praise, good evaluations, and ultimately promotion might be quite acceptable to Alice if the self-esteem hypothesis is correct.

Now, for prediction. Again using Maslow's work, what would you expect to be the result of a staffing change that, through no fault of Alice's, places her under close, direct supervision again? One might speculate that the close attention could be viewed as satisfying if the operating need were self esteem. But, an equally plausible notion is that close supervision could imply a lack of trust and confidence in Alice by her supervisor and that she could find that decreases rather than increases the satisfaction of h er self esteem need. Thus, it is evident that prediction is not precise even though the idea of a hierarchy of needs seems simple and clear.

Given the ease with which Maslow's theory is understood, one might expect that it could provide clear-cut direction for understanding self and others in a variety of situations. However, there are some who have criticized the hierarchy of needs theory. Douglas Hall and Khalil Nougaim analyzed data collected from a group of managers at American Telephone and Telegraph.[8] These data were collected over a five-year period and therefore provided a longitudinal test of hypotheses derived from Maslow's theory. These authors suggested that one would expect need satisfaction at a lower level to be positively correlated with need intensity at the next higher level. Further, they anticipated that strength levels of needs would change over time with correlated satisfaction level changes for the same periods. Using this longitudinal method, which reflects the nature of the theory, the researchers found no support for their hypotheses. However, when the first- and fifth-year data were treated as separate groups, the results, were similar to other studies that have been cited as support for the "needs hierarchy." That is, the older, higher job-level men (fifth-year) were more concerned with affiliation, achievement and esteem, and self-actualization, and less

[8] Douglas T. Hall and Khalil Nougaim, "An Examination of Maslow's Need Hierarchy in an Organizational Setting," *Organizational Behavior and Human Performance 3 (1968), 12-35.*

concerned with safety than were the younger, lower job-level men (first-year).

This conclusion, however, takes into account only need strength rather than need satisfaction. These same researchers asked some thoughtful questions in the discussion section of their report. For example, Can people go down the hierarchy if they become dissatisfied at a higher level? Or, what time interval elapses between lower level need satisfaction and increased potency of a higher need? Is the change momentary or of long duration? The authors stated,

> *In a recent personal communication to one of the authors, Maslow has indicated that he conceives of a long time period between the emergence of the various need levels. He suggests that in the fortunate life history the safety needs are salient and satisfied during childhood, the affiliation needs during adolescence and the esteem needs during early adulthood. Only as a person nears his 50's generally, will the self- actualization needs become strongly salient.[9]*

This information is intriguing in its implications for the work setting. For example, age, if it predicts need level, might become an important factor in employee selection for particular positions.

Maslow himself indicated that management principles based upon his work may well need critical examination. This is because his hierarchy describes the emergence of the mature personality. However, not every individual in the work setting is proceeding toward such maturity. In a personal journal published as a book, Maslow wrote,

> *But now we can also add what should be the proper principle of management for a person who is not satisfied in these various ways? How about people who are fixated at the safety need level, who feel perpetually afraid, who feel the possibilities of catastrophe, for instance, of unemployment, etc.? What would management be like with people who could not identify with each other let's say as seems to be the case among the different classes in France, Germany, Italy, etc. at least much more so than in the United States?[10]*

Thus we can see that although Maslow's theory holds some worthwhile ideas, it is essentially *normative*, describing what the author believed could

---

9 Ibid., p. 32.
10 Abraham Maslow, *Eupsychian Management, A Journal* (Homewood, Ill.: Richard D. Irwin, Dorsey Press, 1965),p.16.

be true under ideal circumstances. It has also been viewed by some as *universal*, although comments by its author as cited above would question that view. For such reasons his theory cannot serve as the complete guide to understanding motivation or deriving management principles. But it can help us as we consider our own behavior and changes over time in those things for which we strive. And the idea of the needs hierarchy can help us recall that each of the employees with whom we work is different, if only by motivation, from each other.

Herzberg's Two Factor Theory

Frederick Herzberg, Bernard Mausner, and Barbara Snyderman proposed a theory regarding motivation and job satisfaction that has gained relatively wide acceptance.[11] Their work proposed that satisfaction and dissatisfaction on the job are the result of two entirely different sets of factors. The first group of factors, the *hygiene factors*, are those that, if present, can prevent dissatisfaction with work. But continued additions to these factors do not result in job satisfaction. The most that can be gained through attention to "hygiene" is the reduction of dissatisfaction, since satisfaction and dissatisfaction are viewed as varying along two separate continuums. The hygiene factors are those related to wages, physical surroundings, fringe benefits, policies, supervision, and job security.

The second group of factors, *motivators*, relate to job content. These are achievement in the job, recognition, the nature of the work itself, responsibility, and opportunity for advancement. These are factors that are theorized to promote job satisfaction and to serve as motivation to work. Thus it follows that the important activities of management should be directed toward meeting hygiene needs and toward increasing opportunities for the employee to participate in those activities that supply the "motivators." One method suggested for providing such opportunities is "job enrichment." This means that the responsibility or scope of function of the individual should be increased. There should be changes in the individual's job so that he can take part in the planning and control functions of the activity. Herzberg, Mausner, and Snyderman theorized that in this fashion the self-realization or actualization needs of the worker are met. [12] This is often confused with the practice of "job enlargement," which is effected by adding varied tasks at the same level. However, it is felt that enlargement is not particularly motivating for any length of time. Another method of

---

[11] Herzberg, Mausner, and Synderman, *The Motivation to Work*.
[12] Ibid., pp 132-134.

promoting satisfaction is to provide frequent recognition for individual achievement throughout the performance of the job.

Perhaps you can recall settings where you worked that you considered lacking in some of the "hygiene factors." Was this dissatisfying to you? Was it sufficiently dissatisfying to affect your performance, or were other factors motivating you to work there and to do your job well? Another question is whether your perception of what was an adequate level of those hygiene factors was the same as your coworkers. Again, taken alone, this theory leaves much behavior unexplained or unanticipated, possibly because it implies that motivation to work well arises entirely from factors in the work setting. But, we can each recall times when our work performance has been affected by factors at home. This illustrates that this theory, too, must be used for guidance, not as the basis for prediction of precise individual responses to organization conditions.

Theory X and Theory Y

The work of Douglas McGregor has also been widely cited.[13] In his book *The Human Side of Enterprise*, published in 1960, he attempted to support the assertion that the ideas that managers maintain about the "nature of man" determine the ways in which an enterprise will treat its workers. In developing this thesis he described the then current views of workers held by many managers. Although he had no statistical data, he said that management literature was filled with materials that support certain assumptions about human behavior that he labeled "Theory X." These assumptions were the basis for what he characterized as "restrictive practices," which cause workers to be unmotivated toward high-quality performance. Essentially, these assumptions view the worker, the "average human," as innately lazy, likely to avoid responsibility, and seeking security at all costs. Because of his dislike of work and of responsibility, the individual must be coerced, threatened, and directed in order to get work accomplished and obtain organizational objectives.

McGregor offered Theory Y as an enlightened basis for deriving managerial behavior. He did so with a cautionary note, one that has frequently been overlooked. It was contained in the conclusion of the book. He said,

It is not important that management accept the assumptions of Theory Y. These are one man's interpretation of current social science knowledge, and they will be modified- possibly supplemented by-new knowledge within a short

[13] Douglas McGregor, *The Human Side of Enterprise* (New York: McGraw- Hill, 1960).

time. It is important that management abandon limiting assumptions like those of Theory X, so that future invention with respect to the human side of enterprise will be more than minor changes in already obsolescent conceptions of organized human effort.[14]

He also acknowledged the normative nature of his work when he stated,

Theoretical assumptions such as those of Theory Y imply some conditions which are unrecognizable in practice (like the perfect vacuum implied by physical theory). This is not a handicap; it is a stimulus to invention and discovery.[15]

The essence of McGregor's theory assumptions centered on an innate human desire to work and to be productive. Rather than requiring coercion, the human actually will work voluntarily and seek responsibility under the right work conditions. Further, he posited that at that time current industrial life required (or encouraged) the use of little of the intellectual and creative ability of workers. In the right atmosphere, according to Theory Y, workers willingly commit to the objectives of the organization when they perceive those objectives to be related to personal rewards.

It is noteworthy that McGregor's rationale for this view depended heavily on the orientation Maslow proposed, which cited a need hierarchy. McGregor's ideas about the "appropriate" assumptions regarding human nature encouraged extensive suggestions about managers' behavior. For example, to capitalize on the workers' willingness to commit themselves to organizations whose objectives are congruent with theirs, the workers are to be more fully informed of plans and objectives. Managers should learn to communicate fully and to encourage workers to do the same. The manager should design methods to provide positive rewards that will stimulate achievement and meet higher needs for the accomplishment of work.

Management literature and practice have been profoundly influenced by this humanistic view of human nature, so eloquently propounded by McGregor. Louis Allen wrote of this influence,

The current crop of MBA's[16] *about to enter business organizations has been more thoroughly indoctrinated than any previous groups, and they are bringing*

[14] Ibid., p. 245.
[15] Ibid., p. 245.
[16] Ibid., p. 47.
*Master of Business Administration. [Allen's footnote]

with them an implicit belief that traditional "authoritarian" methods are ineffective and obsolete. As sincerely as they urged diversification, the virtues of the conglomerate, and quantitative methods a few years ago, many managers returning from advanced management courses are recommending Theory Y and its concomitant sensitivity training or 'O.D.,' self- actualization and job enrichment.[17]

Theory Z

Most of the assumptions about individual motivation are implicit rather than explicitly stated in the work of William Ouchi which he entitled Theory Z.18 While his work focuses on description of Japanese industrial management as related to its high productivity, certain elements of the Japanese method convey certain assumptions about the worker. These assumptions are derived from key factors such as the concept of mutual commitment of worker and the company; an almost organic relationship between the worker and h is fellow workers and managers; creating a shared culture in which superordinate company goals are shared and become intensified; extensive participation of all levels of workers in discussing and examining decisions in process; and the use of problem solving groups of workers of all levels (which have come to be cailed Quality Circles). The use of these approaches along with the high productivity of representative Japanses firms suggest that workers are motivated to work toward company goals when:

1. They are secure in knowing they have long term security in their jobs and

2. Their compensation includes bonuses based on company productivity and

3. They have the opportunity to participate in extensive discussions of decisions in the process of being made.

Since all industry, including health care is keenly interested in high productivity, a great deal of interest was generated by Ouchi's work. Quality Circles have been included in many hospitals. Other facilities have made changes in their decision processes. But, as with other theories, which deal with "how people behave at work and/or why" caution is needed in its application. The major concern is that the issue of culture must be addressed. The Japanese culture and the predominant American culture are different. That cultural aspect is probably a determinant of the fact that in the U.S., mobility from company to company is often viewed as positive for

[17] Lewis A. Allen, "M for Management: Theory Y Updated," *Personnel Journal* (December 1973:, p. 1062. ['O.D.' is the acronym for Organizational Development--author's note.]

both worker and company, consistent with our emphasis on individualism and personal mobility. Because of that cultural difference, the strong mutual lifetime commitment of worker and company is not a major factor in the work life of many U.S. workers. But with caution in mind about "wholesale" application of assumptions and methods, a manager can examine both and find them instructive.

Contingency Models

In a more recent attempt to provide a theoretical basis for both administrative structure and managerial behavior, a body of work called *contingency models* has been developed. More descriptive than normative in its foundation, this approach also speaks to human motivation and its interaction with organizational structure and the nature of the work task as influencing behavior in work settings. This followed the work of Paul Lawrence and Jay Lorsch which brought together a number of ideas regarding how successful organizations in several fields could vary widely in structure and managerial practice.[18] The results were the beginning of "Contingency Theory." Developing this theory from its organizational focus to include concerns about the individual, John Morse and Jay Lorsch stated new assumptions about human beings. [19] In a manner similar to McGregor, they suggest that accepting these assumptions would pave the way for improved organizational functions. The assumptions are shown in Table 1.1.

TABLE 1.1   Contingency Theory Assumptions

---

1. Human beings bring varying patterns of needs and motives into the work organization, but one central need is to achieve a sense of competence.
2. The sense of competence motive, while it exists in all human beings, may be fulfilled in different ways by different people depending on how the need interacts with the strengths of the individual's other needs-such as those for power, independence, structure, achievement, and affiliation.
3. Competence motivation is most likely to be fulfilled when there is a fit between task and organization.
4. Sense of competence continues to motivate even when a competence goal is achieved; once one goal is reached, a new and higher one is set.

From John J. Morse and Jay W. Lorsch, "Beyond Theory Y," *Harvard Business Review, 68, No.3 (May-June, 1970), 67.*

[18] Paul R. Lawrence, and Jay W. Lorsch. *Organization and Environment* (Homewood, Ill.: Richard D. Irwin, 1969).

[19] John J. Morse and Jay W. Lorsch, "Beyond Theory Y," *Harvard Business Review*, Vol. 48, No. 3 (May-June 1970).

In relation to the individual-you or those with whom you work-this notion of motivation can be very important. Note that, unlike Maslow's, this contingency theory states that the need for a *sense of competence* is perpetual in its ability to stimulate action. The presence of other motives is acknowledged, and the writers warn against reading this to mean that all individuals are alike in their motivation. Rather, although each person will meet the need in his own way, the need for a sense of competence is possessed in some degree by everyone.

Using this set of assumptions, consider a work situation with which you are familar. Can you recall encountering a worker who seemed uncomfortable with being *unable* to do the work? When choosing a job, do you tend to seek one that you believe you can perform or one that is likely to be impossible for you? Your answers will help you evaluate the usefulness of the theory's assumption from a personal, empirical standpoint. Further study of research on this topic will provide a more scientific basis for your choice of action.

As you can see from the previous paragraphs, the subject of human motivation is extremely complex, yet very important in learning how to function in work relationships. Given the numerous theories, their similarities and major differences, it is useful to attempt to extract some general guidelines.

1. Human behavior is meaningful, is motivated by needs and desires. There are wide variations among individuals in their pattern of motivation.
2. Values and beliefs affect what a person views as appropriate or as achievable means to meeting needs, as well as influencing the priority placed on various needs.
3. The culture or subculture of the individual has an effect on the values and beliefs of the individual and therefore upon need-related behavior.
4. Work and the work setting can provide means instrumental to meeting some of those needs and desires.
5. The work assignment and the physical and social environment of work can be organized in ways that will increase the possibility of the workers' gaining satisfaction of needs and desires through work.
6. Because of differences in motivation (needs, desires, work, and environment), it is *not* true that any individual can "fit" any organization and vice versa.
7. The idea of general, long-term goals' being incentives related to motivating needs must be connected to the notion of specific "today" needs and

related activity. Long-term and present goals may reflect conflicting motives. We are not always entirely logical in our behavior.

In subsequent chapters, the use of these ideas as the basis for action as manager or as one who is managed will be explained in greater detail.

You as Manager
or as One Who Is Managed

At this point it is worthwhile for you to take a few minutes to consider your own motivation. What has prompted you to choose professional nursing as a career? Has the activity or goal (nursing) remained the same, or has the motive changed at any time since you began school? Are there more immediate needs that interfere with your motivation to become a nurse? Can you project what might interfere with your motivation to practice as a nurse? Time spent in introspection is time well spent. As you function in the work setting, you will find that as your understanding of self increases, so does your ability to understand others whose patterns of motivation and behavior may be very different from others. So stop for a few minutes and actively consider yourself.

The answers to the questions posed above can be viewed from two perspectives. As one responsible for the work of others, you may be able to develop analogies from your own experience to understand the behavior of coworkers. From that basis of understanding you can help to choose assignments, share information, evaluate positively, and possibly even recommend transfer or termination to help the worker see that his work can meet his needs.

As one who is managed by others, you can also be aided by this knowledge of motivation. Aware of the needs that have priority for you, you can request work assignments that will help you meet your goals. For example, you can be candid with your supervisor about the fact that you are presently having some interpersonal problems with your spouse, and you could indicate that although you do not intend in any way to let your performance deteriorate, you would appreciate not being asked to present staff development conferences for a few weeks. Or, because you understand your own desire to achieve, you might ask to be assigned as primary nurse to the newly admitted patient with Reyes Syndrome. Through caring for this challenging patient you may be able to increase your own self-esteem.

Roles

The fact that you have chosen to become a professional nurse indicates that you are aware that there is a need for various individuals to fulfill different primary functions. There is a need for specialization and differentiation. In our complex world, there are few who can claim the ability to meet all of their own needs without any assistance or support. Even the most reclusive person, one who is purposely avoiding the support of either friend or family, will have need of food or other items produced by other persons. As a result of the interdependence our would creates, we live and work as specialists, in some sense of the word. We come to expect that others will do the same, thus providing for our mutual benefit. This is, at the societal level, the basis for the idea of "roles." Each of the jobs that individuals hold carries with it certain expectations both within its own work context and in the society at large. Attorneys are expected to know the law, to be able to reason clearly, and to provide legal counsel for their clients; and society at large tends to expect leadership to accrue to these persons. Thus, the individual called "attorney" is cast into a certain role by the public.

Similarly, the professional nurse has a number of expectations cast upon her as she begins to enter practice. These *role expectations* are defined not only by "others" but also by the person who is the "actor." There is no reason to assume that both parties will have entirely similar expectations of what the term *nurse* means. The manner in which the individual performs is called *role performance.* The individual's performance will reflect not only his own conception of his position but also the conception of what he feels to be the norms defined by society for that role.

When there is disparity between the conceptions of the role held by two parties (one the actor), the result is *role conflict.*

Abraham Zaleznik gives an example of an interpersonal role conflict as that which results when "two or more individuals fail to establish a reciprocal role relationship," such as between a parent and an adolescent child who is testing independence.[20] In that same chapter, Zaleznik also points out that *role ambiguity* is another source of discomfort for a person.[21] This exists when the role is relatively undefined in general or undefined in relation to a particular situation. The nurse functioning in an ambulatory care setting, such as in a chronic disease clinic, provides an example. In the

---

[20] Abraham Zaleznik, "Interpersonal Relations in Organizations," in James G. March, ed.,*Handbook of Organization* (Skokie, Ill,: Rand-McNally, 1965,p. 589.
[21] Ibid., p. 589.

past, the nurse's role in such a setting was rather circumscribed, coordination and basic data collection. The development of nurse practitioner roles changed the view of what might be appropriate roles for nurses in primary health care. The fact that these roles have been demonstrated to be both beneficial for health care recipients and for nurses has firmly placed them in the health care delivery system. Their success has prompted additional exploration by other nurses who are now exploring different ways of using their knowledge and akills. Where the role of nurse practitioner was once the source for role ambiguity, now there are also nurse case managers developing a role. This continuing development and the resulting ambituity can make practice both exciting and uncomfortable. An interesting accompaniment of ambiguity is the attempt to cope through "naming"; the ambiguous role is given a new title that signifies the opportunity to attach new meaning. The new title generally carries some element of the name applied to the role from which the position grew or was derived. In the situation just mentioned, the role is entitled *nurse practitioner.*

Thus role theory, explained here only in its most elemental form, provides an excellent means for analyzing much social interaction. One further concept from the body of theory is that an individual generally functions in *multiple roles.* This means that one may be variously and simultaneously nurse, parent, city council member, and spouse. It is easy to imagine ways in which these roles can create contradictory demands. The result again is *role conflict.* This type of role conflict tends to create a *tension within the individual,* rather than interpersonal role conflict as discussed previously. The natural reaction to this is to develop or utilize some tension-reduction mechanism. Dysfunctional tension-reduction efforts may take the form of panicky flight from the situation, physically and/or mentally, or development of psychosomatic ailments or depression- to mention a few of the less desirable reactions. The tension certainly represents a motivating force. Depending on which theoretical view is used, it might represent a threat to self- esteem (Maslow) or a threat to the sense of competence (Morse and Lorsch). The action taken to reduce the tension of role conflict is probably related to a number of factors, which include past experience in similar situations, personal ideals, and interactional style.

A person whose situation and style are such that he/she wishes to resolve role conflict in a productive manner has a number of options. Suppose that you have recently been married. Your spouse works 8 a.m. to 5 p.m. weekdays. Your position is in a long-term care facility where your hours are 7:30 a.m. to 4 p.m. and you rotate days off, working every other weekend. Increasingly, recently, your spouse has begun to make comments about your not being home on weekends to enjoy sports activities and to be together as a couple. You find yourself dreading a work weekend and note that you are increasingly irritable both at work and at home. *Multiple roles* are conflicting in the demands placed on you by others defining the roles. Perhaps there is some *ambiguity* in one or both of your roles as well. Does your spouse view your proper role performance as requiring that you be available for recreational activity all day every weekend? Does your definition of your role require that? Does your definition of the nurse's role include working on weekends? Obviously, the long-term care facility's definition does.

Now for the options. Assume that you wish to maintain both roles. *Explicit negotiation* is one alternative for dealing with role ambiguity. Perhaps it would work in this situation. This assumes that some changes, compatible with some of the parties involved, can be made. For example, can your spouse make some change of days off or plan for hobby activity on your work weekends? Will discussion help to clarify the importance to you of this particular position in your professional career? Only careful thought on your part, along with an effort at negotiation, can help resolve the problem.

Or take another approach. Is this particular position important to your career? Can you develop to your satisfaction in another environment with different scheduling? This represents another tactic, which is to *abandon* some function or mode of *behavior* of a role in order to reduce the conflict. An extreme example might be to abandon your spouse in the situation. The choice of such change to reduce conflict is related, obviously, to the importance attached to that activity within the role as well as to the role itself and the other roles with which there is conflict. This example also demonstrates a situation where *role clarification* could have been useful as a preliminary activity. That is, before a particular role is assumed, the expectation of the important parties can be made explicit. The "actor" can then determine whether difficult conflicts will result from the combination of roles. The choice to assume multiple roles can then be made with a clearer understanding of the tension that may be encountered.

Another potential for role conflict arises from the expectation related to sex roles. As with certain other roles, sex role performance varies among cultures. For example, in India, the traditional female role in relation to males has been one of dutiful submission. That sort of role definition would be at odds with the expectation of assertive behavior currently encouraged for professional nurses in the United States. The Indian female nurse coming to function in the United States thus may suffer conflict and be dysfunctional in one or more of her roles. Can you identify any other examples of cultural differences in role expectations?

Generalizing about roles is a form of *stereotyping*; that is, one assumes (1) that his own conception of a particular role is accurate descriptively, and (2) that all persons in that role will (should) perform the role in that fashion. Stereotyping is a behavior that is not specific to ideas about role. As a rather convenient form of conceptual categorization, we tend to form sterotypes about many things, such as ideas, racial or ethnic groups, and places. It is probably a mental response representing an attempt to sort into convenient "storage bins" the huge amount of stimuli we receive daily. The fallacy in relying on stereotypes is that they represent generalizations that are frequently based on limited experience about the target-idea-role-group. Unless it is tempered with objectivity, sterotyping can lead to unfair judgment, which can hamper the realization of individual potential. Sex role stereotyping is an example. Many people still hold a sex role stereotype that nurses are female and that males do not behave in the "soft" ways a nurse uses for some nursing care. As a result, that person may not accept care from a male who is a nurse or might discourage a male family member from entering the nursing field. Knowledge of concepts of role theory will not necessarily solve all of the problems that theory helps one to identify and understand. However, there are some possibilities for using theory to develop interactions. Marlene Kramer's book *Reality Shock* is a description of efforts to deal with still another type of role conflict.[22] This is the conflict resulting from the nurse's holding a "professional" role conception while working in a setting that values a bureaucratic role for the nurse. The difference between the two points of view is described as resulting in *role deprivation*. When the person is unprepared for the experience of deprivation, there is a tendency to suffer from what Kramer labels "reality shock." There is a careful distinction made between role deprivation and the reality shock response. "Reality Shock is not completely analogous to role deprivation. It is quite possible for a nurse to feel and report role deprivation and not be shocked by it."[23]

Using role theory and other social and psychological constructs, Kramer generated an eclectic theory. From that theory several hypotheses were developed and subsequently tested. These hypotheses resulted in the generation of extremely useful knowledge regarding the use of educational experience to prevent "reality shock" and its sequela. The educational experience is designed to acquaint the nurse-to-be with a variety of potential

[22] Marlene Kramer, *Reality Shock* (St. Louis, Mo.:C.V. Mosby,1974).
[23] Ibid., p. 24.

assaults to professional role values that will be encountered in the bureaucratic work setting. In addition, the student has opportunities to develop strategies to help integrate conflicting role demands. This is accomplished through a series of seminars, lectures, and written assignments in a fourphase program presented during the student's basic nursing education program. The effort is likened to an immunization, which in this case protects against "reality shock" and its accompanying negative effects.[24] This is a prime example of how knowledge of role theory can be helpful to you as a professional nurse.

Rights and Responsibilities

In choosing to become a professional nurse, you have assumed a special set of responsibilities, both legal and ethical. At the same time you retain your rights as an individual, as guaranteed by the Constitution, the Bill of Rights, and subsequent legislation. Among those rights that affect your professional function are the right to equal access to employment opportunity regardless of sex, race, or religion, and the right to due process of law in situations where one is terminated from employment. A further right is that of collective bargaining representation if you choose it. Other guarantees important in the work setting are the provisions of the Fair Labor Standards Act, which set requirements for overtime pay and a minimum wage, among other things. It is beyond the scope of this book to describe and explain the legal aspects of nursing practice, but it is important that you recognize that both privilege and responsibility are accorded to you as an individual and as a nurse, by the Constitution and by statute. The privileges and responsibilities of the professional nurse specific to each state are defined by the Nurse Practice Act of the state. It is to each nurse's benefit to be acquainted with the content and current interpretation of the state's practice act. Further, it is important to recall that law is not written in stone. As practice changes, both interpretation and law can change. Although law protects and directs, it need not confine practice absolutely since development of new statutes tends to follow rather than precede changes in practice. Changes in practice acts which follow the development of primary care nursing roles are examples of this.

Rules and regulations or statutes exist in many states to assure appropriate quality in advanced nursing practice. The focus of this type of regulation can include some or all nursing specialty roles, particularly those

24 Ibid.

which require post-basic education such as a Master's degree. Thus, the use of certain titles such as clinical specialist, nurse practitioner, and nurse clinician may be restricted to those meeting specific educational requirements. A clinical agency may designate job titles which describe particular roles. Often the titles relate to organizational management functions (e.g. head nurse, nurse manager, clinical director). Other titles describe particular clinical functions (e.g. clinical nurse specialist, clinical case manager). Each job title has its organization's specific responsibilities and qualifications. These organizational titles and requirements legally must be consistent with the Nurse Practice Act of the state and its related rules and regulations.

Ethical responsibilities carry a different sort of weight than legal ones. Accepting professional responsibility implies that one has recognized and continues to consider the dignity of human beings and the relationship of that concept to actions performed in the practice of nursing. Further, entering a professional field like nursing places one in the position of dealing frequently with ethical dilemmas, situations where one ethical concern counterposes another, producing a situation in which there is no clear right answer. In judgment in professional matters, one is guided by philosophical and religious principles developed throughout life. The profession of nursing in the U.S., through its professional organization, the American Nurses Association, has developed the Social Policy Statement This document declares the responsibility of nursing to affect individuals and groups as members of a society and to do so both through acts of direct care and through acts affecting the society at large. In addition, the organized profession produces and frequently reevaluates a Code for Nurses. It is reproduced in Table 1.2 for your consideration and discussion. Discussion is recommended since comparing one's views against another's is a technique helpful in clarifying personal positions on issues.

TABLE 1.2   Code for Nurses

Preamble

The *Code for Nurses* is based on belief about the nature of individuals, nursing, health, and society. Recipients and providers of nursing services are viewed as individuals and groups who posssess basic rights and responsibilities, and whose values and circumstances command respect at all times. Nursing encompasses the promotion and restoration of health, the prevention of illness, and the alleviation of suffering. The statements of the *Code* and their interpretation provide guidance for conduct and relationship in carrying out nursing responsibilities consistent with the ethical obligations of the profession and quality in nursing care.

CODE FOR NURSES

1. The nurse provides services with respect for human dignity and the uniqueness of the client unrestricted by considerations of social or economic status, personal attributes, or the nature of health problems.

2. The nurse safeguards the client's right to privacy by judiciously protecting information of a confidential nature.

3. The nurse acts to safeguard the client and the public when health care and safety are affected by incompetent, unethical, or illegal practice of any person.

4. The nurse assumes responsibility and accountability for individual nursing judgments and actions.

5. The nurse maintains competence in nursing.

6. The nurse exercises informed judgment and uses individual competency and qualifications as criteria in seeking consultation, accepting responsibilities, and delegating nursing activities to others.

7. The nurse participates in activities that contribute to the ongoing development of the profession's body of knowledge.

8. The nurse participates in the profession's efforts to implement and improve standards of nursing.

9. The nurse participates in the profession's efforts to establish and maintain conditions of employment conducive to high quality nursing care.

10. The nurse participates in the profession's effort to protect the public from misinformation and misrepresentation and to maintain the integrity of nursing.

11. The nurse collaborates with members of the health professions and other citizens in promoting community and national efforts to meet the health needs of the public.

Reprinted from American Nurses' Association, *Code for Nurses with Interpretive Statements* (Kansas City, Mo.: ANA, 1985). With permission of the American Nurses' Association.

SUMMARY

Views of the nature of human motivation form the basis of most theories of management. This chapter has begun this book with the perspective each of us finds most important, the self, by considering theories of motivation. Further, the expectations and obligations that belong to each one who is a professional nurse are discussed using role theory as well as the prescriptive statements of the Code for Nurses issued by the professional association.

Additional Reading

Billings, Carolyn V., "Employment Setting Barriers to Professional Actualization in Nursing", Nursing Management18, 11 (Nov., 1987)69-71

Callahan, Carol and Louise Wall, "Participative Management: A Contingency Approach" Journal of Nursing Administration 17, 9 Sept. , 1987) 9-14

Christman, Luther, "The Practitioner Teacher" Nurse Educator 4, 2:8-11

MacPhail, Janetta "Implementation and Evaluation of the Case Western Reserve University Unification Model" in Aiken, L. (Ed) Health Policy and Nursing Practice New York: McGraw Hill 1980, 229-241

Strader, Marlene "Adapting Theory Z to Nursing Management" Nursing Management18, 4 (April, 1987) 61-64

Ulrich, Robert "Herzberg Revisited: Factors in Job Dissatisfaction" Journal of Nursing Administration 8, 10 (Oct., 1978) 19-22

Wine, Julie and John Baird, "Improving Nursing Management and Practice Through Quality Circles" Journal of Nursing Administration 13,5 (May, 1983) 5-10

Chapter 2

Other health care workers

In the past several decades, health care has changed drastically. The changes in nursing have paralleled changes in medicine, in concepts of health, and in the expectations of the general public regarding health care. Many new occupational groups have been created. These health care groups have been created as a result of a recognition of two types of needs. The first type of need is that of support for the physicians and for other health professionals in the performance of their functions. Examples of the new groups are those frequently called *allied health* personnel. These include respiratory therapists, laboratory technologists, radiology technologists, and an array of others. Each of these groups provides assistance in the diagnostic or therapeutic activities of the physician or other health professionals.

The second type of need is that of specialized types of services for patients or their families or the arrangements to deliver those services. These specialized services have grown out of the tremendous increase in knowledge of science and technology that is now available for improving health and treating illness. This increase has created a sometimes narrow specialization in which members of an occupational group become expert in the treatment of one body system or part, such as podiatry, or one type of problem, such as speech pathology. The health care administrator is an example of one response to this proliferation of occupational groups. This person's function is to create and manage the systems that coordinate and deliver health care services to individuals and groups.

The very fact that these groups exist and that all deal with aspects of health services creates a potential for synergy for excellent health services. At the same time, it creates the possibility for conflict and misunderstanding between groups, based on conflicting goals, on territorial disputes, and on misperception based on lack of information about purposes, about functions, and about educational qualifications of each group. As a professional nurse, concerned with providing care and promoting the total well-being of the patient or family, you will have many occasions to collaborate with other health care personnel or to refer individuals to them for treatment or assistance. The following descriptions of the functions and background of selected groups provide only an overview. A yearly perusal of a professional journal in each field is an excellent way to stay informed of the trends in each field, as is discussion with members of the various fields. This sort of inquiry will make even clearer than can this text that there are many similarities among the groups and that there is a common concern for providing for all aspects of health care.

A further factor of the complex situation of health occupations is that the various stages of development of the different fields have created intraoccupational concerns that can limit the influence that the involved groups have on health care at any particular time. Finally, it is also possible that continued proliferation of new health care groups may serve to further fragment care and increase costs. The fragmentation may well be the by-product of increasingly narrow specialization, with the individual, family, or service becoming less and less relevant as a total entity. The increase in costs will be the result of increased institutional costs related to educating the specialists and to employing the graduates.

"Credentialing" Definitions

The method by which a person is designated as qualified for practice varies from one field to another. This variation is a source of confusion due to the fact that the various purposes of licensure and/or certification of individuals and accreditation and approval of schools are easily confused or misunderstood. A report on the issues related to various forms of "credentialing" in nursing has furnished the following definitions that will help clarify these concepts:[1]

Licensure: A process by which an agency of state government grants permission to individuals accountable for the practice of a profession to engage in the practice of that profession and prohibits all others from legally doing so. It permits use of a particular title. Its purpose is to protect the

---

[1] "The Study of Credentialing in Nursing: A New Approach," *Nursing Outlook* (April 1979), pp.266-269. (All definitions given here are based on this source.)

public by ensuring a minimum level of professional competence. Established standards and methods of evaluation are used to determine eligibility for initial licensure and for periodic renewal. Effective means are employed for taking action against licensees for acts of professional misconduct, incompetence, and/or negligence.

Registration: A process by which qualified individuals are listed on an official roster maintained by a governmental or nongovernmental agency. It enables such persons to use a particular title and attests to employing agencies and individuals that minimum qualifications have been met and maintained.

Certification: A process by which a nongovernmental agency or association certifies that an individual licensed to practice a profession has met certain predetermined standards specified by that profession for specialty practice. Its purpose is to assure various publics that an individual has mastered a body of knowledge and has acquired skills in a particular specialty.

Accreditation: The process by which a voluntary, nongovernmental agency or organization appraises and grants accredited status to institutions and/or programs or services that meet predetermined structure, process, and outcome criteria. Its purposes are to evaluate the performance of a service or educational program and to provide to various publics information upon which to base decisions about the utilization of the institutions, programs, service, and/or graduates. Periodic assessment is an integral part of the accreditation process in order to ensure continual acceptable performance. Accreditation is conducted by agencies that have been recognized or approved by an organized peer group of agencies as having integrity and consistency in their practices. (Note: In some states, a governmental agency conducts accreditation processes also. In those cases, the process usually is the basis for the agency's approval for the school to operate and prepare graduates elegible for licensure or registration.)

Approval: A process whereby one agency assesses the practices of another agency for consistency of procedural practices and for evidence of integrity in its conduct of business.

A requirement for individual licensure is designed, as noted above, to protect the public. It also assures for the occupational groups some degree of exclusivity and protection for the practitioners of the field against encroachment by unqualified persons. Depending on the state statutes, licensure can also provide for legal sanctions for improper practice. For these reasons many groups not originally required to be licensed have sought this requirement for their group. And, because of the need to balance the concern for protection of the public against the concern for the privileges granted to those licensed and the resulting reduced access to practice and potential economic effects on health care, state legislatures are slow to create additional categories of licensure.

Other Health Care Workers

The list of occupations involved in health care is extensive. The following sections contain descriptions of those that are most frequently encountered by nurses in various employment settings.

Doctors of Medicine and Osteopathic Medicine

More than 500,000 practitioners of medicine in the United States serve the function of diagnosing illness or prescribing appropriate therapy. Of the total number, approximately 40 percent are considered generalists, with the remainder practicing as specialists in the diseases of some body system (e.g., nephrology) or in some particular approach to diagnosis or therapy (e.g., radiology). Some medical schools admit students with fewer than three years of preprofessional education, but more than 90 percent of entering freshmen have completed four or more years of college. The preprofessional subject requirements vary by schools but usually include biology, organic and inorganic chemistry, and physics. The medical school curriculum is typically 149 weeks, arranged by varying calendars, with the first two periods (academic years) devoted mainly to basic natural and physical sciences and the latter two periods (academic years) primarily clinical. Upon awarding of the M.D. degree, the physician is eligible for national board examination and state licensure. Most physicians then enter residency training, also known as graduate medical education. These programs prepare the physicians for practice in a specialty and may be from three to seven years long.

The movement of medical education into universities and health sciences centers in the United States has been extensive only during the twentieth century. Although medicine as a profession is old, the confinement of its education to specified curriculum is a product of this century, with greater specificity in purpose and rigor in evaluation in the preclinical years than in the clinical phases of programs. A strong element of professional socialization exists in the programs, resulting in a sense of obligation and responsibility for all aspects of the diagnosis and treatment of the patient. It is not surprising that this socialization would encourage the perspective in the physician that he or she is in charge of directing and controlling the practice of all who engage in health care. If the socialization has been intense in this regard, the physician may encounter conflicts rather regularly as other practitioners attempt to function with a degree of autonomy and/or collaborativeness.

The same basic pattern of education holds for the osteopathic physician, although the number of schools is small. There are approximately 25,000 active practitioners, some 65 percent of whom are general practitioners. The academic program averages four academic years and has similar early requirements to those of schools that grant the M.D. degree. The major difference is that the osteopath practices manipulative therapy designed to correct musculoskeletal disorders in addition to using other diagnostic and therapeutic techniques used by physicians. The manipulative therapy is based on the premise that the function of the musculoskeletal system is basic to the function of all other body systems. As with M.D. programs, there is a strong element of professional socialization; in osteopathy there is also a strong emphasis on primary care as a practice focus. After receipt of the basic degree, graduates take a rotating internship and may then enter a residency program in a specialty.

Both physicians and osteopaths must be licensed after passing licensure examinations before they can begin practice or graduate training.

Physician's Assistant

The realization that it is possible to provide certain medical services at lower cost when provided by less expensively educated persons is not new. However, the creation of the physician's assistant is an unique approach based on the concept that rather than perform only a certian series of tasks, such as medical technologists, these individuals should be educated in all phases of medical diagnosis and therapy. The distinguishing difference between the physician's assistant and the physician in practice is that the physician's assistant is not expected to deal with other than the routine or relatively uncomplicated cases. Also, the premise is that the assistant is supervised directly by the physician, even in selected instances of these cases. The educational preparation reflects this purpose in that common problems and basic diagnostic and therapeutic skills are the major content. Some physician's assistants are educated to deal in the problems associated with one medical specialty. Others are more broadly based in general primary care.

Some physician's assistant programs accept only students with previous health care backgrounds, such as medical corpsmen or nurses. Others accept students with some general college-level background work, usually at least two years. Programs vary in length, although all must conform to guidelines issued by the American Medical Association.

The greatest acceptance of these individuals has come in medically undeserved areas where there is no economic threat from their existence to private physicians' practices. Although some private physicians and group practices have successfully integrated the physician's assistnat into practice, widespread acceptance has been much slower than was originally antici- pated.

Health Service Administrator

The complexity of modern health care organization, including govern- mental and other regulation of all aspects of health care, has increased significantly in the last several years. One result is a need for coordination and quality control of the entire enterprise, such as in hospitals, health maintenance organizations, and long-term care facilities. The health care administrator serves that function. Education for this field is mainly at the Master's degree level, although there are community college and Bachelor's degree level programs preparing individuals for long-term care administra- tion, an area that now generally requires licensure. Licensure is not pres- ently a requirement for administrators in other types of facilities.

Medical Technologist

The designation *technologist* is used for the individual with college-de- gree level preparation in laboratory methods and techniques designed to determine the status and function of human body systems. Educational programs are either four or five years long and require a strong background in chemistry and mathematics.

There are other workers in the clinical laboratory field who are expected to function under the direction of the medical technologist or physician. These individuals are designated as *technicians* and generally perform relatively routine or specialized functions, designed by the technol- ogist or physician. In hospitals, a pathologist (physician) is legally respon- sible for the setting of standards and overall quality control of the labora- tory, although operational management is usually the technologist's respon- sibility.

Radiology Technologist

The radiology technologist performs the technical activities required to produce the radiological studies used in medical diagnosis. Programs preparing for this field, as with the medical technology field, are varied, but tend in all cases to focus on the necessary technique and quality control required to assure high-quality diagnostic procedures, which the radiologist (physician) interprets.

Respiratory Therapist

Respiratory therapy as an occupational field arose with the increase in knowledge of respiratory physiology and the related therapeutic interventions which have been created. The respiratory therapists have direct contact with patients because they administer oxygen and other gas mixtures as well as aerosol medications. They also perform respiratory function tests and provide treatment designed to improve respiratory function. As a developing field, respiratory therapy does not have a single educational pattern, but there is movement toward making the program uniformly a Bachelor's degree. The course of study includes among other subjects, respiratory physiology, pharmacology of respiratory drugs, physics, chemistry, and therapeutic methods. The respiratory therapist provides service reflecting the medical plan of treatment and therefore acts upon physicians' orders. There is a national certifying examination for these individuals, but no uniform licensure requirements.

Occupational Therapist

The occupational therapist is concerned with purposeful activity in the rehabilitation of persons with physical or emotional disabilities. They typically work in hospitals, long term care facilities, rehabilitation centers, or psychiatric facilities. Education for this specialty is at the Bachelor's degree level.

Physical Therapist

Physical therapy, in contrast to occupational therapy, is focused on treatment, particularly of the musculoskeletal system. The usual patient or client is one who has experienced injury or illness and for whom adaptation or muscle reeducation is necessary to return to function or to achieve the greatest possible adapted function. A Bachelor's degree in the field is the basic requirement to function as a physical therapist, although there is movement in the field toward requiring the Master's degree.

Each of the occupational groups mentioned immediately above is among those sometimes classified as "allied health" personnel. Although the degree of direct involvement with patients may vary by group, they have in common the fact that their practice is entirely dependent on intiation of a request, referral, or prescription for their services by a physician . This is in contrast to nurses whose practice is not entirely dependent upon physician prescription.

Dentist, Dental Assistant, and Hygienist

The dentist, like the physician, is usually in private practice, providing prevention, diagnosis, and treatment of disease and/or malfunction of the oral cavity and associated structures. As a nurse you may have cause to refer patients for dental care such as children with cavities or elderly persons needing adjustment of dentures. You might also have the opportunity to collaborate in prevention activities, using dentists or information they provide in group teaching activities for patients.

Education for dentistry is a four-year program built on two to four years of undergraduate work. The first two years of the dental curriculum are primarily basic sciences and the final two years are mostly clinical work. Dentists are licensed by the state, and those who practice oral surgery may have hospital privileges.

Assisting the dentist, there may be dental auxiliary workers and dental hygienists. The education for these occupations is not uniform nationally, varying from on-the-job training for some dental assistants to Bachelor's degree programs for dental hygienists.

Dietitian

A basic undergraduate preparation in food and nutrition prepares a person for the year of study in therapeutic nutrition, the major thrust of a dietitian's education. Supervising the preparation of special diets and working directly with patients and their families to improve their understanding of therapeutic diets or to encourage their selection of a healthful diet is the function of the dietitian. When a patient is hospitalized and the medical plan of treatment requires a therapeutic diet, the dietitian acts in response to physician's orders to develop a suitable diet and supervise production of the necessary nutrients. When a person is not hospitalized and is merely interested in learning to choose a healthful diet, the dietitian functions relatively independently. The issue of whether a dietitian can legally prescribe dietary modifications when consulted by individuals arose in one state when suit was brought against a dietitian by a state medical society charging that this constituted unlicensed practice of medicine. Thus, in this field, as in nursing and others, the tendency toward expanded function and increased autonomy has produced some conflict.

Pharmacist

Pharmacy is a field in which much recent concern has been directed toward increasing the involvement of the practitioner directly with consumers. Since modern technology of compounding drugs has eliminated much of the original functions of individual pharmacists, the pharmacist's role seems to have shrunk, and is now largely reduced to pouring, counting, and labeling prescription items. It is clear that the pharmacist's extensive education, requiring at least five years and culminating in the Bachelor of Science in Pharmacy or more recently the Doctor of Pharmacy, prepares one for larger functions. One effort at role redefinition has been to develop a clinical role that will involve the pharmacist as a consultant to physicians regarding choices of drugs for particular illnesses and potential interactions among drugs. In the community, this clinical role has been achieved by the preparation of drug profiles for individuals who purchase medication through a particular pharmacy. As subsequent medications are added, the pharmacist can identify any potential negative drug interaction and can counsel the patient or consult with the physician. These changes have met with limited success but are evidence of ferment in this profession. Like physicians and nurses, pharmacists are licensed following examination by the state in which they practice. Approximately 73 percent of practicing pharmacists are in community pharmacy with the remainder in hospital practice, teaching, and research.

In this field, as in other health fields, the use of technicians has been introduced as a way of reducing the cost of pharmacy operations with a resulting move of pharmacists into the supervisory and managerial activities.

Social Worker

Nurses and social workers have many concerns in common, the uppermost being the ultimate promotion of the highest possible level of health for individuals and families. The histories of the two groups have some commonalities as well. As Idunn Haugen has noted, each group was developed initially to serve a relatively confined purpose, in a specific practice site, nurses mainly in hospitals and social workers in social agencies.[2] Each

2 Idunn Haugen, "A Comparison between the Social Work Profession and the Nursing Profession, Philosophy, Theory, and Practice" (Minneapolis, Minn.: Systems Development Project, n.d.).

group was founded on a charitable religious premise. As time has passed, there have been points where nurses (especially community health nurses) and social workers have seemed to be in conflict over where their lines of responsibility were drawn, with each performing activities the other viewed as theirs. That dispute, similar to some between other health professions, signals the potential for collaboration, especially since it demonstrates that there are areas of mutual concern.

Education for social work at the professional level is the Master's degree. A national certification program acknowledges professional preparation and experience. Some social casework activity, like some nursing activity, is performed by individuals with different educational backgrounds. Usually these social caseworkers are graduates of a Bachelor's degree program in sociology or social welfare studies. The efforts of social workers are directed toward helping individuals and families solve personal and social problems that inhibit their ability to function in daily life.

Audiologist and Speech Pathologist

Specialists in audiology and speech pathology function relatively independently, although frequently on referral from other health professionals, in diagnosing and treating disorders of reception and production of language. Their education is at the Master's degree level, and they participate in a national certification program rather than state licensure. Some of these professionals operate private practices. Others are employed by large health care institutions. They are especially helpful in speech rehabilitation with patients who have aphasia for various reasons and with teaching speech and other communication methods to those with hearing disabilities. Their education backgrounds include general studies, anatomy, physiology and functional patterns of the organs of speech and hearing, and special methods and techniques in diagnosis and therapy.

Clinical Psychologist

Clinical psychology deals with the diagnosis of personality disorders and the use of psychotherapeutic methods to promote improved personal function. Psychiatrists also provide psychotherapy but are licensed as physicians and may therefore prescribe medication as a part of therapy. The psychologist, in contrast, although not licensed to prescribe drugs, may make extensive use of psychometric tests in diagnosing the patient's problem. The psychiatrist is not typically educated to perform this type of testing. The function of these two can, as a result, frequently be complementary. Licensure for practice is required in clinical psychology. In some states, licensure can be granted to persons with only the Master's degree, but the trend is toward the Doctorate as the required credential.

Problems of Expansion and Layering in Health Occupations

The several health professions mentioned above are those with which the nurse most frequently has the opportunity to work.

As new knowledge is produced and new functions are identified, there may be new occupational groups created or new expansions and shifts made in the functions of various existing groups. The natural tendencies toward expansion and exclusivity are not peculiar to any one group, and they frequently tend to produce conflicts, conflicts that may result in less than optimum cooperation among groups toward the common goal of high-quality health care. A danger related to expansion is that in the glow of assuming new activities or functions, the core reason for the development and continuance of the occupation is given less emphasis than it deserves, both in practice and in education. Nursing is a good example of this. The role of nurse practitioner was created originally because in the care of children, well child care and care of minor, routine illness occupied the majority of the time of pediatric physicians. Since their background focused on diagnosis and treatment of illness, the assumption of the more routine management of minor illness and parent education by specially educated nurses was viewed by many as a desirable development, particularly in areas where a shortage of pediatricians was present. An early term to describe these nurse practitioners was "physician extender", a term which made the medical aspect of the role prominent. Early work in developing this role also emphasized that the use of good nursing skills in prevention, family guidance, and patient education would benefit the patient beyond what they usually experienced when cared for only by the physician. Subsequent application of the nurse practitioner idea to other patient populations has often emphasized the physician extender aspect. Expanding function in medical management of chronic illness has caused some to overlook the basic nursing function of providing physical and emotional comfort and promoting a return to normal function as soon as possible and to the extent possible. The diagnosis and therapy become "the thing." This is not to suggest that expansion of function is not appropriate in many cases, but rather to note that it should not constitute abandonment of other aspects of nursing function. The potential result is that the newly expanded function, many times a "give away" from medicine, supersedes the original function, with the result that there is no longer a separate occupational identity for the whole original occupational group and therefore a questionable need for it when funding is limited.

Another tendency that seems to exist is to create a "not quite professional" group within each field, which is then made responsible for certain tasks. These assistants, aids, or technicians are assigned, at least in the beginning, to tasks that are considered routine. In fact, it is evident that some physicians and some members of the general public perceive nurses to be an example of this type of assistantship in relation to medicine. It is reasoned that it is more economical to have some tasks performed by persons with less extensive (and less expensive) education and with lower salary rates. Perhaps this is true under some conditions or in some fields, but no systematic evaluation has been done of arrangements reflecting this principle across the variety of fields in which this layering has developed.

SUMMARY

There are several occupational groups providing health care services, some with direct patient care responsibilities and others with functions designed to aid physicians and other health professionals in diagnosis and therapy. This chapter briefly describes the functions and education of those groups most frequently encountered by nurses. Some of the issues and concerns common to all health care occupations are discussed.

Additional Reading

Webster, Denise. "Medical Students' Views of the Role of the Nurse" Nursing Research 34 (Sept./Oct., 1985) 313-317

Chapter 3

Types of health care agencies

As the number and types of health care agencies have increased, so have the options for nurses' employment. This chapter describes the principal types of agencies that provide health care and their major characteristics.

TYPES OF AGENCIES

Hospitals

By far the majority of registered nurses (RNs) in the United States work in hospitals. Some 68 percent of RNs are employed today in these institutions.[1] Hospitals have often been a subject of study by sociologists and by other social scientists because they are complex organizations, have some aspects in common with other organizations as well as some that are unique to a hospital. By definition, a hospital is:

an establishment that provides-through an organized medical or professional staff, permanent facilities that include inpatient beds, medical services, and continuous nursing services-diagnosis and treatment for patients...Hospitals are further classified as general or special, depending on whether the provision of care is limited to patients in any particular medical diagnostic category [2].

Each hospital has its governing board, which reflects the control of the agency by a particular level of community authority, as in various types of government-controlled agencies, or by a special interest group such as a church or a group of investors. In each case, the governing board constitutes

1 American Nurses Assn.*Facts About Nursing* Kansas City: ANA 1987,191
2 American Hospital Association, *Classification of Health Care Institutions* (Chicago: American Hospital Association, 1974), p. 4.

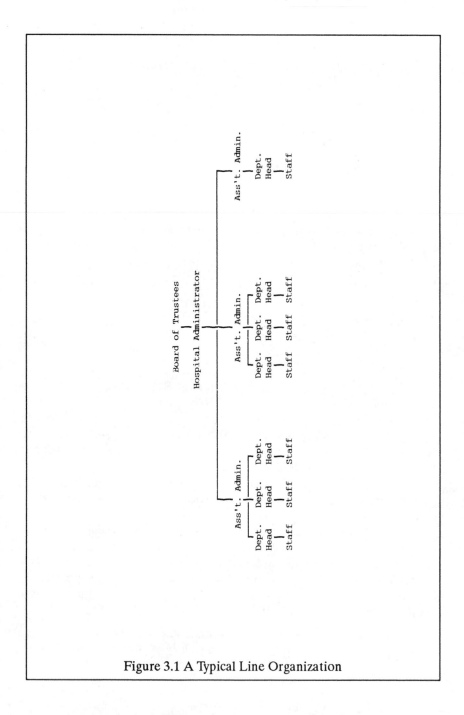

Figure 3.1 A Typical Line Organization

the legal final authority and has responsibility for the operation of the agency. The board then delegates operational authority and responsibility to an administrator. The title of that person may vary from administrator to president depending on whether a corporate model is used. In each case the administrator is charged with with responsibility for the total operation of the hospital. The complexity of health care today and the problem of coordinating the variety of services needed in giving health care make the administrator's job a complex one.

Even small hospitals today must deal internally with providing a variety of specialized services, offered by persons trained in the various health disciplines, and must meet accreditation requirements, in addition to finding adequate funds to meet the hospital's financial requirements. Externally these hospitals must assure good community relations and deal effectively with third-party payors including the federal government and private insurance companies as well as regulatory groups including city and state health authorities. And, of course, the overriding concern behind all of these must be the provision of high-quality health care to patients.

Larger hospitals or those affiliated with teaching institutions become even more complex with the addition of students and faculty; programs for basic, continuing, and graduate education; and research. These hospitals also become more complex as the range of services becomes increasingly specialized to offer tertiary-level care, that is services that provide highly specialized treatment and require technologically advanced equipment and facilities.

One way in which organizations are structured in order to assure that such complexity is coordinated is an hierarchical line organization. This structure places the board of trustees of the hospital (or whatever title is used) at the top of the structure. The line of authority and responsibility descends to the administrator, then to one or more assistant or associate administrators, then to department or division heads, and finally downward to the first operational level. In the nursing department, the operational level would be at the direct patient care level. At each sucessive level, there is a group of individuals reporting to and responsible to a person at the next higher level (an organizational superior). This very orderly arrangement can be depicted on an organizational chart such as that shown in Fig. 3.1. In smaller hospitals,there may be no assistant administrators. In larger hospitals the person in charge of nursing is often both an assistant administrator and the functional head of the nursing department. Although the structures may vary, the principle is the same; that is, defined lines of authority are created, and the power attributed to the employer to cause employees to perform work according to those lines is related to the employer's or supervisor's ability to reward or to withhold rewards such as salary, promotion, and other benefits.

Some hospitals have adopted a corporate structure model and have titled the administrative head as Chief Executive Officer. This person's immediate top assistants in the line organization are often titled Chief Operating Officer (in charge of a variety of daily operating issues) and Chief Financial Officer (in charge of all financial affairs). Where this is the case, the line hierarchy is essentially the same as depicted, only the titles are changed, primarily reflecting the movement to view health care as a business.

There is, however, one aspect of hospital organization that does not fit this pattern. This is the relationship of the physician(s) to the hospital structure. It is this aspect that makes the hospital different from most other complex organizations. The medical staff of a hospital does not function as a part of the regular line organization. Rather, the professional staff is organized as a separate entity with its own officers and committees. The medical staff, communicating officially through its chief of staff, is viewed as being attached to the organization at the level of the administrator in a consultative and collaborative relationship. In some hospitals, expecially large teaching hospitals, the chief of each medical service is also a faculty member and is viewed as being responsible for the conduct of graduate medical education (residency) programs on that service. This physician is also frequently the chairman or associate chairman of the corresponding department in the associated medical school. Many large hospitals have a position with the organization called Medical Director or Director of Clinical Affairs or other similar title. This position is salaried and may be part time or full time. The responsibility of this position usually relates to providing continuity with the medical staff, whose chief usually holds a relatively short term and who is typically in full time practice or who holds a full time academic appointment. Other responsibility often includes advising the chief administrator on medical practice standards and overseeing quality assurance activities for medicine.

On initial consideration, this "outside the line" placement of the medical staff seems staisfactory since it is a way of managing the professional responsibility of the physicians as a group, rather than their being supervised by some non-physician. The primary difficulty created by this arrangement is that because physicians have a legitimate concern for the total care of their patients, they may attempt to exercise control or supervisory authority over a variety of personnel whose responsiblity and authority are already defined within the line structure. Nurses are one of the more frequently chosen subjects for such interaction, nurses at every organizational level. When this is the case, a role conflict is often produced since the physician's organizational authority, although relatively small, is augmented by extensive informally attributed power. After all, in the final analysis, the physician controls input of patients to the hospital. Therefore, the greater the individual physician's control of input (patients), the greater is the potential to successfully wield authority. In situations where the medical staff is relatively mature and is well established and has worked out its own relationships, such forays into the line organization are relatively limited. The net effect, though, is a very complicated series of potential interactions that have fascinated sociologists for years.

The medical staff organizes to serve its functions by the use of committees. Although there is no set number of committees required, most staffs will include at least the following :[3]

1. *Executive Committee*: Acts for the staff to implement its policies and other related duties overseeing the other committees and their function.
2. *Credentials committee*: Considers the qualifications of applicants to medical staff. This group recommends type of appointment and privileges. The governing board officially makes all medical staff appointments upon recommendations of this committee. The appointments will be to one of the following five categories, which describe the privileges of the appointment:
   (a) Active Staff: May vote, hold office, deliver all services; bulk of the total medical staff.
   (b) Associate staff: Being considered for active staff; may not vote.
   (c) Consulting staff: No vote nor office; are not regularly seeing patients in the agency but will do so upon request or as consultants.
   (d) Courtesy staff: No vote nor office; those who only wish to admit an occasional patient to the hospital.
   (e) Honorary staff: Former staff members whom the staff wish to honor.
3. *Medical Audit or Medical Care Evaluation Committee:* Responsible for assuring the quality of care through audit procedures.
4. *Utilization Review Committee:* Considers for appropriateness the type and level of use of hospital services by individual physicians.
5. *Joint Conference Committee:* A combined committee of medical staff and hospital governing board to provide liaison between the two groups.

[3] Beaufort Longest, Jr.*Management Practices for the Health Professional*Reston, VA: Reston, 1976, 19

5. *Joint Conference Committee:* A combined committee of medical staff and hospital governing board to provide liaison between the two groups. As with all functions, the performance of the roles of medical staff officers may also change. For example, some researchers have discussed the possibility that professional nurses might function as independent practitioners rather than line employees, with a relationship to the hospital similar to that of the medical staff. One wonders if this is compatible with maintaining the 24-hour continuity of care that has been a hallmark of nursing's importance in hospital care. The future remains open to experimentation.

Nursing Homes

Nursing home is the common term for what is classified as a nursing care institution, a facility that provides "diagnosis and treatment for patients who are not in an acute phase of illness but who primarily require skilled nursing care on an inpatient basis.[4] Association,*Classification of Health Care Institutions,* p.4.Nursing homes may either be *general,* caring for all types of patients; or *special,* catering to the treatment of certain categories of patients.

Another set of categories classifies nursing care facilities by type or level of care. These include:

1. Domiciliary care facility - a facility which provides room, board, and basic supervision for persons who are able to care for themselves with minimal assistance.

2. Sheltered housing - a special environment to accomodate the limitations of the handicapped. Special services may include meal service or dining rooms and assistant services. Residents are able to function without continuous supervision.

3. Intermediate care facility (ICF) - Facility designed for persons who require some nursing care but do not require professional level of service of a skilled nursing home or hospital. Intermediate care facilities must have health personnel present around the clock and regulations require registered nurses on staff daily.

4. Skilled nursing facility (SNF) Persons needing skilled care must require the services of a registered nurse and other therapists and the skilled nursing care must be needed on a 24 hour basis to require the level of care in this type of home.[5]

4

5 Charlotte Eliopoulis *Caring for the Nursing Home Patient* Rockville, MD: Aspen Publishers, 1989, 13

facilities are elderly persons who require assistance due to weakness or infirmity or who are alone and need the assistance that a spouse or family member might otherwise provide. Some of these institutions may combine wings or units for different levels of patient need, thus producing a facility with a range of types of care. The primary therapy provided in all of these facilities classified as nursing care institutions is general nursing care, although there may also be occupational therapy activities, therapeutic diet supervision, physical therapy, and pharmacy services available either on a regular or consultative basis.

The advent of benefits through Medicare and a state-level program of old age assistance have increased the utilization of nursing care facilities. With this expanded use have come regulations for establishing certain standards in physical facilities and checking that adequate levels of staffing and quality of care are provided. Although facilities that do not accept Medicare patients are not subject to this supervision, the effect of it has been to provide some basic assurance to the public regarding minimum standards that homes must meet in order to receive payment and to continue operation.

Ambulatory Care Institutions

Ambulatory care institutions, which include clinics and physician's offices, provide diagnostic and treatment services to patients who are ambulatory. The services required by those using ambulatory care are typically episodic, that is, not occurring regularly and not requiring extended periods of nursing care and observation, as in the hospital or nursing home. The purpose of the institution will define the type of client or patient population, whether it is a specific age group, diagnostic category, or a general population seeking general care. As payment mechanisms have changed, there has been a steady increase in the number and types of services which have become outpatient activities. Services have developed around types of procedures and/or equipment. They include hemodialysis centers; radiology/radiotherapy centers; chemotherapy treatment centers; urgent care centers, where minor emergencies are treated; and outpatient clinics which may be operated by a medical group practice, a health maintenance organization, or a hospital or university health sciences center or medical school. The description, names, and organization arrangements are numerous and seem limited only by the imagination of the health care entrepreneur and the third party payors. In some university health science centers, an ambulatory clinic may be an organizationally separate activity housed in the hospital building. Another variation is that the outpatient clinic is a department within the hospital's overall organization. Many of these operations are relatively small and therefore are not highly complex in their organization, although some ambulatory facilities in health maintenance organizations or in large health sciences centers are quire extensive. Nurses' functions in these settings vary widely, from actually performing a large portion of data collection and initial assessment for medical diagnosis and nursing diagnosis and therapy, to "directing traffic" and points on the continuum between. Often the nurse's role is primarily technical and task focused, not because a more comprehensive role would not be useful, but because the service has been developed around the delivery of some specific medical therapy or diagnostic techniques.

Day care institutions are an area in which there is considerable development, particularly due to the increasing numbers of elderly persons. The expense of nursing home care can often be delayed or avoided altogether if an elderly person can participate in a day care program while family members are at work. Nurses are important in day care for health supervision, program planning, individual care planning and agency management. Because of the concern about the costs of care for the increasing elderly population as an element of health care expenditures, this aspect of health care delivery is certain to continue to increase.

Another developing area of non-institutional health care is home care. Procedures such as intravenous therapy, complex dressing changes and respiratory care procedures which were once performed only in hospitals are now performed in the home. Because of the high degree of uncertainty resulting from intermittent versus constant observation; differences in availability of equipment and support services and personnel, the home environment is a special challenge for the nurse. Add to these environmental differences between home and hospital and variables created by the presence of family members who are affected by and participating in care, and we find created a health care situation which demands the highest level of professional skill. These same variables, plus the geographic distances between home care sites make the management of home care nursing an even greater challenge.

Health Maintenance Organizations

The Health Maintenance Organization (HMO) is not really a category in the classification scheme because it is not a separate type of facility. Rather it is an organization designed to provide care, based on the concept of prepayment at a predetermined rate for all specified health services for an individual or group. In providing health services, the HMO may develop, own, lease, contract for, or otherwise arrange for health care in any one or all of the types of facilities listed in the classification scheme below. The basic concept is to encourage the use of preventive services in order to reduce the use of more expensive acute care services. The prepayment element is thought to be an incentive to both the enrolled members of the HMO, to use the preventive service, and to the provider, to keep costs down by preventing acute episodes.

Classification Scheme

The several institutional settings in which health care is delivered, and which most nurses practice, have been organized into a classification scheme, primarily to standardize definitions for collection of information on health care. This classification system is outlined in Figure 3.2. Institutions may be classified further according to their governance. That set of categories is listed in Figure 3.3.

I. Medical Care Institutions
   A. Inpatient care institution
     1.Hospital
      (a)General
      (b)Special
     2.Nursing Care Institution
      (a)General
      (b)Special
   B. Ambulatory Care Institution
     1. General
     2. Special
     3. Day Care Institution
      (a) General
      (b) Special
   C.Home health institution
     1.General
     2.Special

II. Health-related care institution
   A.Intermediate care institution
   B. Resident care institution

Figure 3.2 Outline of Classification Scheme of Medical and Health-related Care Institutions. Reprinted with permission of Reston Publ. Co. Inc., a Prentice-Hall Co., 11480 Sunset Hills Rd., Reston, VA.

I.Government institution
Institution controlled by an agency of government.
A.Federal institution
Institution controlled by an agency of federal government.
B.Nonfederal government institution
Institution controlled by an agency of state or local government.
1.State institution
Institution controlled by an agency of state government.
2.Local government institution
Institution controlled by an agency of local government.
(a) District Authority Institution
Institution controlled by a political subdividion of a state created solely for the purpose of establishing and maintaining medical care or health-related care institutions.
(b) County institution
Institution controlled by an agency of county government
(c) City-County institution
Institution controlled jointly by agencies of municipal and county governments
(d) City institution
Institution controlled by an agency of municipal government

II. Nongovernment institution
Institution controlled by a nongovernment association or organization operating on a not-for-profit basis or by a corporation, partnership, or individual operating on a for-profit basis.
A. Not-for-profit institution
Institution controlled by an association or organization operating on a not-for-profit basis.
B. Investor-owned institution
Institution controlled by a corporation, partnership, or individual operating on a for-profit basis.

Figure 3.3 Classification by Control in Health Care Institutions. Classification by control is determined by the nature of the organization responsible for the fiscal and legal operations of the institution. Reprinted with permission of Reston Publ. Co., Inc., a Prentice-Hall Co., 11480 Sunset Hills Rd., Reston, VA.

Control and Regulation
of Health Care Agencies

Because health care institutions affect the well-being of the public, certain types of these institutions are subject to legal requirements and monitoring for various aspects of their physical plant and for the services rendered there. The regulations and mechanisms vary from state to state, but the general purpose of such regulations is to assure, to the extent possible, that certain minimum standards of safety and quality are met. Other regulations are imposed upon agencies participating in Medicare and state-level welfare assistance programs. In order to receive reimbursement for their services from these programs, the institutions must meet regulations regarding utilization of services, costs, and quality of staffing and services.

Another form of control is that engendered by voluntary accreditation. The Joint Commission on Accreditation of Healthcare Organizations is the major accreditation body for health care facilities. While participation in the accreditation process is voluntary, JCAHO accreditation is a powerful incentive in that it is the basis for agencies' being able to receive certain types of funding from third party payors and to participate as sites for clinical education in medical, nursing, and allied health programs.

It is an interesting activity to ask staff members at various levels in a health care facility about their experiences with accreditation procedures and their practice. Frequently the answer of individuals at upper organizational levels will demonstrate that what lower level staff recognize as the expected level of practice is, in fact, a result of supervisory efforts to move practice into line with accreditation requirements.

The Nursing Service of the agency is scrutinized as one aspect of the review for the entire facility. There are standards [6] which are the basis for certain required characteristics which must be present in an accredited nursing service. These standards relate to the structure of the nursing service, its standards and processes of care, staffing, and quality assurance activities.

Nursing departments may also seek accreditation through the National League for Nursing. This type of accreditation is less widely sought, probably due to the lack of the incentive of reimbursement requirement. However, the National League for Nursing has achieved the status of official

[6] C.H. Peterson, D. Kranz, and B. Brandt, *A Guide to JCAH Nursing Services Standards* Chicago: Joint Commission on Accreditation of Hospitals, 1986

accrediting body for home health agencies. It is likely that this will result in an increase in this accrediting service for the growing home health industry.

SUMMARY

A classification scheme has been presented as a way of recognizing the various types of health care institutions. There are brief descriptions of the institutions in the various categories and of the several regulatory forces that affect the operation of these institutions. As a nurse, functioning in a health care agency, you are affected by the general purpose and specific intents of the facility as well as by external forces that affect the operation of the agency.

Chapter 4

Focusing
on specific aspects of the agency

Entering a health care agency for the first time can be a bewildering experience whether you enter as a patient, a student, or a new employee. Aside from general information for classifying the facility, more specific information can be useful in helping you as student or staff nurse to better understand the environment you are entering.

Philosophy

A statement of philosophy can usually be found in the printed information that the agency provides for employees and the public. Such a statement will generally speak to the major purpose of the institution; for example, it will specify that the agency provides service to indigents or service and research in cancer. Next, it will describe the level of responsiveness to the community, that is, whether this is a facility dedicated to the care of persons in a certain neighborhood of the city. Then it will discuss any special approaches to care, for example, an osteopathic approach or a family-centered care approach. And finally, it will state any particular beliefs regarding patients and/or employees, such as a belief in their individuality and dignity regardless of race, sex, or religious preference. Although the statement may not be labeled "philosophy", a statement of purpose or statement of belief is usually available. Ask to see the statement. The statement may also include objectives or specific aims, such as "to reduce and stabilize the perinatal mortality rate in neighborhood X," or "to provide a facility for the clinical educational activities of nursing students."

An important consideration in examining this statement is whether there is a logical consistency between it and the type of authority under which the agency operates. For example, a statement implying a belief in the responsibility for providing continuity of care from hospital to home would be consistent with a government-controlled Veterans Administration hospital's scope of authority.

If the agency does not have a written statement containing its philosophy, there are three possible explanations. First, there is the possiblity that there is, in fact, no explict guiding purpose or philosophy for the agency. Second, there is the possibility that the purpose is in the process of change. The third possibility is that although the governing board may be of one mind on this issue, there has never been any effort to actually state the philosophy. In this case, the guiding purpose may be inferred from policy made by the board and from the range of programs that are developed there. However, even with a published statement, one must compare it with the operational programs as well as with the type of authority to determine whether there is a logical consistency between the stated purpose and the agency's operation. A lack of consistency between these should prompt you to look very carefully at the other elements of the agency.

Philosophy and Objectives-
Nursing Department

From your perspective as a nurse, the philosophy and objectives of the nursing department will be an important concern. In addition to looking for logical consistency as above, it is also useful to question a sample of staff members to determine their understanding of and agreement with the department's philosophy and objectives. For example, a situation where family-centered maternity care is a prominent objective would be falling short of its purpose if the evening shift personnel were systematically turning away all sibling visitors. The point to keep in mind is that what is important to the patient is what actually occurs, not what the statement of philosophy says. Likewise, it is what you and your colleagues are expected to do, the type and extent of care, that is the evidence of the philosophy, not only that which is contained in the nursing philosophy statement. For that reason, one cannot accept on faith that the intent is equal to the outcome. Careful questioning and observation are necessary.

As a student, you may use the information to help you understand the situation in which you have your clinical practice. For example, hostility from patients may not be surprising when they expect sibling visiting in maternity and are denied it. As a graduate, this type of information may help you to decide whether you wish to work in a particular agency or to identify areas for possible improvement in the agency's function.

Standards of Practice

Another level of concern is with the standards of practice in the nursing department. The first question is whether standards of any sort have been adopted. The concept of standards as very specific requirements about the level of care given to patients is a relatively recent development. These standards provide a sound basis for audits or other evaluation techniques. Even when agencies have not yet formalized standards as explict as those for evaluation, there should be some evidence of basic expectations of care. One type of query to determine what those expectations are is, "What routines are there here, or what procedures are used to assure good basic care?" One would expect answers to mention such things as the minimum frequency of home visits to patients in community health, specified intervals for rounds in inpatient settings, basic plans of care for specific patient or family problems, and supervisory concern for patient care activities, as well as certain requirements for the content of inpatient records.

Again, the best information is gained by asking questions and observing activities at both supervisory and operational levels. If supervisory level personnel believe standards exist and operational staff are unaware of them, then there may be a gap in the training and supervisory cycle, although improvement is possible in this situation. If neither level is definite about the existence of any standards, it is questionable whether much improvement is possible without intervention at a higher administrative level.

Benefits and Obligations
of Employment

The most personally relevant aspects of a health care agency are the employee's obligations and the benefits of employment. As a new nurse, or as you consider a change of jobs, you may find that the recruitment efforts of the facility will be designed to address many of your typical concerns about a position. In times of nursing personnel shortages, there is an emphasis onmaking a position attractive to enter. As you consider positions, you should analyze the items that will make the position initially attractive and which will make the position continue to be attractive after several years.

The typical concerns are salary, assignment, and shift rotation policy, and procedures if these are relevant in the facility. Although you may receive information about some of these features without asking, it is worthwhile to probe past the initial information. For example in relation to salary, are there any special rates for intensive care units, evening or night duty, or any differential for education or experience? Further, at what frequency are salary increases provided, and are they "across the board," merit only, or some combination of the two? Is unit assignment made on the basis of interest and experience, or is there a method to seek transfer when openings occur? Do shift rotations seem equitable, and do they allow sufficient time for adjustment to new sleep patterns between shift changes? Each of these factors will prove to be important to the nurse employee as time is accrued on the job.

The orientation that a new employee receives is another characteristic unique to each facility. Both length of time committed to orientation and the content are worth asking about, as is the degree to which orientation can be an individualized program. As the content of some orientations is examined, it may be noted that little attention is given to professional expectations but much to specific procedural activities like narcotics procedures, fire drills, etc. Both professional expectations and procedural activities are important, so the ideal would be to find a balance in content between the two.

Other aspects of concern are retirement programs, insurance programs, and other benefits that are, in effect, additions to salary. For example, is the retirement program one to which the employer contributes as well as the employee? Is it required or optional? Is there group (lower cost) insurance for health care, death, and disability? Does the employer contribute to the premium payment? Some agencies also provide child care for employees' children. Since each of these benefits represents money saved, the actual dollar value to each employee could be viewed as nontaxable income.

The other common element in benefit packages is the amount of vacation/annual leave and sick time/personal leave available to each employee. Very limited leaves may imply a lack of recognition of employees' needs for recreation and for relief from the stresses on the job. Realistically speaking, the nature of the benefit package probably represents a combination of the economic situation in the area, the market for jobs in the particular field, and the agency administrator and governing body's beliefs about how employees should be treated. In a tight job market, with relatively good availability of personnel, the benefits package may be slimmer than would be the case in situations where personnel were in short supply.

Another factor that will influence benefits and is important to assess is whether a bargaining agent represents the interests of some or all of the employees of the facility. If you agree with the purposes of a union and the general premise of collective bargaining, you may consider this a positive factor. Where unions are present, one of their major concerns will be to bargain for improved salaries and benefits.

Position Descriptions

One factor which will have a lasting effect on a nurse's performance is the description of the position for which she/he is employed. Seeking specific information about the position requirements as included in the job description can benefit the nurse who is making decisions both about specific employment and about long term career development.

The most direct information supplied by the job description is the general set of minimum expectations for the category of worker. Both what is included and what is absent are important to consider. For example, do the position descriptions indicate that you will function in a manner consistent with your education and experience? Not only should you attempt to identify whether you meet the minimum requirements of the position, but also, you should look at whether you will be expected to perform up to your capabilities, by using a variety of elements of your education and experience background. As health care facilities become appropriately sophisticated, they attempt to differentiate the types of functions expected of nurses with different education and experience. This is crucial to economically efficient and effective care. You can request information about different position descriptions or career levels. Determine whether these are based solely on education, length and type of experience and certification or whether they also identify different performance expectations. A "career ladder" which does not include specifications of differences in performance is essentially a reward incentive plan. While that is attractive, it may not be sufficiently attractive long term if performance expectations are not differentiated, because it offers little incentive to excell in one's area of practice.

When you review the materials provided by a potential employer and read the job description, look for the following elements:

- General function of the position
- Duties and responsibilities
- Experience and education required
- Lines of authority and accountability
- Date of most recent review of the description

Job descriptions for professional positions tend to be in rather general terms, describing functions and relationships rather than specific tasks, since there is a need for professional judgment in selecting the correct action from a variety of possible actions. Compare the agency's description with generally accepted standards of professional functions and with your own preparation as a professional nurse.

Two other elements that are agency specific which may affect the nurse's long term satisfaction with a position are 1) opportunities for professional development and 2) opportunities for career advancement. Critical questions in this regard are, "What policies exist for time for travel to professional meetings, for tuition reimbursement, and for internal staff development opportunities?" To elicit the career development opportunities one might ask, "What is the route for advancement for persons with my background? Is there a specific plan to help each staff member develop along either the clinical or supervisory path if they desire? Are there written policies and procedures describing how one can advance?"

Policy and Procedure

Another area of interest for the professional nurse is the health care agency's policy and procedures. These documents are important and have relevance for their practice. In effect, the agency's written policy defines that facility's expectations in relevant areas of nursing care. A brief review can help you determine if there are major inconsistencies between the policy or procedure manual, the Nurse Practice Act of the state and/or relevant standards of professional practice to which you personally adhere. Any existing disparities could point to potential difficulties. The nurse's practice will be held legally to the standards defined by the state's Nurse Practice and subsequently to the agency's policy if it is not inconsistent with the state's law.

Using the Information

The final step in making use of information about these specifics of the agency is to put the information into some useful perspective. As a professional nurse, deciding whether to begin or to continue to work in a particular agency, the best guide will be your own values and preferences. If you have some particularly strong belief about, for example, care of the dying, the position description, and other aspects of work mentioned above should be considered in relation to that belief to see if they are compatible. Also, do you have requirements or expectations about salary and benefits that are met or not met by those offered by this facility? Finally, does the position as described make full use of your professional ability, or does it demand functions beyond your capabilities? Will your reintegrated professional role be facilitated by the position and by the agency's goals?

This type of self-questioning suggests the ways in which the information about a health care facility can be made relevant to the individual nurse's perspective as she/he develops a better understanding on the information needed to function as manager and managed as a reintegrated professional.

SUMMARY

Several specific aspects of an organized health care facility's operation can be examined in order to better understand the agency as an environment for work. Your perspective may be as a student, examining this information as a part of the study of the agency where you have clinical experience, or as a graduate, considering a new position. In either case, your function will be enhanced and/or your choice of positions improved by understanding as much as possible about that environment.

Additional Reading

American Nurses Association, <u>ANA Standards</u> Kansas City, Mo.: The Association. 1986

Creighton, Helen, "Legal Implications of Policy and Procedure Manual - Part I" <u>Nursing Management</u> 18,4 (April, 1987) 22-25

"Legal Implications of Policy and Procedure Manual - Part II" <u>Nursing Management</u>18,5 (May, 1987) 16-18

Poteet, Gaye and Alice Hill, "Identifying the Components of a Nursing Service Philosophy" <u>Journal of Nursing Administration</u>18, 10 (Oct., 1988)29-33

Trexler, Bernice, "Nursing Department Purpose, Philosophy, and Objectives: Their Use and Effectiveness" <u>Journal of Nursing Administration 17,3 (March, 1987) 8-12</u>

Chapter 5

Power relationships and politics

Power. Politics. What is your first reaction to those words? Is it distress, disgust, or dismay? None of these reactions would be surprising since so many negative experiences come to be labeled as "the result of an exercise of power" or "an encounter with politics." Or perhaps your reaction is not negative but rather disinterested because you consider both power relationships and politics as the province of those who are in major businesses, in elected offices, or are the very wealthy. They seem not to be the direct concern of ordinary people. If any of these reactions describes your response, you may find the approach to the content of this chapter difficult to accept. This is because the emphasis will be on viewing both power relationships and political behavior as phenomena of human social interaction, phenomena that are neither categorically good nor bad. The *intent* and the *consequences* of the relationships are the causes of negative or positive reaction. Therefore, this chapter attempts to impart an understanding of these phenomena so that the negative consequences you may encounter will be minimized and the maximum benefits can be realized in your professional interactions.

Definition of Power

The very use of the term *power* to describe a social concept implies that an analogy can be drawn from the physical sciences; one that will help to clarify the meaning. Examine first a couple of definitions and then consider the analogy.

J. D. March states that power is the *potential* of one individual or group, the agent, to affect or influence the behavior of another, the actor.[1] A similar definition is presented by D. Mechanic.[2] He calls power a *force*, one that results in behavior that would not have occurred if the force had not been present. Both definitions call to mind properties of electricity. The analogy is simple. Electricity is a force, a potential. Until it is directed,i.e., a circuit formed, there is no change or effect produced by its presence. To continue the analogy, one might note two possible results: (1) electrocution can result if the *power* is used unwisely, or (2) current can operate many of the machines that make modern life comfortable. Either result of the realization of the potential (creating a current) is possible and is defined *not by the electricity but by the user.*

The same analogy can be used with social power. It is neither positive nor negative on its on, it exists as a potential. Some individuals want to operate many machines for convenience, for production, or simply for fun, and therefore seek large amounts of electricity. So also some individuals may wish to have the potential to product large amounts of work, to accomplish a variety of actions, to "get things done," for convenience, for production, or for fun. Logically, then, these individuals or groups would be interested in having or gaining the social power to do this.

Other authors have developed theoretical models involving power as a central concept. These concepts differ from one another, although sometimes only subtly, primarily in the refinement of terms. For example, for Robert Bierstedt, *influence* is used as a noun with many properties similar to March's noun *power.*[3] In March's work, *influence* is used as a verb. The result is very different meanings for the term *influence.* Such distinctions are important in understanding the author's perspective and in considering the validity of the theoretical proposition and subsequent research. Therefore, as you read this text or other literature on this topic, it is useful to identify and clarify the terms basic to the model(s) discussed. In this text, the use of key terms may be illustrated by Fig. 5.1.

[1] D. Cartwright, "Influence, Leadership and Control,"in J. D. March, ed., *Handbook of Organizations* (Chicago: Rand McNally, 1965),p.4.

[2] D. Mechanic, "Sources of Power of Lower Participants in Complex Organizations," *Administrative Sciences Quarterly* (December 1962), p. 349.

[3] Robert Bierstedt, *The Social Order*, 4th ed. (New York: McGraw-Hill, 1974), p.350. See also March, *Handbook of Organizations, p.6*

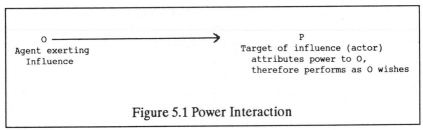

Figure 5.1 Power Interaction

Given this perspective, there are several questions that can yield important answers for the person who is manager (agent in the interaction) as well as the person who is being managed (target in the interaction). Some of those questions are: Why is the power or potential element of this model so important, rather than the means or acts used to produce the desired behavior? What are the sources of power? Is the power of a group simply equal to the sum of the power of each of its members? Does power exist as an absolute entity, or is it relative and/or relational? Other more directly practical questions are: How can I estimate the power I possess in certain situations? What can I do to increase my power? Should I? The list could continue indefinitely. The following section will provide some answers to such questions.

Bases of Social Power

The attributes, assets, or resources of an agent (individual or group) provide the bases of social power. It is the perception by the target that the agent possesses one or more assets, *and* is able and willing to make use of them, that creates the power, the potential to influence. As you consider the various bases of power, remember that it is not simply the possession of the resources that creates the power, but rather the *perception*, by the target, that (a) the resource is possessed, and (b) it can and will be used. It is this perception that makes social power relational, and it explains why the same resources produce differing amounts of power in relation to different targets.

Perhaps you can recall a situation in which the same individual's power is estimated very differently by two persons. One sees the powerholder as neutral, having no ability to cause him to act in any way at all. The powerholder is simply a person he sees on the bus. The other person estimating the power is the employee of the powerholder. He knows that Mr. Power has the ability to increase his salary for good performance. And, based on past experience, he knows that Mr. P. will, on occasion, do just that. Mr. Power is the same person, but because he is perceived differently by these two people, his power in regard to each of them is different.

One comprehensive classification of the bases or sources of power was developed by John French and Bertram Raven.[4]The categories of power bases in that classification include reward power, coercive power, legitimate power, referent power, and expert power.

Reward Power

Reward power is that which is generated by the target's perception that the agent has the resources and willingness to provide him with something he values in exchange for his complying with desired behavior. The resources relevant in this case may be money, materials or goods of some sort, or some less tangible resources such as compliments or praise, affection, and job promotion or enlargement. If this is the only base from which an individual derives power, it is possible that when the more tangible assets are depleted (the money, for example), the target's desire for the less tangible rewards will not be sufficient to produce the desired results. This is especially true in a work situation because although work may be the primary source of monetary "rewards," the supervisor who can affect that reward is seldom the main source from which an individual seeks the greatest part of his life's praise or affection.

As you examine these ideas, you will notice that the idea of a reward as an incentive to behavior is similar to material discussed in Chapter 1. You considered several views of motivations in that chapter. Further, the notion of a particular type of need motivating behavior at one time and not at another reflects a point of view similar to Maslow's.[5]The major difference in this chapter's information is a widened perspective. The view has moved from a focus on a single individual and his or her behavior to an interaction between two or more persons, as perceived from one side of that interaction, the "actor's"(or target's) perspective.

Coercive Power

Coercive power is that which is based on an individual's fear. It depends on the application or, in most cases, on the threat of application of

4 John R. P. French, Jr., and Bertram Raven, "The Bases of Social Power," in D. Cartwright, ed., *Studies in Social Power* (Ann Arbor: University of Michigan, 1959). pp. 150-167.

5 Abraham Maslow, *Motivation and Personality* (New York: Harper & Row, 1954).

physical sanctions, such as the infliction of pain, restriction of movement or freedom, death, or control by force that prevents one from meeting basic physiological or safety needs. The more obvious examples of physical threat are ones that are direct and are aimed at producing physical and/or mental discomfort, whereas the measures related to interfering with basic needs may be either direct or indrect. For example, depriving a person of water and food is a direct method that would be the basis for coercion; whereas an indirect method would be depriving a person of the job that is his primary source of income, which would mean interfering with meeting his basic needs and thus be a basis for coercion.

The actor (or target) acknowledges that another has this sort of power when he (the actor) behaves in a certain way due to the implied or real threat of beatings, embarrassment, verbal abuse, loss of job, or other potentially undesirable and/or painful possibilities. Holding such power depends on the agent's keeping the actor in proximity in order to assure that the threat of receiving the punishment or deprivation is realistic. For example, if the would-be power wielder is 100 miles away and is speaking to you by phone, the threat of direct physical violence rendered by that person might be relatively weak, and the subsequent power to cause you to "eat spinach" might be quite small.

Legitimate Power

Legitimate power is attributed to an agent or source when the actor's values indicate that the agent has a legitimate right to influence him and that he (the actor) in turn, has an obligation to accept that influence. Those who have strong religious beliefs may attribute such power to their priest. In the work setting, legitimate power is generally attributed to persons based on their position in the organizational hierarchy, although this expectation may or may not be made explicit by the organization.

The basis of the legitimation of another's power arises, as mentioned above, from the values and/or norms that the actor accepts. These values may have their basis in the broad cultural values such as those affecting attitude toward persons of various ages or sex. A more specific source of legitimation is the individual's acceptance of specific social structures, such as a hierarchy in a business organization or a series of ranks in a club. Some would argue that these examples are, in effect, only institutionalized and/or internalized examples of reward or coercive power. It may well be true that the potential for reward or punishment is directly related to this type of power. However, there is, in these cases, a certain lack of explicitness regarding outcome. The power is attributed even though there is no clear indication that the individual occupying a position would use either reward or coercion, but rather simply because the position is "expected" to have power.

As cultural values and norms change, the legitimate power attributed to some will shift. For example, in some cultures, the elderly are honored for their wisdom and have considerable power afforded them in decision making because of the status conferred by age. In most Western cultures, the value of age is relatively lower, and if countries are "Westernized" as well as industrialized, the power attributed to the elderly may decline. In the United States, until relatively recently, females tended to be less "legitimately" powerful than men, based on the predominant values in our society. As a result, women in our society attribute more power to men than to other women in almost every type of endeavor. Surely this has affected the way in which nursing, as a primarily female occupation, has developed. The change in women's perspective of themselves that is emerging in our country and elsewhere will very likely produce changes in male-female power attribution as well.

Referent Power

Referent power arises from a desire for oneness with an individual or group, which can subsequently influence the actor. One who admires and wishes to identify with a person, a favorite teacher for example, will be influenced by that person in many aspects of behavior. Some social groups hold this sort of power in relation to those who wish to be members. One has only to consider the many ridiculous actions that sorority or fraternity initiates are willing to perform in order to cite an example of this type of power affecting behavior.

Expert Power

Expert power is based on the actor's perception that the agent holds greater knowledge than he holds or than others hold. In this case, it is as though the agent is evaluated by the actor on two scales: (1) a relative one, "He knows more than me," and (2) an absolute one "He knows almost all there is to know about obstetric nursing." The degree of power seems to be related to a combination of these estimates of expertness. Expert power typically is limited to actions related to the agent's area of expertise. Amitai

Etzioni states that power is sector- or base-specific.[6] That is, to have power in one sector does not automatically mean having power in others. For example, one would not necessarily expect persons to comply with the directions of an accountant (expert in tax matters) in regard to health practices, although those same persons would probably perform as the accountant directed in regard to record keeping for taxes.

Assets That Create the Power Base

The previous section on bases of social power discussed potential sources of influence. Continuing the analogy of electricity, wecould point out that various resources or assets might be used to generate this electricity. Water might be the resource used, or cobalt, or oil. Likewise, in the case of social power, the basic resources or assets are also varied.

In our modern society, *money* is for many people a potential reward. It serves many purposes. Money can be the means to meet basic needs through purchases of food, shelter, and clothing. It can also represent status and achievement, which are in themselves rewards to some. Thus, money is a major asset in creating a reward power base. The ability to withhold money or to deprive persons of money they posess can be the base for coercive power as well. Money can also be a mediator in achieving a referent power base. This is because money and the real and symbolic goods it can purchase are frequently cause for admiration and subsequent attribution of power by some who may aspire to have similar wealth.

Groups seeking to gain power frequently depend on *people* as the assets from which to derive power. Although it is true that people are an asset from which power can be generated, at least one author has noted that this is a widely variable asset. Morton Deutsch stated that the utility of people as a resource of power is a function of their numbers, their personal qualities, their social cohesion (trust and mutual goals), and their social organization (effective coordination and division of labor).[7] This variability could explain, for example, why simply "having a lot of people on your side"

6 Amitai Etzioni, "Organizational Dimensions and Their Interrelationship: A Theory of Compliance 70 in B. P. Indik and F. K. Berrier, eds.*People, Groups and Organization* (New York: Teachers College Press, 1968), p.94.

7 Morton Deutsch, *The Resolution of Conflict* (New Haven, Conn.: Yale University Press, 1973), p. 395.

may not help to produce the power needed to influence policy or procedure in health care in your country. The possession of a mass of interested persons does not necessarily create an asset sufficient to develop power. In many ways, nursing as a profession is an example of how a very large group can wield relatively little power in many areas. Perhaps one explanation lies in the lack of cohesion and lack of strong social organization within nursing as a profession.

Social status is an asset in developing both a referent and a legitimate power base. A certain "ability to get things done" seems to be conferred on those who achieve high social status. The achievement of high social status is very complex and apparently is related to a number of factors that may vary according to culture. The factors include economic status of self and family, sex, age, education, and occupation. Although the elements prompting high social status vary among cultures, its function as an asset in creating power is constant although not always highly potent. The degree to which it is a factor is, as with all power bases and the assets that create them, dependent on the target (actor).

Knowledge or information is another prime asset. This asset is directly related to the expert power base. As mentioned above, attribution of expert power is apparently based on evaluation of knowledge both on an absolute scale and on a relative one. Therefore, simply knowing a lot will not necessarily create power for the knowledge holder. It is paradoxical that in teaching personnel with whom we work, we may bring them to a knowledge level similar to our own. In doing so, we may be simultaneously dissipating our own power base. This observation is not to suggest that continuing development of staff or education of patients is undesirable, but rather that one must rely on multiple assets and bases for power to accomplish goals, and one must continually analyze assets as they relate to potential targets of influence.

Perhaps at this point it is useful to reiterate that although discussion of power may evoke negative feelings, there is no real reason to perceive power as other than a neutral force-the potential to get things done. It is the uses of power that require examination for negative or positive intents.

Power - Who Needs It?
How Much is Needed?

On observing a variety of individuals, you will notice that they seem to vary widely in their ability to prompt others to act. That difference can be viewed as a difference in levels of power attributed to them by others. As mentioned above, power is defined in relative terms, depending on both the actor and the agent. Therefore, individuals will have varying levels of power, depending on the target or actor with whom they are dealing. But you can probably think of someone who seems powerful in many areas. Or, conversely, you might be able to identify a person who is unable to affect the behavior of anyone at all. The direct reason for the latter situation is a lack of assets to create any of the power bases mentioned above.

The reason for that lack of assets should be examined. Why do some people seek to accumulate the assets that are the basis for power, whereas others appear to be indifferent or to actively avoid gaining a power base? Social and cultural factors can be identified as possible contributors to this difference. Until the relatively recent past, women as a group in the American culture have tended to wield far less power than would have been expected. Culturally and socially, their sphere of concern and interest was more limited than that of males. Whether by choice or by unthinking adherence to norms and mores, American women have been traditionally less likely to seek the assets upon which power is based.

Ethnic and cultural minority groups have been in a similar position in regard to power in the United States. In the past several years, a national concern for equal treatment and for equal rights for all has awakened the concern of many who have subsequently come to realize that the ability to influence others is a key element in achieving equal opportunities.

Another approach to understanding differences in power is psychological. This considers factors within the individual (rather than group attribution) that may affect the level of aspiration or degree of success in gaining bases for power. James Tedeschi, Barry Schlenker, and Thomas Bonoma in early attempts at theory development on this topic have addressed the question, Who wields power?[8] They identified self-confidence, a generalized expectancy of success, as one factor. Those who are high in self-confidence will estimate high probability of obtaining rewards and avoiding costs in using power. These authors also noted that the higher a person's status, the more deference he expects. That person, then, is more self-confident in terms of the possibility of gaining and using power. This information implies that early learning toward developing the self-concept

---

[8] James T. Tedeschi, Barry R. Schlenker, and Thomas V. Bonoma, *Conflict, Power, and Games* (Chicago: Aldine, 1973), p.97.

will affect a person's predispositon toward seeking power. It does not, however, imply that these attributes are fixed and do not continue to vary throughout life. Consider your own perception of yourself. As you learn more about nursing, do you gain confidence about yourself as a nurse and as a person? Or, conversely, do negative experiences in some activities decrease your confidence both specifically in those activities and in general?

Another aspect of the theory developed by Tedeschi, Schlenker, and Bonoma suggests that the question of why levels of aspiration for power vary can be explained in terms of the relative expectation of costs and utility of gaining and using power. Combining concepts from game theory and economic theory, these authors state that a person's subjective expectation of utility in regard to any social behavior will be the basis for deciding to act. Choosing to gain and use power is one specific type of such social behavior. If the expectation of utility (gain or rewards), based on subjectively defined values and preferences, is high, one will choose to seek and use power. If the expectation of utility is negative (costs are great and rewards are low), or the expectation of positive utility is low, then the agent will choose not to seek or use power.[9]

The following example illustrates how this theoretical statement might explain behavior:

> You are a staff nurse in a rehabilitation center. On your unit there are two nurses aids (NAs). Their usual functions are limited to basic patient assistance in activities of daily living and some assistance to the staff nurses in general unit activities. You have a patient, an above-the-knee amputee, who is interested in beginning to take some short trips off the unit, with supervision, to gain confidence in his mobility with his new prosthesis. You would like to have the nurses aid accompany the patient on trips on the hospital grounds. There is no prohibition against assistants performing such tasks, but there is no precedent either. The choices you make about asking the NA to do this can be related to (1) the utility you have assigned to the action and (2) the expectation of success (the NA agreeing to perform the action). Suppose, for example, that you are convinced that this activity is important for the patient and you believe that the NA will find it satisfying to be helpful in this way. The utility is thus relatively high from your perspective. If you are self-confident and are aware that you have a legitimate base of power in your position and are aware also that the NA attributes expert power to you; and since you have had a good working relationship with the NA in the past, you will have a relatively high expectation of achieving the utility you have assigned to the action. Therefore, you would choose to ask the NA to take on this new task.

9 Ibid.,p.93.

In reality, we seldom are so thorough in our reasoning about choices to attempt to influence others, as in the case example above, but the concept of subjective expectation of utility is a useful one in analyzing decisions to use power.

The most obvious examples of power use in organizations are those where one (the source) possesses a legitimate power base as the superior in a superior-subordinate organizational line, such as in head nurse-staff nurse or staff nurse-nurse assistant relationships. However, the legitimate base is not the only relevant base, nor is it a necessary prerequisite for the exercise of power. You can probably think of examples in which a staff nurse or a group of staff nurses has influenced a supervisor to change some procedure or to make some decision favored by that group. In this case, bases of power other than the legitimate base prompted the action.

Thus, although social power is not finitely quantifiable, it is probably true that different power bases are acknowledged in varying degrees by different individuals. For example, someone's legitimate power, especially if I perceive my own to be nearly equal to his, may carry "very little weight" with me. However, if he possesses reward power in the form of ability to increase my salary, that may very well cause me to attribute considerable power to him. Because of this individual difference in attribution of power, it is sometimes difficult to determine "how much is enough" to accomplish the desired end.

As you analyze situations where you wish to influence others to act, and where you are the subject of influence attempts, it will become apparent that there are advantages to understanding how power is gained, how it may be dissipated and the effects of lack of power-all of which are discussed in the next section.

Gaining, Using, and Being without Power

Since power is created from assets, in abstract terms, one gains power by amassing assets. Confining the question of assets to the professional situation you are involved in, there are several possible ways to increase assets and therefore potentially increase power. One major asset is position; that is, to increase the status and authority of position is to increase the legitimate base. Another asset is the ability to provide praise (most of us have that ability if we use it wisely), to recommend salary increases and other forms of tangible rewards, and/or to make work assignments. These and similar assets create the reward bases.

Gaining the opportunity to provide some of these rewards is usually related to position definition. Frequently, however, opportunities to gain and use these assets are overlooked. For example, if you have authority by position description to make personnel evaluations, you have defaulted on gaining assets for power if you have let that become a ritual rather than a meaningful opportunity to provide reward. The converse of the ability to reward is the ability to punish, by withholding rewards or by more direct and physical means. Although a strong ethical sense of individual rights and a belief in the ability of people to improve and achieve when rewarded may discourage the actual use of coercive power, there are some for whom coercive power is the only sort they will acknowledge.

The primary asset for expert power is the possession of information or skill. Increasing assets for this base requires an increase in knowledge or skill by the agent and probably also requires some effort to make the target aware that the expertise exists. The referent base is one for which it is difficult to amass assets since the attribution of this type of power is largely based on attraction to a person or group conceived by the target. Physical attractiveness is frequently an influence in creating this base, but is not the only element.

Another consideration in accumulating power is the possibility of combining bases; that is, rather than relying on reward power alone, combine the reward base with the expert base or use other combinations of bases. In this way, the potential of accumulating power is maximized. Even though one base may have little relevance for an individual target, the other base or the combination may. When the target is a group, a combination of bases can help appeal to the responses of various members of the group.

Still another option to increase power is coalition formation. This strategy is frequently used by individuals or groups with relatively little power vis-a-vis their target. Two or more parties combine their assets and thereby combine power bases toward accomplishing a particular goal. The coalition is not a permanent nor total partnership. The only real necessity is that the partners agree that both can benefit from the alliance and that they make clear to the target that they are united in this purpose. This is a common strategy in situations where decision making is based on votes, such as in legislative activity. Combining single votes from a variety of disparate sources can produce a necessary majority on a particular issue.

In organizational settings, although not as obvious as in legislative activities, coalitions may be formed by lower power individuals or groups in order to gain desired ends. The power base resulting may be any of those mentioned above. An example would be when staff nurses in a community health clinic form a coalition with a local women's group to gain power in seeking additional funds for equipment. The staff nurses may possess a small coercive base and a moderate expert base. These bases could be combined with the reward base represented by the women's group's continued financial support of special projects of the clinic. This example also illustrates that coalitions are not limited to participants in the formal organization, even though the target and the desired behavior are within the organizational context. As a group that has traditionally held relatively little power in most arenas, nurses could make good use of coalition formation in seeking to accomplish goals in health care.

Although it is possible to learn about power and subsequently to make definite efforts to gain the assets to increase power, some individuals or groups may never gain much power. This may be because their level of aspiration does not require it or because they are able to meet their own needs without dealing with other people. For those who are without power yet wish to receive rewards (or prevent pain), there is little other open as a course of action except: (1) to comply and consistently be a target rather than a source of influence, or (2) to ingratiate themselves with those who do hold power. Ingratiation, according to Tedeschi, Schlenker, and Bonoma, is "deliberate and illicit strategies people employ for the purpose of increasing their attractiveness in the eyes of others and in the hopes of thereby acquiring subsequent rewards."[10]. This may produce satisfying results if one wants to be dependent upon the wishes of others. But this characteristic seems inconsistent with the expectations that a professional person or group should be decisive and able, when necessary, to cause things to happen, that is, to exercise some power.

Another more satisfying strategy when one is relatively powerless is to set about to offset the power of others by reducing the dependence on others for some rewards. This requires the ability to evaluate oneself and grant "good feelings" for positive accomplishments. Another effort at such decrease in dependence for rewards might be to seek a work setting where a fair and impartial system for merit evaluation and subsequent promotions is in operation. Reducing dependence on others for information also offsets those persons' power over to you. When you can use or gain direct access to

---

[10] Ibid., p.85

primary sources of information, you do not depend on others for that information or their interpretation of it. For example, if you seek and use the personnel manual to answer your own questions about policies, you have offset a bit of the power a long-term organizational member may have in relation to you.

The Cost of Using Power

One final idea among the general concepts about power is *cost*. Power is created from assets which are finite. It is possible to exhaust the assets through "spending" just as with strictly tangible assets like money. Some assets are less tangible than money and are more difficult to quantify, yet they do form expendable items both absolutely and relatively. For example, in the absolute sense, it is possible to exhaust the supply of new information you possess in holding an expert base. If you do not maintain and update your knowledge and skills, those with whom you deal can attain the same knowledge level. In the relative sense, it is possible to exhaust your store of relevant rewards in relation to a particular target if you "run out" or if the item ceases to be rewarding to that target. Suppose that I am rewarding a child for running errands by giving him candy. I can "run out" of candy, or he may decide that he no longer likes the candy and would prefer apples or money instead.

Tedeschi, Schlenker, and Bonoma described costs of influence (the use of power) as falling into two categories: source-based costs and target-based costs.[11] The example above can be used to illustrate both types. A source-based cost is one that is voluntarily incurred by the source. In the example, I chose to use some of my asset-candy-to gain the influence I desired. I chose to do that on my own. A target-based cost is one incurred by the source as a result of responses by the target. If the child resists my efforts to use candy as a reward to get errands run, I may find it necessary to use some other resources to accomplish the same end. Although I retain the choice in whether to expend the asset or to forget about the errands, the target has changed the cost to me. Thus, as either party to an influence effort changes, the power equation changes also. If you are to use power wisely, it is

[11] Ibid., p.95.

necessary to monitor such changes carefully in any attempts you may make to influence others.

Politics in the Work Setting

Just as with power, politics has come to carry some negative connotations for anyone who does not enjoy complicated interaction among persons in their professional activities. Consider the following example as a preliminary to further discussions of the concept.

> You have just arrived at work, the first day of the second month on your first job. As you arrive you notice that two other staff nurses are engaged in a very animated conversation. You overhear bits of it-"I've only had one weekend off a month for the last three months." "Short of staff.""Admitting patients that should be in CCU (coronary care unit)." "Never enough linen.""Rotate to nights with only one day off between changes." As you approach, one of the staff nurses looks up and says, "Are you interested in working with us? We're going to organize a staff nurses unit and get the state nurses association to represent us. No one is taking care of us and we can't take care of patients as a result."
>
> "Well," you say, "I need to think about this a little, but I surely do believe that nurses need a voice in decisions about what happens to them and their patients."
>
> Then imagine this next scene. It is four days later. You are just emerging from Mrs. J's room where you have just managed to get her to help feed herself after weeks of depressed dependence. The smile of accomplishment you are wearing turns to dismay when you look about and see that six of the ten patients for whom you are responsibile have call lights on and there is no one in sight. Where, you wonder, have the personnel gone? You mentally set priorities and quickly begin answering the lights. Just as you emerge from the fifth patient's room, you see two nurse's aids emerge from a vacant room. With them is the ward manager from your unit. The ward manager is carrying the personnel schedule, which he develops for the head nurse's approval. You hear one aid say to the ward manager; "I know Mrs. Parsons won't even notice the change and it really will help me. Head nurses don't pay that much attention. To them an aid is an aid. Thanks, I'll see you at lunch." The other aid then says to the ward manager, "I'm sure glad that you're in charge of scheduling now. You understand our schedule change problems lots better than Mrs. Parsons did. But that's no surprise."

Does this seem real to you? If it does, perhaps we can now examine what was really happening in this situation. At first glance two things are evident: (1) the staff nurses are organizing, and (2) there are at least two nurse's aids who have found a way to get their schedule as they like it, possibly at the expense of paying close attention to the patients. An example of *good* and *bad*? Perhaps, but the evaluative terms *good* and *bad* might be used quite differently, depending on your perspective. For example, suppose that the perspective we take is that of the nursing supervisor, not a newly licensed staff nurse. Do you suppose the supervisor's response might be different to the first scene? Or suppose that you were one of the aids, who has what she thinks is good reason for getting a specific day off each week. The perspective makes the difference, because in each case the individuals involved were acting in what they believed to be their own best interests. That is the very core of what is called *politics*. It is a very human, very interesting, and possibly very frustrating and potentially damaging phenomenon. It is also one that most of us are not well equipped to deal with on other than an emotional basis.

In order to examine politics from a theoretical perspective, a first step is to define the term. Stephen Robbins defines politics as "any behavior by an organizational member that is self-serving." He goes on to say, "It is *functional* when that behavior assists in the attainment of the organization's goals. It is *dysfunctional* when it hinders these goals."[12]

Political behavior can be totally individual, the action of one person, for that one person's ends. It can also be group behavior directed to goals a group views as in the best interest of its members.

It is evident that one of the natural consequences of self-interest behavior is potential conflict. Since the self-interests of one individual and those of another do not always correspond, the possibility exists that at some point the individuals will perceive that their interests are antagonistic. Conflict will then ensue. To use the above example, when the registered nurses organize as a group to promote their interests, the nurse executive may see that particular political behavior as in direct opposition to her desire to maintain a good public image. Each party to the interaction has defined her own interests, and these interests may conflict with each other. It is interesting to note that seldom does anyone actually publicly admit aloud that self-interest is the issue when such a conflict arises. Values, ethics, organizational integrity, the care of the patients-all of these are the reasons given for one's position. The staff nurses may be deeply interested in some professional value that prompts concern for the ratio of staff to patients. Or, from the other point of view, perhaps some organizational loyalty prompts the director's position. Once the position is taken it becomes the person's own-an element of self-interest.

[12] Stephen P. Robbins, The *Administrative Process* (Englewood Cliffs, N.J.: Prentice- Hall, 1976), p.64

Although conflict is a potential result, this is not to suggest that *all* political behavior results in conflict. Sometimes political behavior will result in a person's position, extent of power, scope in performance, or recognition being enhanced. Furthermore, this may not be at the direct expense of another person. Of course, if we view power, participation, and recognition as being finite in quantity, then we can reason that one persons's gain is someone else's potential loss, for the quantity is no longer available to them for potential increases in their own power or recognition. Therefore, some political actions will cause considerably more conflict in an organization than others. For example, you can predict that an action will cause major difficulty if you can determine whether either or both of the following conditions exist: (1) The action is performed deliberately by a large or organized group. (2) The total organization (not just individuals in it) is at risk of losing money, prestige, or operational capacity as a result of the action. Examples of political activity can be viewed as existing along a continuum, from small one-person "shows" to large major campaigns, with a variety of maneuvering between these two points.

Another key point in understanding politics is that the less structure in the organization and the less clarity in roles, the greater the chances of political activity taking place. Robbins notes that a well-run bureaucratic structure discourages political activity.[13] This seems logical, since the power, scope of decision making, and other parameters of each position in a bureaucracy are spelled out regardless of who fills the position. The result is a highly structured built-in certainty of routine. But it is also proposed that a tight bureaucracy may be antithetical to the development of creative work and so it is best suited to routine kinds of work. Therefore, since much of nursing, especially in less structured settings, requires creative activity, the development of a tight bureaucracy hardly seems to be a logical solution to reducing political activity in an organization. This last statement might imply that when political activity exists, it needs to be stamped out. Is that necessarily true?

Robbins in his definition of politics, as noted earlier, spoke of functional and dysfunctional political behavior. The dysfunctional conflict-producing politics has been discussed above. He also calls some politics *neutral*. *Neutral*, he says, is that behavior in one's interest that is essentially passing

---

[13] Ibid., p.65.

the buck.[14] The individual does nothing overt, neither does she or he state an opinion. Rather the person protects *self* by being noncontroversial. Although this may be somewhat frustrating, it is generally not worth the effort to get the person to take a stand on the issue, unless, of course, that person is supposed to be making decisions regularly.

What then is functional politics, a form of behavior that may need to be encouraged rather than discouraged? The definition said that self-interest behavior that promotes the goals of the organization is called *functional*. Given the meaning, performing well on the job, thereby seeking a good evaluation and promotion and obtaining salary increases, is functional political behavior. It promotes the individual's self-interest while furthering organizational goals.

Political behavior then can certainly be either a negative or positive force for the organization as well as for individuals. Since that is so, your concern as a person entering a work setting in a new role is not necessarily how to stay out of politics, or how to keep from being a target. Rather, your effort should be directed toward understanding the political behavior present in an organization and making wise choices about when and how you will participate.

As mentioned earlier, formal organizational structures, especially the extreme form of the bureaucracy, are designed to reduce or eliminate uncertainty and should as a result reduce politics in the organization. However, humans, being what we are, generally find ways of getting past formal structures when we want to. In organizations, the result is the unofficial network of communication and decision making often referred to as the *informal organization*. The example of the nurse's aids' going directly to the person developing the schedule rather than to the head nurse as prescribed by the formal organization is an example of the informal structure in action.

The key to understanding institutional politics is understanding the organization's informal structure. It might well be said that small groups are the key to holding the informal structure together. How then does the new nurse in the situation identify where these groups are and what their functions are? One of the best ways is to note who spends time together at work. Who helps out whom, without being requested to? Who takes coffee breaks or mealtimes together? In these groups that consistently form at

14 Ibid., p.77.

social times, who seems to be at the hub? To whom do the members seem to defer in conversation? That person is a leader in some way. Take note. That group provides communication for its members. If you are astute, within a month you can recite all the pairings and other groupings that develop on your unit and division. All you need to do is watch, listen, and make mental notes. This activity in itself is preparatory. It is much like learning the rosters of the football teams playing in a game. You will need the information later, whether as a spectator or as a player.

Once you have begun to identify how the informal communication and decisions seem to flow, you must remember that the "nonstructure" is quite fluid, potentially changing as new members come and go. So you need to periodically validate your observations. The next thing with which to be concerned is your own position in this structure. Your first political act may well be deciding how to respond to or participate in the informal structure. Will you seek the safety of a group headed by someone else? There is a risk here that the group's interest may not reflect yours. Will you be a full-time loner? The risk in this situation is of being so marginal as to lose communication in both informal and formal structures. Perhaps you will align yourself with another "rookie". There is a certain comfort here. But will your own development be retarded by remaining peripheral in this way? One suggestion is to try to find out, by accepting invitations and by making intentional efforts at gaining proximity, what the interests of various groups and individuals are. You can do this by identifying recurrent themes of conversation. You can ask, "What do you think?" kinds of questions. Then you can look past the superficial reasons and rationale to identify possible reasons why those interests are someone else's self-interests.

You must remember that interaction among your coworkers goes on all during the work itself. All that interaction has meaning. If you want to manage the politics that will affect you, you will need to be acutely aware of both the work and those with whom you work, because both elements are inextricably related.

At the point when you have become somewhat aware of the social groupings and their defined self-interests, you can then begin to make intelligent choices. You can become a part of those activities and groups that you see as functional, in the sense mentioned earlier, and satisfying for you.

It will take vigilance to avoid having your interests dictated by group pressure. A very important step toward preventing yourself from being submerged in the work group and risking loss in integrity of personal choice is to build a strong personal support system. This system can only provide support *when needed most* if it does *not* depend on your being defined by your work alone. The people in that support system must relate to you as friend, piano player, skier, spouse, or whatever, and only incidentally as nurse. Having that kind of wholeness can make you even more valuable as a nurse because it provides balance and perspective and the basis for empathy.

Now, to reiterate, in order to manage the politics you encounter, it is necessary to:

1. Understand it in specific terms-people and issues.
2. Make intelligent decisions about how to participate and with whom in *functional* self-interest activities.
3. Remember that doing an excellent, consistently visible job is,in itself,one of the most functional self-interest activities anyone can perform.

One other issue regarding politics needs consideration here. What do you do when you are the target or are about to be a casualty in another person's political moves? The first thing to do is to try not to put yourself in that position. That is, do not be so naive as to believe that everyone is acting in *your* best interest. It is not a typical human trait to be constantly altruistic. There is no need to be angry or to feel betrayed by this statement. In fact, it is placing a terrible burden on our fellow humans to expect them to be super-human at all times.

We would all like to think that we could depend on our colleagues to sort out whether any act they perform will infringe on another person before proceeding. Many people will. But just because *you* do not intend to drive into the back of the car in front of you is no reason to throw away your rear-view mirror, assuming (because *you* have good intentions), you won't be rear-ended. Thus it is with the world of work. Realistically it is better to be aware of human temptation and identify to whom you may be a threat or a convenient stepping stone. You can make yourelf an ally of someone you may be a threat to, by providing willing assistance and helping them know that you as an ethical person will not advance at their expense. For those who might use you as a stepping stone, confrontation is a healthy way to inform them that you are not to be so used. That confrontation can be growth-producing for both of you.

Again, it is important to note that everyone legitimately has self-interests, and there is no reason why he or she should feel uncomfortable for advancing his/her interests in an ethical, functional way. Identify what you want to accomplish, and whether you can accomplish it within the framework of a particular organization's goals and in the company of its personnel. If you find through examination, either from interview or experience there, that you cannot accomplish your goals, your choices are to either

surrender your interests, leave the organization, or try to change it (which is ultimately an attempt at advancing your interest).

As you grow and learn, you will reexamine your self-interests. Where once your greatest concern was with your position providing a learning experience, perhaps you will reach a time when you are concerned with how you can develop new strategies for providing care. A careful self-inventory at regular intervals is important. At the same time, it is prudent to recognize that other than functional forms of political behavior exist and will probably continue to do so. Political behavior, like social power, exists; it is neither good nor bad in itself, and only becomes so from certain perspectives. Politics needs to be understood and dealt with competently if one is to survive and flourish in the work setting.

SUMMARY

Social power has been examined here as a construct for analyzing and understanding interaction designed to produce influence. Examples have been cited to illustrate how understanding power relationships can be a useful tool in professional situations. The related concept, politics, was presented, relatively briefly, along with suggestions for using this information for successful personal interactions in the work setting.

Additional Reading

Damrosch, Shirley, P. Sullivan and L. Holdeman, "How Nurses Get their Way: Power Strategies and Nursing", Journal of Professional Nursing (Sept./Oct., 1987) 284-290

del Bueno, Dorothy, "Power and Politics in Organizations" Nursing Outlook 34,3 (May/June, 1986) 124-128

Gorman, Sheila and N. Clark, "Power and Effective Nursing Practice" Nursing Outlook 34,3 (May/June, 1986) 129-134

Lamar, Edie, "Communicating Personal Power Through Nonverbal Behavior" Journal of Nursing Administration 15,1 (January, 1985) 41-44

Langford, Teddy, "Impotence May be Curable: An Essay" <u>Nursing Leadership</u> 1,1 (June, 1978) 29-32

McClelland, David and D. Burnham, "Power is the Great Motivator" <u>Harvard Business Review</u> 54,2 (March/April, 1976) 100-110

Chapter 6

Conflict and its management in work relationships

Building quickly, like a thunderstorm, some conflicts can develop rapidly into major disturbances. Other conflicts build slowly, taking weeks or months to develop. Either type can result in discomfort for the persons involved. When the conflict affects work relationships, it can be doubly troublesome since it not only affects the individuals and their emotional state but also the work output. This chapter examines conflict as a social phenomenon, its outcomes, and techniques for resolving or managing it.

Conflict Defined; Dynamics Identified

Stephen Robbins states that conflict "refers to all kinds of opposition or antagonistic interaction. It is based on scarcity of power, resources or social positions, and differing value structures."[1] This definition, like this chapter, does not refer to psychological conflict but rather to social conflict, either interpersonal or intergroup. There is no single pure form of conflict. Instead there are numerous conceptions of conflict presently used by social scientists developing research on the topic. Some theorists argue that if one person perceives himself to have a conflict with another, it exists whether it is realized or not by both parties. Another useful concept is that conflict can be covert or overt. Covert conflict may result from antagonistic psychological realtionships vis-a-vis another party or group. These such antagonistic

---

[1] Stephen Robbins *Managing Organizational Conflict* Englewood Cliffs, NJ: Prentice-Hall, 1974, 23

relationships exist when there are incompatible goals and interests or incompatible value structures. In any one of these cases, one could be in conflict long before any overt signs were visible. Overt conflict, on the other hand, can range from verbal skirmishes to all-out warfare.

An example of covert (social) conflict might be your feeling antagonistic toward another staff member in response to her stated desire to be head nurse, even though you may not speak to her about the issue. Since covert conflict is not visible, it is not amenable to the same type of resolution techniques that can be used in resolving overt conflict. In this example, the conflict might be based on your concern with the staff member's standards for performance, that is, a differing value structure, or it might be because you want the position (status) yourself. Or perhaps there are a combination of the sources of conflict operating.

Another view of conflict in an organization is that it exists along a continuum from concensus (no conflict) to violence (extreme conflict). Sexton's model is shown adapted[2] below as Figure 6.1. In this view, when conflict moves from polarization ("Taking sides" in a rigid way) toward impasse (This cannot be solved using ordinary methods), participants have moved toward pathological levels of conflict. When pathological levels of conflict occur, external controls (such as restraint by authorities) are necessary. The idea of a continuum of conflict is valuable. It suggests that different levels of conflict are not fundamentally different, but are differences in degree or extensiveness.

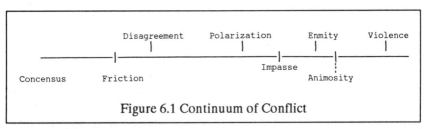

Figure 6.1 Continuum of Conflict

The usual response to the mention of conflict is that it is a negative situation. Robbins has taken a different position, stating that what he characterizes as the *interactionist's view* of conflict in organization is the more productive approach. Contrasted with two other approaches to conflict, the *traditional* and the *behavioral*, the characteristics of the interactionist's view are shown in Table 6.1. This approach is, according to its author, normative, a prescription, rather than descriptive as are the two

2 adapted from Dorothy Sexton,"Organizational Conflict: A Creative or Destructive Force",*Nursing Leadership* 3,No.3 (September, 1980)p.18

other approaches. The traditional approach assumes rather simply that conflict should be eliminated, whereas the behavioral approach focuses on acceptance of conflict as "built in" to human interaction. The interactionist approach further assumes that conflict can have positive functions but does not seek in any way to create conflict. Although I do not agree with Robbin's view as to the value of manager-created conflict, there does seem to be merit in admitting this as one possible method for improving function in some organizations.

Robbins also states that conflict can be functional or dysfunctional.[3] In an organization, conflict is functional if it supports the goals of the organization. The rationale here is that change and innovation are stimulated by conflict. Dysfunctional conflict is that which does not further the organization's goals. However, this may not be directly functional for the individuals involved.

A final element in defining conflict is an indication of factors that lead to the creation of conflict. Three such sources are listed by Robbins. They are communication, structure, and personal behavior factors.[4] A key source of difficulty arising from communication occurs when communicators are operating at different levels of abstraction. For example, one nurse's interpretation of "we adhere to standards of excellence in practice" may be that the hospital has a formal statement of standards and that supervision is directed to those standards. This interpretation of the message is at a much more detailed level than the actual abstract statement. A conflict could ensue if the nurse places high value on having explicit standards and they do not exist in the agency.

Structure of an organization can produce conflict when the reward system seems unfair or implies that rewards are limited and therefore must be competed for. Complexity can also produce difficulty with access to information and subsequent conflict. Personal behavior factors related to conflict generation include low self-esteem, dogmatism, and authoritarianism. The low self- esteem person tends to see practically everyone as a threat of some sort. Therefore, the implication that the threat means loss of current possessions, status, or power is a strong stimulus for conflict. Whether the conflict will be overt in such a situation depends on a number of other factors, including other personality attributes. The dogmatic individual will be frequently at odds with others over value structure questions. That is because his own interpretation of values tends to be narrow, quite specific, and rigid, usually implying not only that his is the appropriate view, but that

3 Ibid.,p.23.
4 Ibid.,p.25

it is the *only* view. One can be dogmatic in "any direction." That is, one who holds what are characterized as liberal views may be just as dogmatic about these views as the conservative, although the usual association with dogmatic is conservative.

Reflecting on personal experience, we can identify that there are typical circumstances under which conflict can logically be expected to develop. They include:

- Situations where resources (money, time, space, etc.) are limited.
- Situations where communication is hampered by language differences (either different languages or different vocabularies are used or there are physical impediments to communication such as deafness).
- Situations where parties have major differences in values, goals, or ideas about methods related to the issue at hand.
- Situations where one party is not allowed participation in decision making which affects them (if they expect to have this input).
- Situations where one party attempts behavior control over another.
- Situations where one party is more dependent on another than he/she wishes to be.

Some literature implies that all conflict can be resolved. This is not necessarily the case. In an organizational conflict, the manager can usually take some action to reduce conflicts but not necessarily to successfully eliminate every one. Some factors are beyond the manager's control. Carla Mariano wrote,

A major factor in maintaining conflict at high intensity occurs when protagonists define a negotiable conflict (the focal issue is over a divisible resource, like money, which can be made available to the entire group) as non-negotiable (the focal issue becomes a non-divisible resource, like status or success, when there can be only one winner if winning is to have any value).[5]

In such a case, if the manager were trying to mediate this conflict, the escalation would be beyond her control.

Conflict Escalates

Whether you are a participant in the conflict (a disputant), or are a manager concerned about conflict between or among those with whom you

5 Carla Mariano, "The Dynamics of Conflict," *Journal of Nursing Education*, 17, No.5 (May 1978), 7.

work it will be useful to know how serious a conflict is. Being able to identify whether one or both parties has moved far toward the extreme pole of the conflict continuum (see Fig. 6.1) will help you be effective in either of those roles.

As an observer, you can detect changes in behavior of the conflict parties as conflict escalates. Changes include:

• Arguing heatedly.
• Increasing loudness of speech.
• Interruptions.
• Making personally derogatory comments.
• Broadening the conflict to other issues.
• Seeking allies.
• Breaking rules of common courtesy.
• Making physically intimidating gestures.
• Initiating actual physical violence.

As a party to a conflict, you can probably identify escalation by your own emotional and physical reactions. Even if you do not feel personally threatened by the conduct (because you believe you are winning?) you can detect the heightened awareness and accelerated sensory input which is typical of the early stages of the stress response. After all, the stress response is to ready us for *fight* or *flight*. But, because many of us perceive conflict negatively in all cases or at least when we believe we are losing, you may experience escalation of conflict as increase in "bad" feelings. These include negative emotions such as anger and physical sensations such as nausea, stomach pain, diarrhea, headache, and/or dyspnea.

Reaction to Conflict

Much that goes on in our Western culture discourages open conflict between individuals and groups, probably because the potential high point on the conflict scale is annihilation of some or all participants. Families, the churches, and many schools tend to expect conformity and do not tolerate conflict. The suppression of all conflict suggests that since some forms of conflict are deadly, all disagreements are bad. This is no more logical than to say that since automobiles are involved in deadly accidents, all autos should be banned or at least made inoperable. Conflict is a natural protective response. One typical reaction to the *conflict state itself* is anxiety at some level. The degree of anxiety will depend on the extent to which our culture has created distaste for conflict in us as much as the actual extent of conflict. If anxiety is allowed to increase without being identified and dealt with constructively, it can be personally detrimental, causing emotional discomfort, inability to concentrate, and possibly resulting in the use of even less satisfying coping mechanisms. For these reasons it is useful to gain understanding of conflict and of useful interventions that will prevent either yourself or those whose work you supervise from being affected negatively by conflict.

Groups tend to react to conflict with other groups by becoming more cohesive among themselves. This, too, varies depending on the commitment of individual group members and the degree to which they identify their self-interests as being affected by the conflict.

Managing Conflict

A number of authors have identified methods used to deal with conflict. Although they do not speak to this issue, one legitimate concern for you as manager or as one who is managed is the perspective or role you play in the conflict and how this may affect your use of any of these techniques. As each of the methods is discussed below, it will be considered from these two perspectives.

Fred Luthans suggests three strategies that can be used in dealing with intergroup conflicts.[6]. In each case, the perspective is that of the manager or top administrator, with the further assumption that he or she is functioning as a third party rather than as one of the protagonists. The first strategy is to *erect buffers*. This means to place intermediate persons, procedures, or physical space between the two groups so that necessary interaction between them is reduced. This is especially helpful if the basis of the conflict is concern about status.

The second strategy is *creating better insights*.[7] This refers to group training or human relations training or other similar activities designed to help the individuals involved change their behavior by helping them have new understanding of their own needs and motivation. Since this is a learning approach, the hazard is that the individuals will not be receptive enough, nor intelligent enough, or both, to perceive the relationship of the "new insight" to the old situation. In cases where there are relatively

---

6 Fred Luthans, *Introduction to Management* (New York: McGraw-Hill, 1976), p.298
7 Ibid., p.298

open-minded, positively motivated group members, the approach has a good chance of success.

The third strategy is to *redesign the organizational structure*.[8] This, in effect, is a cure by excision. The source of the conflict is identified and is either moved out of the organization altogether or is placed in a new relationship to different groups. If the conflict is clearly group-group, the groups may be reconstructed with new members, based on a new structure for the organization. For example, a nursing home might use a version of team nursing that places a registered nurse (RN) over two licensed vocational nurses (LVNs), each of whom works with two nurse's aids. Suppose that the two teams are constantly in conflict over who is to do the cleanup chores in areas of common use, who will give report first, and other similar status and resource-related concerns. The RN is not willing to terminate any of the personnel since each is a good worker. Therefore, the RN restructures the organization, making each individual responsible for a group of patients, and having one rotating functional assignment for the LVNs giving medication and treatments.

Several other techniques are listed by Robbins.[9] *Expansion of resources* is a logical choice when the source of conflict is scarce resources. For example, when each nurse can have all the linen she wants, conflict over linen no longer occurs. This technique, like many others, assumes that the conflict manager is not one of the protagonists, so the nurse would be acting in her manager role if she chose this method, since it requires some level of authority and discretion for use of resources.

Avoidance is another very common technique. This may be a nurse's choice, no matter what managerial or professional role she is in, if she becomes a party to conflict. Simply put, one either withdraws from the situation or avoids it. Although this may sound cowardly, not taking sides, as a matter of fact there are some conflicts that with time will simply dissipate on their own. If the conflict has been avoided, there will be some degree of saving of energy. This method is effective only if withdrawal actually does reduce or eliminate the conflict. For example, if you have a conflict with another person, avoiding speaking to that person, in effect, may not be avoiding the conflict if you are carrying it around with you while it grows larger. Avoidance is useful only as a protagonist manager when you can effect the same for others who are in conflict.

Smoothing is another technique that is expecially useful if the persons involved will not be interacting continuously over a long period of time. It

---

8 Ibid., p.298.
9 Robbins, *Managing Organizational Conflict*, p.67

will not be useful if long-term team building is one of your goals. Smoothing is the "oil on troubled waters" solution of emphasizing common interests among the combatants and playing down differences that may exist. It can be used by an individual in either a participant or nonparticipant role, although it is probably more easily done by a nonparticipant. An example of this technique is when, in a meeting of a temporary committee, a conflict arises over an element of the planned new patient chart form. The "smoother" points out that "we are all interested in good care and in meeting accreditation requirements, and the matter in question is really a minor difference; so surely we can agree, especially since we only have one more meeting."

Compromise can be generated among the individuals or groups in conflict or may be suggested by an arbitrary other. This compromise method is one that acknowledges, especially in resource disputes, that everyone cannot have what they want. Therefore, rationing the desired resource or substituting others for it are the compromise solutions. A common example of compromise is the union-management bargaining sessions, where each party wants to keep or to gain the available resources such as wage money. The agreement reached is always a compromise. The compromise in union-management disputes has become almost ritual, but in other cases it may be a novel solution to a conflict. There are some people for whom compromise is not acceptable. It represents a "Solomon's solution"-a resource that to them should not be divisible is being divided. The degree to which a person or group may take such a position, that compromise is untenable, probably depends on the expectation of success and the degree to which acceptance by the other person or group is valued.

The fact that some individuals are granted authority to supervise the performance of certain functions by others makes *authoritative command* another possible technique for conflict resolution. "Stop that, right now," is the message conveyed, which, of course, could be used effectively only if the person giving the command is not one of those in direct conflict. You might have occasion to use this technique in your manager role, but you should not assume that it is more than a temporary measure, for if the conflict is serious, it will recur.

Another method which can help make positive use of the conflict situation is *rational problem solving*. The intent is to assemble those in conflict and to get them to agree to focus on the problem and a rational solution to it. This assumes that there is a rational solution available, although for conflicts over values or status this may not be true. In cases where problem solving can work, the technique is to have either the most objective protagonist, or preferably a third party, lead the group through the following problem-solving steps:

- Definition of the problem.
- Collection of facts and other pertinent information.
- Suggestion of alternative solutions.
- Choice of a solution.

The final choice is best reached by consensus rather than by a simple majority since the conflict is embedded in "not agreeing" with something; and when the majority rule is used, the minority have no reason to agree. Further steps will include a decision or a plan for action and some method for follow-up or evaluation.

Another method for positive conflict management is the *development of superordinate goals*. This method is most appropriate when the individuals or groups involved are going to be interacting continuously over time. In this case, the action is to help the group, again probably best done as a nonparticipant, to choose some goal on which everyone can agree, in order to divert them from the source of conflict to a more productive effort.

R. Tappen suggests that *confrontation* is a direct and honest way to make conflict a productive experience, since the individual or group involved receives direct feedback on the other individual or group's thoughts and feelings about the conflict situation. She lists six techniques used in confrontation.[10]

1. *Confrontation through information:* Each one tells what is seen or felt from her perspective.
2. *Direct challenges:* This demands that the other person change his/her behavior.
3. *Calling the other's game:* Where game playing is a diversion producing conflict, a statement is made indicating that the game is recognized.
4. *Processing:* This means interrupting a group's function and evaluating it, examining the conflict.
5. *Videotapes and tape recordings:* No interpretation is provided. Simply present the person or group with the feedback.
6. *Collective bargaining:* This technique involves group feedback either by formal union-management activities or by other group action designed to deal with a conflict felt by the group.

[10] R. Patten, "Strategies for Dealing with Conflict Using Confrontation," *Journal of Nursing Education*, 17, No. 5 (May 1978), 50-52.

Mediation Skills

Each of the methods of dealing with conflict mentioned above can be useful no matter whether you are a party to the conflict or a manager of it. Another series of techniques is especially useful for the manager. These are mediation skills. Mediation is the process by which an external party is allowed to help those in conflict reach a resolution. Mediation is *not* arbitration, which occurs when a third party solves a conflict on behalf of the participants who are then bound by the solution. As a manager, you should avoid becoming an arbitrator with your employees' conflicts since you can then become a convenient target for blame by both parties. The arbitration also tends to relieve the conflict parties of responsibility to develop problem solving skills. They are free to "Take it to Dad" to settle the issue. The long term result can be detrimental to their personal and professional growth.

If you choose to attempt to mediate a conflict, a special version of the problem solving process will be useful guide. Be aware that mediating is a time consuming task which requires patience and objectivity. Steps in mediating include the following:

Gather data about the conflict from those who are parties to it. Because each party to a conflict has a unique perspective on the situation, each must be interviewed, separately, but with knowledge of the other that this is occurring. Your purpose as mediator is to help each person make a clear statement of what the issues are, to determine if the parties have any goals in common, to check whether the disputants are willing to deal productively with the conflict, or if they are receiving pleasure or gain from continuing the dispute. Other questions to answer from each person's perspective are, what is my potential loss in this situation? Why is this *personal* to me?

State the Problem(s) in the conflict. The mediator should analyze the data which have been gathered and decide at least the following as elements of the problem he or she is to help solve: Is the conflict over facts, methods, goals, or values? Is there evidence of *any* common goals? Would a new definition of this conflict help in generating solutions? What is likely to occur if the conflict continues?

Bring the parties together to begin a mutual effort to resolve the conflict. This aspect requires careful "stage setting". Find a neutral site and make the room comfortable. Provide some light refreshments such as juice or soft drinks if you believe this helps lower tension. Have a plan of *process* in mind which includes each of the steps in this problem solving process. As the mediator, you are responsible for setting the structure in which the parties can work to solve their conflict. State the purpose of the meeting and clearly indicate that you *will not* be the person to resolve the conflict, the disputants will. (If you are the manager or other organizational superior of those in conflict, you may choose to use some of your legitimate power to *require* that they do work toward a solution. If you do not have that organizational authority, you will need to rely on their mutual desire to conclude the discomfort caused by the conflict.)

Gain agreement in definition of the problem. Based on your earlier assessment describe your perspective of the problem. Be objective and make the statement in a way that places no blame or indicates no "good side" in the conflict. The statement could take the form, "Mr. X, you believe that you should be allowed to care for as many AIDS patients as possible since you want to become especially competent in their care. Ms. Y, you believe that the AIDS patients would be better cared for if you also were assigned to some of them." If each agrees to your statement of their main concern, you can then begin to seek a single problem definition to which they can *both* agree. For example, "Would you agree that a conflict has arisen over the best way to make assignments to care for AIDS patients?" This makes it possible to reference the issue at the level of a common goal - in this case good care for AIDS patients. Both can then address themselves to a possible solution to accomplish that superordinate goal.

Explore Possible Solutions Prompt the participants to create as many possible solutions as they can generate before they begin to evaluate them. As the solutions are evaluated, be certain each person identifies there personal thoughts *and feelings* about each. Encourage open communication so that each can begin to see the other's view point.

Choose a Solution After the parties have explored possible solutions, they must choose one to implement. One way to make the choice is to have the parties develop a description of the characteristics of a desirable solution which can then be used to evaluate the possibilities they have identified. For example, they might agree that a desirable solution would have the following characteristics:
1. Require no changes in shift or schedule assignments.
2. No interference with the school schedule of Mr. X or the committee meeting schedule of Ms. Y.
3. Make it possible for each to earn merit points for promotion.
4. Emphasize continuity of care and development of nurse-patient relationship for the AIDS patient.

These criteria can then be used to screen the "possibles". The mediator may choose to set a follow up meeting to make this decision. A period of time for reflection and further consideration can help reduce tension if the parties feel that they are making progress.

Make Explicit Agreement to a Solution and Plans for Subsequent Action. In this case, the mediator is best served by writing a summary for all participants that specifies the agreement reached. In addition to the solution selected, as part of this phase, the mediator may address any individual behaviors by the parties which have contributed to solving the problem, for the purpose of positive reinforcement. For example you might say, "As I am writing this, I would like to comment on what I saw when Mr. X began to not interrupt Ms. Y when she was explaining her ideas. Ms. Y began to relax and lowered her voice. I think that these actions by each of you helped reach a solution. I would like to include something about that in this summary. What are your thoughts on that?" A focus on the positive is important for positive reinforcement. To find the positive, you may have to look for absence or reduction of a negative behavior. The agreed choices will be evaluated. Assuming that agreement on a course of action will settle the conflict may leave too much to chance. Follow-up is important to indicate the importance of the issue and its solution.

Implement. This stage is entirely the responsibility of the participants. They must act as they have agreed to. The fact that they have made the agreement with the participation of a mediator encourages compliance, since the agreement is to some extent more public than if made only between the parties.

Evaluate. Based on earlier agreement, the mediator can call the parties back together, if only briefly, to review their satisfaction with the outcome.

The mediator's role in this process is to facilitate not to dictate or to solve. To provide facilitating structure a mediator should use the following guidelines as the basis for choice of action:

- Encourage safe ventilation of feelings.
- Rephrase statements if clarification is needed.
- Rephrase statements to reduce personal threat.
- Take action to equalize the power of the parties.
- Promote focusing on common goals.
- Reduce tension by verbal comments, jokes, by changing topics to areas of likely agreement, by calling for cooling off period.
- Ask objective questions to help parties identify their implicit assumptions.

- Help parties create alternatives by emphasizing "both-win" or "no-lose" versus "limited loss" choices.
- Remain calm.

Conflict-Making the Most of It

The potential does exist that conflict in the work setting can produce discomfort and that that discomfort can produce positive change. In order for that to happen, there must be a number of individuals in influential positions who recognize that potential. Otherwise direct authoritative command and smoothing or other "stop the conflict now" methods will be the only ones chosen to deal with conflict, and the positive potential will be reduced.

As a new professional in a health care setting, it will be uncomfortable to be in conflict and dismaying perhaps to be expected to deal with others' conflicts. For these reasons, the following questions are suggested to guide your decision making in dealing with conflict.

As a Manager

1. Am I the person responsible for helping work out this conflict or is it "their" problem?
2. What is my goal in dealing with this conflict?
3. Which approach is most likely to produce the kind of outcome I want?
4. Am I able to do what is required in the approach I think is best?
5. Are the people in conflict ready or able to do what I plan? This is critical if you have chosen a group problem-solving activity. Some people are made very anxious by direct confrontation or open conflict and may need to learn about these techniques some time when they are *not* direct participants.

As a Participant

1. If I am feeling conflict, am I dealing with it effectively?
2. Can I, because I understand something about conflict, take the initiative to help resolve it now, or am I too involved?

The Difficult Person - Conflict as a Way of Being

A special challenge for the nurse is the sort of person who seems to engender conflict, no matter what the topic. While the term "difficult person" is not very specific, most of us can think of at least one person whom we would characterize this way. The difficult person seems to find turmoil necessary, to have a "chip on the shoulder", to be consistent only in being negative. If the difficult person were a patient or a patient's family member, one might select a nursing diagnosis of Ineffective Coping and set about to attempt to help the person deal effectively with the health situation creating the response.

But, in one's role as a nurse manager, it is not appropriate to enter a therapeutic role with staff. Not only does this type of nurturing/therapeutic interaction create confusion for staff, it can render the manager ineffective in attempting to provide leadership and discipline. For this reason, when a nurse manager identifies a trend in a staff menber's behavior which could be characterized as "difficult person", realizing that conflict and negativism are a way of being rather than a specific response for this person, a managerial rather than a therapeutic nursing response is appropriate.

Specifically, the manager must identify the unacceptable behavior, document its repeated occurrences (after dealing with each separate incident) as a trend, identify in specific terms the effects on patients and other staff, and identify the elements of the position description which are not met when this behavior is occurring. Then, a counseling session should be held to indicate to the staff member the desired behavior, feedback on unacceptable performance, consequences of not changing the behavior and a time limit. Every effort should be made to offer the employee assistance with planning how to change the behavior and with referral for assistance if personal problems are mentioned as being the basis for the negative attitude. Perhaps the individual actually is unaware of how she or he is viewed by others. Perhaps a series of crises has resulted in a pessimistic outlook. In any case, the manager's concern must be with creating a work group and work situation which results in high quality care. The "difficult person" is a problem which a manager must solve. The manager's own responses to "difficult people" can role model for others to learn that one does not need to allow others to involve them in a conflict if they do not choose it. The following illustrates this situation:

Martha Kelsey, Director of Nurses in Francis Nursing Home hears yet another series of remarks from Erline Cahill, Nurse Assistant, speaking to coworkers. Today's complaints center on how another nurse assistant on the prior shift has left work undone. Erline is encouraging her group to write a letter to the administrator to see about getting the other aid "fired". Martha decides to review the growing file of notes on counseling sessions and anecdotal notes about Erline's performance. While several anecdotes describe good direct patient care with unconscious patients, there are five items over the last 3 months which reflect consistent negativism and being at the heart of conflicts. She also notes frequent illnesses on Erline's attendance record. Martha decides to call Erline in for counseling.

The next day, when she talks with Erline, she begins by describing the reasons for her concern, the expectations for positive staff interactions and teamwork and the effect of continuing staff conflict on patient care. Erline sits in stony silence and when Martha asks if she has any thoughts or feelings about what she has said, Erline suddenly breaks into tears. "Am I going to lose my job? I can't do that. Then he really make me sorry. You just don't understand."

Martha suspects that Erline has an abusive marriage and is tempted to begin to counsel her in this regard. But, she recalls that in this situation she is manager first. She responds by focusing on seeking counseling as a means of problem solving, offers the names of several counselors including low cost services, repeats the expectation for change and sets a date for a follow-up counseling.

This example may make dealing with a "difficult person" seem simple. Definitely that is not the case. But the principles are simple.

- Remember you are a manager to the staff, not their nurse.
- Identify unacceptable behavior and make note of it.
- Provide immediate feedback on behavior, positive or negative.
- If a trend in behavior represents continuing negative or conflict -causing behavior, do disciplinary counseling.
- Be consistent and persistent.
- Seek your supervisor's consultation on the problem and your plan for solving it.
- If problem behavior is not corrected, use the standard procedures of the facility to recommend termination.

Assertiveness and Conflict - Nurses' Choices

A final concern is that as nurses we should not allow our value of understanding and accepting others to cause us to assume responsibility for conflicts that do not belong to us. Further, as Tappen warns,[11] because we are nurses we may choose soft therapeutic techniques based on a "conflict = illness premise" when other methods requiring individual responsibility

[11] Ibid., p.47.

of the conflict participants would be more growth-producing for all involved. There is no illness per se involved in disagreeing or in producing social conflict. Therefore, we are not "nursing" the participants. We are, if we are productive, acknowledging that it exists and are working to resolve and manage it.

Assertive communication skills are often *not* the usual skills practiced by nurses in their nurturing role. More often the soft therapeutic techniques become habitual and are used in other than therapeutic situations. Adding assertive communication skills to your repertoire can help make the distinction between the therapeutic role and the manager role clearer for you, your colleagues, and those whom you supervise. Assertive communication techniques are just that, skills. The skills are intended to make clear and direct the wishes of the speaker. Because being successful in conflict situations demands the ability to clearly state ones own concerns, assertive communication skills can increase your ability to deal with conflict in ways other than avoidance, smoothing, or accomodating.

The assertive communication techniques are simple. It is their active use which requires practice, and the willingness to state ones own desires and wishes relies on acknowledging that your wishes are important and legitimate. This opinion of one's self stems from healthy self-esteem. Unfortunately, self-esteem is a commodity which is often in short supply among nurses.

Practicing assertive communication will often prompt responses from others which are surprising in that they do result in respectful acknowledgment of the assertive person's rights. In effect, beginning to use these skills appropriately can benefit one's self esteem.

The basic assertive communication techniques are called: *Broken Record, Fogging, Negative Assertion*, and *Negative Inquiry*. As you consider examples of each technique below, remember that their use is based on the speaker's behaving as if her or his wishes or concerns are equally as important as the other person in the communication. This requires that a person question some culturally encouraged patterns of "polite" behavior that seem to expect that the polite person always complies with the wishes of anyone who is aggressive or attempts to be persuasive.

Broken Record is the verbal pattern to use when a person seems unwilling to accept your message. This usually occurs when the other is attempting to persuade you to do something you do not wish to do and your message is "no". Another occasion for Broken Record is when your message conveys what you believe is a legitimate request or desire on your part and it is not being attended to. The technique is simple, you repeat your message, with little if any variation, until you are certain the other has heard and acknowledged it.

> You: "I understand that you want to make functional assignments in the unit today. It is not our policy and I cannot agree."
> Other: "But, Mrs. J. prefers to pass medicine and not take patients so I'll just do it for today."
> You: "I understand that you want to make functional assignments in the unit today. It is not our policy and I cannot agree."
> Other: "You never let us try anything new. I intend to make those assignments as I want to."
> You: "I understand that you want to make functional assignments in the unit today. It is not our policy and I cannot agree.

Fogging is used to acknowledge that you have heard the other person's message and are accepting without being defensive or counterattacking. It is a technique that may cause some discomfort if you are easily hurt by criticism. But, its use is positive, because criticism is often a tool others use to manipulate us into acting as they wish us to.

> You: "I expect the assignments to be made according to our current policy. It is based on our standards."
> Other: "You have never, ever taken a suggestion I've made and used it. I don't see why I even work here if I'm not appreciated."
> You: "I agree that I have not yet implemented any suggestions you have offered. (Agreeing with the truth) I can see where that might cause a person to feel unappreciated. (Agrees with possibilities)
> Other: "If the policy is the problem, then you need to change it."
> You: "Yes, a change of policy would make following your suggestion possible."

Negative Assertion is used to state, from your own perspective, negative information. It defuses criticism from others and makes criticism from them useless as a manipulation tool.

> Other: "You're just out of date and out of touch professionally. You should change that policy right away to get in the mainstream."
> You: "People have said I remind them a bit of Florence Nightingale. In some areas I haven't reviewed my values against current practice in quite a while."

Negative Inquiry further defuses aggressive behavior by asking the other to be specific about criticism, rather than global. It invites criticism *unemotionally* and, in combination with other asssertive techniques such as fogging, can help to prompt more assertive communication from the other, in place of aggressive, manipulative comments.

> Other: "Florence Nightingale, ha! I'd say more like Sairy Gamp. Your standards are the lowest."

You: "Is it some particular area of the standards that is not suitable?"
Other: "Well, in assignment making for one. We should be able to adapt to the staffing."
You: "Are there any other standards you are concerned are not suitable?"

Three other communication skills are a part of the assertive communication repertoire. They are *Free Information, Self-Disclosure*, and *Workable Compromise*. The first two are statements to help those who are communicating to know one another better as humans.(Giving and seeking Free Information without being asked) and Self-Disclosure (commentary on personal thoughts and feelings in response to another) create a climate which encourages directness and mutual assertiveness.

You: "I've been so tied up recently with recruiting that I haven't had time to review standards and policies. (Free Information) It concerns me that you feel unappreciated here because I value you as a nurse. (Self Disclosure)"

Workable Compromise is communication which offers to reach a point which is mutually agreeable. (I prefer to call this skill *Inviting Collaboration* since compromise implies that neither party will be totally satisfied by the outcome.)

You: "I would like for us to work on this issue together. We could meet tomorrow to begin, at 2:00 p.m. if you will continue today with the current policy. Is there anyone else you think would like to work on this?"

Practice these skills in your communication and review the results. Both responses from others and you will change if you previously have been regularly passive or aggressive rather than assertive.

SUMMARY

Conflict is a social phenomenon that nurse managers must deal with daily. Some techniques for understanding it, resolving it, and managing it productively have been presented, along with a guide for clarifying your choices as nurse-manager when dealing with conflict.

Additional Reading

Beaubien,J. and K. Caesar, "How Well Do You Handle Criticism?,"*Nursing Life*,6,No.5 (May, 1986),p.47-48.

Chenevert, Melody, *Special Techniques in Assertiveness Training for Women in the Health Professions*, 2nd Ed.,St Louis,The C.V. Mosby Co.,1983.

Deutsch, Morton, "Toward an Understanding of Conflict," *International Journal of Group Tensions*,1,No.1 (January 1971) 42-54.

Gustafson David P.,E. Sullivan, and David O. Evans, "Dealing With Conflict" in Sullivan,E. and P. Decker,*Effective Management in Nursing*,2nd Ed.,Menlo Park, California: Addison Wesley,1986 pp. 513-534.

Isaac,S. "Professional Growth: 5 Ways to Resolve Conflict", *Nursing 86*,16 No. 3 ,(March, 1986)p.89-91.

Levenstein,A "What Makes You Mad?", *Nursing Management*16 No.7,(July, 1985)p.57-58.

Nierenberg, G. "The Art of Negotiating",New York: Simon and Schuster, Inc.,1986.

Silber, M.B.,"Managing Confrontations: Once More Into the Breach" *Nursing Management* 15,No 4. (April, 1984)p.54.

Chapter 7

Superior-subordinate relationships

The organizationally defined status of superior or subordinate in a managerial relationship can be difficult to maintain comfortably, no matter which role you are taking. As a new professional, you are likely to be taking both roles almost simultaneously. Therefore, this chapter examines both aspects of superior-subordinate relationships in the work setting.

This superior-subordinate relationship can be defined as one in which an individual (the superior) has a defined responsibility for supervising or coordinating some element(s) of the work and/or performance of another (the subordinate). No matter how decentralized an organizational structure is, when there are organizationally defined levels or varying status and responsibility, there will be some superior-subordinate relationships created. These ranked relationships exist outside the work setting as well, although in social and family relationships there is more of a tendency toward change and development in relationships over time with a move toward less distance and differences between status as both parties age, mature, or change, as the case may be. In organizations, the "rules" governing the relationship may be more formalized than in other situations. For example, there may be a written policy that all workers address one another by *Mr.* or *Ms.* and last name only. Formal evaluations and explicit statements of the connection between performance (as judged by superiors) and rewards (such as pay increases) are often present and represent a formalization of the "rules."

Since there are analogous superior-subordinate relationships in nonorganizational life, it is not surprising that individuals may carry feelings and behavior from these other relationships into the work setting. These intrapersonal concerns may be a reflection of the individual's typical reaction to relationships within his or her family. The pyschologists who have developed transactional analysis have provided a clear description of these modes of behavior, based on different ego states.

The Parent ego state contains the attitudes and behavior incorporated from external sources, primarily parents. Outwardly, it is often expressed toward others in prejudicial, critical, and nurturing behavior. Inwardly, it is experienced as old Parental messages which continue to influence the inner Child. The Adult ego state is not related to a person's age. It is oriented to current reality and the objective gathering of information. It is organized, adaptable, intelligent, and functions by testing reality, estimating probabilities, and computing dispassionately.

The Child ego state contains all the impulses that come naturally to an infant. It also contains the recordings of his early experiences, how he responded to them, and the positions he took about himself and others. It is expressed as the "old" (archaic) behavior from childhood.[1]

If, as a subordinate, one functions from the Child state, it is easy to invoke critical Parent behavior from the superior, or reciprocally, to attempt, because one is in a superior position, to function in the Parent mode, thus gaining Child responses. For some, this mode of behavior may be anticipated, reciprocated, and even satisfying. In this case, what exists is a complementary transaction, each getting what is expected. However, those who prefer to function neither as parent nor child vis-a-vis coworkers may continually be cast in "crossed" transactions, transactions in which the other party's responses are of an unexpected character.

Even if the concepts of transactional analysis are not palatable, the behavioral realities remain. Passive, dependent behavior or angry, petulant behavior by a subordinate frequently invokes critical, overbearing, or demanding behavior by the superior and a continuing reciprocating cycle is created. In this fashion, each person's own personality can directly affect the superior- subordinate relationship.

Besides the tendency to respond in particular ways, which each of the parties may bring to a superior-subordinate relationship, there are some social and organizational norms that affect the general tone of the relationship. One factor so defined is the degree of power attributed to a superior's position, regardless of who occupies the position. If the organizational norm is to attribute extensive power to the position of supervisor; then, without much consideration, subordinates may exhibit deference to that person in decision making and in other elements of their interaction. As a result, this

---

[1] Muriel James and Dorothy Jongeward, *Born to Win* (Reading, Mass.: Addison-Wesley, 1978) p. 17. Copyright 1978. Reprinted by permission of Addison- Wesley Publishing Co., Reading, Mass.

can negatively affect the quality of decision making and the type and extent of information that will be shared. Seldom is limited information or poor decision making in the best interest of an organization, and the "if she wanted me to know, she would ask me" attitude toward a superior can certainly produce this undesirable type of decision making.

The superior and subordinate in organizational positions can be conceived of as roles rather than a fixed, immutably defined elements. When the perspective is taken that these are only roles, then it becomes possible to consider behavior within the roles that may be varied productively, even in light of preexisting individual and social factors. Role function can be negotiated, reviewed, and selectively varied if the individuals wish to do so. Taking this point of view makes it possible to question the tacit rules that may be accepted in the situation and to consider the current effectiveness of behavior based on past precedent for superiors and subordinates in the organization. Careful consideration of one's behavior from each perspective, superior and subordinate, can create relationships that are growth-promoting for both parties involved.

Being Effective
in the Superior Role

The responsibility of the superior in a superior-subordinate relationship can be complex. To be done well, this side of the relationship in an organizational setting requires that the supervisor be able to:(1) analyze the subordinate's style of interacting with the superior, (2) develop a repertoire of behavior suitable to a variety of subordinates, (3) develop a degree of trust, (4) teach the subordinate effective and efficient ways to accomplish work, (5) supervise in order to provide feedback, and (6) evaluate and provide rewards for positive accomplishments. Complicating this responsibility is the fact that the superior usually has responsibility for more than one subordinate. This creates a series of dyadic (two-person) relationships, each with its own unique characteristics, rather than a single superior-group of subordinates- type of relationship. See Figure 7.1 for the two contrasting views of the interactions of superior and subordinates. Neither view is entirely correct alone. Both types of interaction are necessary.

The result is a need to spread one's time equally among all subordinates, which in itself is no small task. Yet the amount of interaction and the degree to which it is dispersed are important facets of creating productive superior-subordinate relationships.

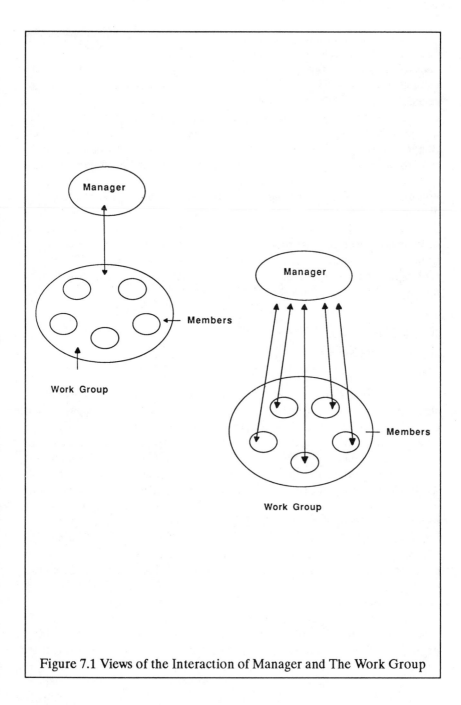

Figure 7.1 Views of the Interaction of Manager and The Work Group

A competent manager focuses on spending time with others as an important part of the job. Just how much is difficult to say. Certainly, it depends on the number of subordinates. Four hours might be too much interaction time if there are only two subordinates. However, the point is clear, the superior must interact with others in order to accomplish the role's responsibilities.

Each superior-subordinate relationship is different becuase each interactive pair is different. The superior can be more effective in the relationship if she has analyzed the way the subordinate tends to interact with her. Questions to consider in the analysis include the following:

- Who initiates most of the interaction?
- What are the tone and content of the interaction?
- When asked to make a decision, does the subordinate seem to defer to her superior?
- Does she ever disagree with her superior when the two of them are conversing?
- Does the superior get "second-hand" information that the subordinate is uncomfortable or unhappy about some aspect of their relationship?
- Does the superior feel she can trust the subordinate?
- Is there evidence of procrastination, intentional omissions, or failure to complete work as requested?

If the superior answers the questions and discerns a pattern of reticence or dependence or extreme compliance and attempts to please in the other's behavior, further work is needed. This type of interaction can indicate: (1) discomfort on the part of the subordinate in interacting with superiors, (2) a negative response to this particular superior, or (3) a culturally or individually derived dislike for disagreeing with or being open in communication with a superior.

Using the transactional analysis concept, perhaps what is occurring is that the subordinate is interacting in the Child mode. If the superior interacts as the Parent and both Parent mode and Child mode are positive, this will cause little conflict since the interaction becomes complementary. However, a continually dependent mode is not growth-producing for the subordinate nor productive for the organization in terms of developing ability and leadership among personnel. The obvious alternative to responding as Parent, that is, as authoritarian, is to move into the Adult mode, to expect open interchange, to make each person increasingly responsible for her own actions, and to refuse to accept dependence or passivity. Although this may be the most obvious alternative, it is unlikely to be the most immediately effective. As you read the following brief case, ask yourself how you might react in either role, superior or subordinate, and whether the superior's approach was a useful one.

When Susan Allison first came to work on 3 North as evening Charge Nurse, she was pleased to have Kerry White, a young licensed vocational nurse (LVN) assigned to the unit. Kerry was thoughtful to patients and completed her work capably. As time passed, Susan began to be a bit uncomfortable that Kerry seemed to ask her opinion too frequently on decisions that seemed routine. "Is it all right to feed this patient now?" Can Mrs. Smith be up in a chair again? It's only ordered once on our shift" Susan decided that Kerry needed to be more confident and not so dependent on her, so she began asking questions in response when Kerry came to her for a routine decision, hoping to help Kerry reason through to the answer. Her plan was to praise Kerry as she began being more decisive on her own. However, Kerry semed to be very uncomfortable when Susan did not respond with a decision, and she would ask Susan the same question again, "What do you want me to do?" After several such occasions, Susan noticed that Kerry was beginning to leave parts of her assignment unfinished. These were never major tasks, just some small details. Kerry also seemed to be asking another LVN who was older than she the same type of questions she had previously been bringing to Susan. The switch from one role or mode of behavior to another by Susan produced a negative reaction in Kerry. Clearly, this was not the type of interaction Kerry expected from a superior in the work setting. Had Susan analyzed the situation from the perspective of what was occurring in the interaction rather than wondering what Kerry needed, she would have recognized that an interaction is affected by both individuals responding to one another. She would have taken into account her own role as superior and how this may have affected the tone of the interaction from Kerry's point of view. She also might have anticipated that Kerry would perceive a change in her from an expected "kind parent" to "rational adult," which could cause a negative reaction becuase there was no advance discussion or negotiated change in role behavior by either party.

In contrast with Kerry another of the staff on the unit, Jane Compton, seemed rather quiet, very competent, able to receive suggestions comfortably, and able to respond with or initiate suggesions of her own in discussing patient care with Susan. It would have been easy for Susan to deal with Jane in the same way she had tried to interact with Kerry, or Susan could have chosen to spend very little time with Jane because she seemed so independent and capable.

Choosing the reinforcing communication mode would have been a good choice in two ways. First, it would appear to be complementary to the subordinate's choice of behavior. (Jane appears to be acting in a rational, relatively deliberate and nondependent manner.) Second, it demonstrates that Susan, the organizational superior, has developed a repertoire of responses and the ability to vary the style or mode of interaction as needed. In working with patients, a nurse would call this recognizing the patient's individuality, "starting where the patient is." The principle is the same in working with personnel.

Much literature in management alludes to the need for the manager (as superior) to develop a particular style of "managing". This implies that, for example, a participative style is most desirable. However, consistent with more recent work on effective organizations and effective managers, a contingency approach is more desirable. That is, the contingencies of the situation affect the choice of the manager's behavior. The work of Blake and Mouton is one of the earliest emphasizing this perspective and the same emphasis is continued in their recent publications.[2] More recent work by Hersey and Blanchard,[3] and Blanchard et al[4] build on the same premise.It is important, though, to distinguish between recommendations about how a leader or manager should interact with a *group*, as leader or manager of the group's function, and how a superior chooses to interact with a subordinate, a ono-to-one interaction. It is consistent to carry the contingency principle from the level of the one-to-one interaction (the focus in this chapter) through to the organizational level. This means that no single style of interaction, or of management, or of leadership, or of organizing is best for all situations.

As research continues, there will be more knowledge available upon which to base "if/then" statements regarding each of these levels of organizational interaction. "If the individual is operating from a dependent mode, then the superior should approach him in an authoritative mode until the person can begin to function more independently" is an example of such a statement. In superior-subordinate interaction,the key is to know clearly what your own expectations are, what the range of acceptable behavior by subordinates is, and to anticipate that each subordinate will vary and that individuals in the group of subordinates will each differ from the others.

The other premise that is important to accept if the superior- subordinate relationship is to be mutually rewarding is that individuals can and do change and that change can be growth toward greater independence and maturity if conditions are conducive. This means that the superior should attempt to create an atmosphere where behaving maturely will be rewarding.

The superior should also attempt to create an atmosphere of trust. Consistency and fairness, considering each person as an individual worthy of an equal share of time and attention, are important in developing trust. Another important factor for developing trust is maintaining confidentiality and respecting the private information that a subordinate may divulge to you. Nothing can destroy developing trust so quickly as hearing a remark made in confidence repeated in public by another person. A part of the ability or willingness to trust that an individual exhibits is related to child-

    2 Robert R. Blake and Jane Mouton, *The Mangerial Grid* (Houston, Tex.: Gulf Publishing, 1984).

    3 P.Hersey and K. Blanchard, *Management of Organizational Behavior* (5th Ed.) Englewood Cliffs, N.J.: Prentice-Hall,Inc.1988

    4 Blanchard et al, *Leadership and The One Minute Manager*,New York: Wm. Morrow and Co.,1985.

hood experiences. Some trust quickly, others seldom trust, if at all. But no trust will exist when one party to a relationship appears to be unconcerned about the dignity and fairness accorded to the other.

Another difficulty is posed when the superior finds it difficult to feel positive toward her subordinates. It is a very natural reaction to be negative to some people simply because they remind you of someone you do not like, or because of some single occurrence. But the responsibility that comes with an organizational superior's position demands that the superior examine those reactions, try to find the reason, and attempt to work toward a positive approach. This is not to suggest that you must like or feel affection for everyone with whom you work. It only suggests that you should attempt an open-mindedness and acceptance of each person, in order to establish a suitable working relationship.

Another part of the responsibility of the superior in a working relationship is to teach subordinates the most efficient and effective ways to accomplish their jobs. To do this, it will be necessary to supervise the person at the job, suggest ways to be more efficient or effective, and provide praise when accomplishments merit it. The only way that one can successfully aid the subordinate in these ways it to first know the subordinate's job well enough to coach her at the tasks and advise on the overall function.

Providing feedback and reward can be relatively simple at the direct person-to-person level. A word, a smile, a gesture will do it. In the long run, though, something more may be needed, like a merit recommendation for salary or promotion. As the superior, it will be important for you to make judicious use of each of the types of reward you control, from the smile (used liberally) to the merit salary increase (used only when actually deserved).

As mentioned above, the relationship of superior and subordinate in an organization can be viewed from the perspective of role theory. The two roles are thus potentially available to be negotiated in the ways described in Chapter 1. Negotiating roles makes it possible to focus on behavior, not on personality, and to have regular intervals for renegotiation completely separate from the formal evaluation of the subordinate by the superior. This formal evaluation is essentially a one-way superior-to- subordinate activity. No matter how it is managed, no matter how much participation is encouraged, the fact remains that it is the superior who makes the recommendation and signs the evaluation form. In contrast, role negotiation can be a mutually defined interchange, with each party identifying the desired behavior for his or her role, and coming to some agreement on the negotiated element.

Being Effective
in the Subordinate Role

Doing well as a subordinate is just as important as being a good superior. Developing in this role requires careful analysis. One of the first activities is to consider your style of interacting with your superior. Just as in the superior role, it is important to be able to vary your interactions as is appropriate to function well with the other party in the interaction. In the subordinate role it will be more difficult, though, to work toward a mature interaction style if the superior is not so inclined. This is because the underlying premise is that, at least in the beginning, your superior has the option to set the tone of the interaction. Think about typical ways of interacting by asking yourself some of the following questions:

- Am I at ease when I talk with my superior?
- Do I state my true opinions when she asks?
- Do I always wait for her to initiate any interaction?
- Do I find myself wanting to get back at her or not wanting to work in the way she expects?
- Do I consider our interaction helpful to me in my work?

If, as you consider these questions, you realize that you are uncomfortable or reticent with your superior, then you should evaluate your reactions. Is this your style with everyone or only with authority figures? If only with superiors, is this because of cues you are picking up from them or because of your own feelings about how you should or must behave? From this base, you should then be able to decide how you might need to vary your behavior, depending on your superior's manner, rather than reacting in a stereotyped way. The person who is your organizational superior is human too. If you are uncomfortable dealing with her, she may not have the opportunity to be as communicative or as helpful as she might be because your discomfort may prompt limited or negative communication from you.

One very important aspect of a subordinate's behavior that can contribute to an improved and more productive relationship is the acceptance of criticism. It is very difficult for even the most confident superior to fulfill her/his complete responsibility if the subordinate always reacts defensively or negatively to any suggestion for improvement. You can take the initiative in seeking assistance and thereby create the opportunity for continuing and helpful interchange. If you have trouble even imagining doing such a thing, why not try it out with a friend, as a role-played experience, before attempting it at work?

The same concern for trust and consistency in a relationship recommended for the superior is important for the subordinate to nurture as well. It is tempting to trade"awful boss" stories with others who have the same superior. It even creates a sort of group spirit. But that same type of interchange, overheard or carried by gossip, can shake the trust the superior holds toward you and will result in an unproductive relationship.

If your superior does not seem to know the requirements of your job or is unable to give helpful suggestions and positive feedback, you may wonder if a relationship even needs to exist. Unfortunately it is true that organizational superiors, like those in subordinate positions, are sometimes not fit for the jobs they are in. There are two possible consequences: (1) the superior is not particularly helpful but does not bother the subordinate, so the situation is tolerable, or(2) the superior is actually a hindrance in work or makes work unpleasant for the subordinate. If the latter is the case, it is quite legitimate for the subordinate to try to improve the situation, just as it is the responsibility of the superior to seek to improve the subordinate's function. The main difference is that this is usually a part of the expected job duties of the superior, whereas the subordinate is acting from a base of personal rights and a sense of concern.

Choosing to act from the subordinate's position may be a difficult decision, but if you value your work and want a helpful relationship with your organizational superior, action may be needed. The first step will be the most difficult. This may mean talking directly to your superior about the situation. It may be a risky thing to do unless you take care to explain the situation from your own perspective. For example, "I really need to have you make suggestions about how to improve my work, not just assume it is o.k." Or, "When we talk, I get the feeling that what I am saying is not important to you." Such statements are based on a recognition that it is your need and your perception that prompt the concern. You are using "I" statements, admitting that these are your thoughts and feelings rather than trying to blame someone else. A conference like this will often pave the way for a better relationship and more open communication.

If there is no change and your concern continues, you are free to go up the organizational line if you really believe that your work is suffering, but it is important to notify your immediate superior that you are doing so. If there is a bargaining agent representing you in your agency, there my be specific procedures that are to be followed in these situations, although it is not necessary to begin immediately by elevating a concern to the formal status of a grievance as many such procedures attempt to do.

An alternative to going farther "up the line" is to ask for a transfer to another unit or section, thereby changing superiors. Any decision to do so must be balanced against potential losses. For example, if you have a good work relationship with all the rest of the people in your group, you might lose more than is gained by the change.

In each relationship, including superior-subordinate ones, problems can occur. These problems will be magnified and will become irritating if both parties are not committed to making the situation work productively. This type of commitment can be generated most easily when there is a basic element of mutual respect and acceptance. If these elements do not exist, considering a change may be the best choice if all other attempts to solve the problems have been unsuccessful.

Do Professionals Need a Superior-Subordinate or a Supervising Relationship?

As nursing has emerged as an influential part of health care, the question about whether nursing is a profession has been discussed extensively. One major concern in these discussions has centered on the hospital as the major employment site of nurses and the fact that most hospitals are organized so that the nursing service is to some extent hierarchically structured. This results in at least one and possibly several successive layers of ascending superior- subordinate relationships within the department. The concern about professional nurses in a bureaucratic (layered) organization is based on the tendency for each succeeding upward layer to consume the superior's time with activities less relevant to the concerns of patient care and more concerned with supervising the activities of those lower in the hierarchy. As noted earlier, there are situations where the certainty provided by such a structure is highly desirable. However, the current situation in much of nursing is that many nursing tasks are performed by other than professional nurses. In these situations, it is important to assure the correctness, adequacy, and coordination of tasks through supervision. This, then, is one type of situation in nursing where a superior- subordinate relationship defined as a *supervisory* relationship is necessary.

As for the professionals and the degree of supervision required for them, it is not entirely clear what contingencies should affect the decision about the number of layers required for supervision. The use of primary nursing as an assignment mode (see Chapter 13) has reduced the need for supervision at the unit level. This structure can increase the autonomy of decision making by the nurse and can allow the major portion of her time to be spent in direct care activiites. Furthermore, it is possible, when the staff is an all-RN group, to change the function of the central coordinating person (head nurse, unit coordinator, or other title) in such a way as to reduce the overseeing activity and produce a mentor relationship with the individual nurses. This is still a form of superior-subordinate relationship.

As long as nursing, especially in hospitals, is an activity requiring coordination among several individuals rather than solo practice, where the individual is entirely self- sufficient, it is likely that some sort of superior-subordinate relationship will exist. This relationship will exist for one or both of two purposes: (1) to provide for the continuing professional development of the individual, as in the mentor relationship, or (2) to maintain coordination and control over quantity and quality of practice. The challenge then, is to become skillful in negotiating these relationships from the perspective of either role and to make them both as satisfying and as productive as possible.

Referring to the transactional analysis concepts presented earlier, we can see that a superior-subordinate relationship which functions in an adult-adult fashion would make colleagueship possible. While the two individuals would have different types of organizational responsibilities, collegial interaction would be based on mutual respect and on adult-adult communication. No matter what the organizational structure, this mode of interaction is likely to be mutually satisfactory.

SUMMARY

This chapter has examined aspects of superior-subordinate relationships as they exist in the work situation. Viewing either side of the relationship as a role that can be negotiated and the total relationship as something potentially beneficial for both the organization and the parties to the relationship was suggested as a premise for productive functioning.

Additional Reading

Darling, L.A.W.,"Becoming a Mentoring Manager", *Journal of Nursing Administration* 15,No. 6,(June,1985) p. 43-44.

Davidhizar,Ruth and Nano Farabaugh.,"The New Manager: Finding Your Place and Theirs",*Nursing Management*,17:4 (April,1986) 43-46.

Chapter 8

Collaborative relationships

The "health care team" is a phrase that is often seen in both popular and professional literature. A related concept is "interdisciplinary collaboration." Both terms imply that some sort of cooperative effort is involved in providing aspects of health care. It is true that for many of the elements of care to be provided, cooperation must occur at several levels. Cooperation is needed for most services that involve two or more providers. However, not all of this cooperation takes the special form that could be called *collaboration*. This chapter examines collaboration as a special type of interaction and its relationship to team approaches to care and other models of practice.

A dictionary definition of *collaboration* is "working together, especially in a joint intellectual effort." The key term in this definition is *joint*. This implies that a collaborative effort is one in which there is not a superior/subordinate, order-giving/order-taking, relationship. Rather, common usage implies an equity among the participants in the relationship, both in working and sharing rewards. Of course, a variety of relationships may be labeled by their participants as "collaboration" or "team work" or whatever. To the extent that one accepts that a term means what those using it agree that it means, their definition would be correct. However, this text's definition is a normative one, describing an ideal form of collaboration, which distinguishes it from other forms of interaction and relationships.

The following expanded definition is needed as a begining toward further discussion and clarification. *Collaboration*, as an interaction, is characterized by activities directed toward an agreed upon goal by two or more persons among whom exists a norm of equity and mutual recognition of complementarity of their knowledge and abilities. There is an underlying assumption that the result of this interaction will be more effective or more efficient than individual action of any participant toward the same goal would be.

The common goal may be one that has been defined by one individual who then assembles others with whom to collaborate. For example, a physician may seek collaborators in the care of a family in which a mother has rheumatic heart disease. The physician has set a goal of not only treating the mother effectively but also of maintaining the integrity of the family. Or the goal may be set by the collaborators as a pair or group, as a result of a situation in which they have a continuing general collaborative relationship. An example might be a nurse, physician, and physical therapist who function as a treatment team in a rehabilitation center. They may discuss together the definition of a goal in the care of a recent stroke patient.

The norm of equity implies that although there may not be constant equality (the same share for each one) in decision making, in any particular activity, the dominance in decision making does tend to "even out" over time. To illustrate, assume that in the case of the rehabilitation team mentioned above, for the care of the stroke patient, the physical therapist may: (1) take the lead in decision making about increasing activity, and (2) may see the patient more frequently than the nurse and physician. Here, the group acknowledges the therapist's special ability with this sort of patient. Her "share" with this patient is larger than with some other patients with whom the others may have greater interest, ability, or interaction. The fact that the norm of equity is established precludes a superior/subordinate interaction because the assumption is that at some point the situation will reverse and change that balance.

The same is true in a more abstract fashion when the collaboration is more situation-specific, as in the first example. Although the group assembled to care for the family may disband after the care is completed, the potential exists that any one of the group may need the others' assistance at some later point. The fact that a call to collaborate may come from various points, not just from the physician, is part of what characterizes this interaction as collaboration.

In each of these examples, a concern with constant equality would probably produce an unworkable situation. Yet an implicit assumption that constant equality in all matters rather than equity should exist is often the basis for conflict and ineffective relationships. Since there is opportunity for great conflict around this concern, potential collaborators would do well to discuss this concern early in their interaction, especially if the relationship is to be a continuing one.

Complementarity of skills and knowledge is a necessary but not sufficient cause for collaboration to exist. Mutual recognition that no one person holds all the knowledge, skill, or resources necessary to meet a goal is required in order for true collaboration to exist. In addition, an underlying willingness to interact regarding a goal must be present. As basic as this may seem, even if skills and recognition are present, without mutual willingness to collaborate, some other form of interaction may occur, most frequently a superior/subordinate interplay.

Why Collaborate?

Although some current literature may imply it, it is unlikely that a collaborative approach is always the best, most efficient, effective way to operate in health care. There are bound to be some situations in which one person, acting alone, can provide the care necessary and can do it efficiently. However, there are two types of situations in which collaboration is most useful. These are: (1) situations in which a general operating mode of the organization brings together the skills most frequently needed for the population served, and (2) specific situations where the goal to be met requires assembling skills or knowledge not held by one member alone.

The first category is best exemplified by primary health care in a high-density, multiple-problem community. In this situation, most problems require more than a single, isolated goal or single set of provider skills to solve them. For this reason, setting up the care delivery system as a collaborative group effort (a team approach) sets the stage for using the approach consistently in a place where the likelihood of need for such an approach is high. There is a growing interest in this mode of delivery of health service as evidenced by increasing references in the literature to "team care." However, caution should be exercised in interpreting considerable interest and certain successful experiences to mean that team practice is the *only* way in which health care can be delivered effectively. Rather, the needs of the population to be served should define the system for delivery.

The practice of some specialists, nursing, medical, or otherwise, is such that many problems that the specialist deals with are clearly within the ability of that one individual when they are presented by the patient or client. For example, a nurse specializing in family planning counseling may see 15 persons a day. Thirteen of these individuals may be there because they know what they want. They simply need to have a bit of information and to have a pap smear. In such cases, the nurse may have little need for collaboration, and can efficiently and quickly provide the care needed alone. The other 2 of the 15 clients may have more complicated needs. Perhaps one has reservations about birth control due to religious beliefs, plus financial difficulties imposed by the recent birth of a fourth child. In this case, a situation from the second category arises. The nurse might call upon a social worker to meet with her and the patient and collaborate in working with the patient. The collaboration is situation-specific and is based on an acknowledged willingness by the parties to collaborate when needed.

In either case, the underlying reason for collaborating is a recognition that this particular mode can improve the solution of the mutually acknowledged problems, not simply the fact that collaboration is a fashionable concept.

Personal, Cultural, and Educational Factors Affecting Collaboration

Those who choose to collaborate and who do so effectively exhibit certain behaviors that can be identified as characteristic of effective collaboration. They:

- Share a mutual respect for the expertise of their collaborators.
- Define a common goal through discussion.
- Accept mutual responsibility in reaching the common goal.
- Participate in mutual review upon reaching the common goal.
- Communicate in an honest, open face-to-face mode.
- Share decision making power as peers, equitably.
- Share knowledge for the benefit of the group of collaborators.
- Offer support to collaborators through positive statements regarding their contributions.
- Understand the common language or terms common to the problem at hand.
- Have mutually acceptable roles.

Perhaps there is a personality type common to individuals who choose to collaborate. One might guess that self-confident, extroverted persons who enjoy interaction and who are relatively articulate might show up more frequently as collaborators than others. This might be an interesting question for research. However, it is clear that whatever configuration personal makeup may produce, many of the interactive skills necessary to collaboration can be taught and learned. Assuming that there is value in some collaborative relationships, we will take the position that any student in a health care profession can learn to collaborate.

Another factor that may influence collaborative interaction is gender. Due to the fact that cultural expectations of males and females differ, early life experiences may have produced differing approaches to peer interactions among males, between males and females, and among females. Popular literature alludes to the American culture's emphasis on team sports for males as one factor that prepares males for effective team or collaborative interaction in other aspects of life. This same train of thought continues with an indication that females, lacking in these early learning experiences, tend to be competitive with one another and not willing to collaborate. This rather dismal view of gender differences, from the female perspective, would imply that it is hopeless for females to attempt to collaborate with other females unless both have played Little League Baseball. Little sound scientific evidence is available to support these assertions of male-female differences in approach to collaborations within gender groups. Therefore it will be assumed that differences that exist are individually variable rather than variable by gender.

A gender-related factor that *may* affect collaborative interaction is that created when male and female attempt collaborative interaction. Until relatively recently, in our culture, the female social role has been less openly assertive in interactions with males. When individuals who have been performing in this fashion in their female-male interaction are placed in a situation where a peer relationship is expected, old patterns of submissive deference, or worse yet, passive aggression, may be difficult to overcome. The game playing that ensues can be relatively minor flirtatious coyness of the female and exaggerated virility and expansiveness of the male; or it may be vicious sort of male put-down of the submissive female who in turn manages to not quite understand and therefore never does what is agreed upon; or it may be that neither party can interpret interaction with members of the opposite sex as anything other than potential sexual advances. Perhaps as successive generations of men and women are reared in an atmosphere of fewer stereotypical expectations, this type of reaction will no longer emerge as a problem. At the present, this gender-related or perhaps socioculturally related behavior can pose problems to effective collaboration. For this reason, specific efforts by leaders of any collaboratiave effort may need to be directed to helping participants identify ground rules designed to create peer interaction. The emphasis should be on identifying the potential problems of typical gender/sociocultural role behaviors.

Another factor that apparently affects the individual's inclination to collaborative activity is professional education. M. G. Nolan, as others, has described the education of nurses, as least in the past, as encouraging conformity to rules and routine and promoting submissiveness.[1]This she attributes to our military-religious heritage and the traditional female role that has been emphasized in this traditionally female occupation. DeTornyay's contrast between traditional medical education and nursing education makes the difference clear. She notes that the long educational and socialization process in medicine prompts physicians to view themselves as solely responsible, legally and morally, for their patients' care. Further, physicians are taught to develop responsibility to carry the burden of decision making alone. None of this predisposes to functioning comfortably in interdisciplinary collaborative relationships.[2] However, the process of medical education does emphasize collegial consultation. This form of consultation differs from collaboration as defined here in that the decision making authority is *not* shared with the consultant. Rather, the relationship is one of sharing of knowledge, freely requested and freely given. Both collegial consultation and collaborative interaction are important methods of augmenting the skills and ability of the sole health care provider. Collegial consultation occurs, at least in medicine, relatively frequently, but collaboration occurs only rarely.

The professional education of nurses has, at least in the past, emphasized tact and diplomacy when dealing with others, caution and tentativeness is decision making, and adherence to proper lines of authority. Seldom has collegial consultation been promoted. Rather, the superior/subordinate channels were stressed as the mechanism for receiving assistance and additional information. As a matter of fact, the "channels" usually kept the individual nurse from having to make a decision and being individually accountable for it. Even as interdisciplinary collaboration has begun to be a fashionable concern, much of the effort in nursing has gone into blaming physicians for not promoting collaboration rather than actively teaching nursing students to collaborate and then rewarding them for doing so.

It seems, then, that neither the professional socialization nor the purely informational aspects of the curricula of medicine and nursing have, in the past, prepared individual practitioners to develop interdisciplinary collaborative activities. Other health professional groups are not any more

---

[1] M. G. Nolan, "Wanted: Colleagueship in Nursing," *Journal of Nursing Administration*,6,No.3,(1976),41.

[2] DeTornyay,Rheba "Doctor and Nurse,Restraining Forces in Team Work"*Hospital Forum*17(May, 1974) pp.5-6.

highly evolved in this respect. The result is that those who wish to collaborate on a situation-specific basis not only will need to find someone of like mind but also must reclarify the "ground rules" of the collaboration each time a new joint effort is developed. If a collaborative practice effort is to be developed as a mode, the individuals must be selected and trained for the effort, and any organizational suprastructure must be examined for support or fit with this mode of delivery. In short, current patterns of education have not predisposed individuals to collaboration as a common behavior, and patterns of practice do not provide a strong support for collaboration among health care providers.

A Climate for Collaboration

An interpersonal interactive climate of openness and trust is conducive to effective collaboration. If there is a continual undercurrent of suspicion or a hint of condescension, then any willingness to collaborate quickly evaporates. What remains instead is what Jack Gibb called "defensive communication."[3] In a classic article, Gibb contrasted defensive climates with supportive climates, indicating that a defensive climate produces distortion in perceptions on the part of the communicators, reducing the efficiency of the communication. Defensive climates are induced in six ways: (1) by communicating in evaluative rather than descriptive terms; (2) by attempting to control the individual rather than focusing on the problem at hand; and (3) by implying that communications and behavior are part of a strategy to manipulate the individual rather than spontaneous reaction or response. Other defense-inducing communications, contrasted with supportive behaviors, are: (4) expressions of neutrality or lack of concern as contrasted with empathy; (5) superiority rather than equality; and (6) certainty ("I have the answer, I always do") rather than provisionalism (Perhaps this answer will work").[4] If only one of these six elements or messages comes through, perhaps defensiveness will not arise. When defense-inducing messages of several sorts coincide, whether verbal or nonverbal, it is difficult not to react defensively and to subsequently communicate the response in the same vein. Such a situation makes collaborative interaction difficult indeed. The only possible solutions once such a cycle has been created are:

---

3 Jack R. Gibb, "Defensive Communication," *The Journal of Communication,* 11 (September 1961), 141-148.

4 Ibid.,pp. 142-148.

(1)abandon the interaction, (2) one person attempts to stop the downward spiral of the relationship and calls the problem to the other's attention, or (3) a third party is called in to help work through the difficulty.

At the organizational level, there are certain elements that can encourage collaboration. Among these are: (1) an emphasis on reward for quality of work not simply for quantity and speed of task accomplishment; (2) personnel selection methods that consider experience in collaborative activities as a positive factor and that examine philosophical beliefs regarding professional interaction as an improtant piece of data; and (3) committee structure within the organization that can serve as a prototype of collaboration. For example, Joint Practice Committees at the unit level or at the hospital level could bring nurse and physician representives to work together on problems of clinical practice policy. In a Visiting Nurse Service, a Clinical Practice Committee, or Quality Assurance Committee could be multidisciplinary. For the above three elements to exist, there must be a commitment at the top administrative level to promoting opportunities for collaboration. Even with this commitment, without careful planning and a strong internal organizational development plan, what exists will be only good intentions.

Creating Collaborative Interaction

When an appropriate problem or goal (one requiring multiple skills) as well as a neutral atmosphere exist, an opportunity is available to collaborate. The elements essential to initiating this collaboration are: (1) a clear understanding of the concept of collaboration, (2)willing collaborators, and (3) an opportunity for the collaborators to interact, preferably face to face.

The first condition can be met by exploring the earlier content of this chapter in discussion with others. Search for examples of collaboration in action. Observe the interaction. All the while, keep in mind that several levels of collaboration exist and that they vary depending on the involvement of one or more persons at the following points: (1) initial discussion of the problem or goal, (2) goal definition, (3) decision making on the plan of action, (4) implementation of the plan, and (5) evaluation. Table 8.1 demonstrates that collaborative activity can take many forms.

Level I involves collaboration only in the initial phase of the activity, with one person subsequently responsible for completing the accomplishment of the goal. With each level, the degree of involvement of collaboration increases, with Level IV being the greatest point of interaction. In Level IV, although interaction may involve all individuals at each phase, a division of labor along disciplinary lines may exist at the implementation phase. This is appropriate in the interests of efficiency and effectiveness. The choice of level of interaction depends on which level will be most efficient in meeting goals with greatest effect, and available resources.

TABLE 8.1 Levels of Collaborative Interaction

Phase of Activity	Number of Persons in Interactive Involvement			
	Level I	Level II	Level III	Level IV
Initial discussion	2 or more	2 or more	2 or more	2 or more
Goal definition	2 or more	2 or more	2 or more	2 or more
Action plan	1	2 or more	2 or more	2 or more
Implementation	1	1	2 or more	2 or more
Evaluation	1	1	1	2 or more

When collaboration is initiated, the relationship, like any other, will evolve and change over time. S. R. Jacobson outlines typical phases in the evolution of an interdisciplinary collaborative group. The phases are the following:[5]

Early enthusiasm: A sense of unity and cooperation pervade.

Warming up: Interest in learning about participants' backgrounds and a need to explain one's own.

Insecurity: A struggle against closeness with each member falling back to "represent one's own."

Tug of war: Participants begin to question the need to collaborate and begin to acknowledge external pressures.

Negatives emerge: Fear of loss of professional identity and status, of exposure of inadequacy, or of criticism become pronounced.

Hostility: Open recognition of negative attitudes toward others in the group and their profession. Negative feelings of hostility and anger are experienced.

Reaffirmation: Definite attempts are made to think, speak, and work in relation to others, to come to terms with conflict of values of group members.

Identification: A resurgence of sureness, freedom, and easy collaboration.

The description of the various phases of collaboration makes it clear that alone willingness to collaborate is not easy assurance of a smooth road for the participants.

5 S. R. Jacobson, "A Study of Interprofessional Collaboration," *Nursing Outlook,* 22 (December 1974), 751-755.

Finding one or more willing collaborators may be a difficult task in some settings. However, the general topic can be discussed as one means of identifying those who are open to the idea. Finally, when those who are to collaborate are identified, at least in the early phases of this type of interaction, a structured role negotiation would be helpful. This activity, described in Chapter 1, clarifies mutual expectations and sets ground rules. One of the rules must be that when conflicts arise, they will be discussed and worked through. This element is essential to any future collaboration and especially if the collaborators function continuously as a treatment team. The more members in the interaction, the more important this norm setting and role definition is. Do not hesitate to initiate the role negotiation. As a peer in the interaction, functioning under a norm of equity, you, as well as the other(s), will assume initiation for various phases of the activity. Therefore, this first step is appropriately taken by the person who thinks of it first.

SUMMARY

Collaboration is a special form of mutual interaction toward specific goals or in pursuit of solutions to problems. In health care, the collaboration among and within disciplines, although potentially beneficial, is also relatively infrequent. This chapter has presented factors affecting the creation of collaborative relationships and has suggested activities to develop them.

Additional Reading

Baggs, Judith and Madeline Schmitt,"Collaboration Between Nurses and Physicians",*Image: The Journal of Nursing Scholarship*,No:3(Fall,1988)145-149.

Cargill,Victoria A.,"Nurses are Colleagues, Not Servants: A Win-Win Proposition for Everyone",*Health Matrix*,(Winter,1986-87)33-35.

Chadwick-Jones, J.K.,*Social Exchange Theory: Its Structure and Influence*,London Academic Press, 1976.

Johnston, Phillipa F.,"Improving the Nurse-Physician Relationship",*Journal of Nursing Administration*,(March 1983)19-20.

Kirk,Roey,"Negotiations: Getting What You Want",*Journal of Nursing Administration*,16:12(December,1986)6-9.

Koerner, Beverly L., J.R. Cohen, and D.M. Armstrong,"Collaborative Practice and Patient Satisfaction",*Evaluation and the Health Profession*,No.3 (September,1985),299-321.

Koerner, Beverly L., J.R. Cohen, and D.M. Armstrong,"Professional Behavior in Collaborative Practice",*Journal of Nursing Administration*,16,No.10,(October,1986)39-43.

Langford, Teddy and Linda Vengroff,"Interdisciplinary Collaboration a Vehicle to Cost-Conscious Health Care"in W.K. Kellogg Foundation, *Stemming the Rising Costs of Medical Care: Answers and Antidotes*,1988,21-31.

Lynaugh, Joan, and B. Bates,"The Two Languages of Nursing and Medicine,"*American Journal of Nursing,73,No.1 (January 1973),66.*

Minard, Faith,"Competition vs. Cooperation Among Nurses",*Nursing Management*19:3(March,1988)28-32.

Pluckhan, Margaret L.,"Professional Territorality, A Problem Affecting Delivery of Health Care,"*Nursing Forum*,11,No.3(1972)80-84

Rubin, I.,and R. Beckhard,"Factors Influencing the Effectiveness of Health Teams,"*Milbank Quarterly*,50,No.3(1972),317.

Chapter 9

Group relationships - Leadership skills

"I've sat in a circle so many times since I came to nursing school that I don't care if I ever am in a group again." More than one student of nursing has made this or a comment similar to this because many educational activities in nursing are conducted in groups. Leaving school will not, however, provide relief from group activity because both our social and work lives are conducted in large part in groups. Because group relationships are a vital part of our work life, this chapter focuses on the nature of groups, especially task-oriented groups, and on your function as a leader or as a member of these groups.

Groups-What They Are and How They Function

A group is:" a number of persons who communicate with one another often over a span of time, and who are few enough so that each person is able to communicate with all the others, not at second hand, through other people, but face to face."[1]

Groups are persons who interact with one another, who are psychologically aware of one another, and who perceive themselves to be a group. Given these definitions, frequency of interaction is not a critical variable in the definition of a group, nor is distance, although at some time the individuals must interact face to face. There is extensive literature on groups relating both to the various purposes of the group (such as therapeutic, socialization, and task accomplishment) and to the dynamics of interaction. The content of this

---

1 Fred Luthans, *Introduction to Management* (New York: McGraw-Hill, 1976), p.279

chapter focuses on only a small portion of the total scope of group theory and practice, that is, groups in the work setting.

There are three types of groups: (1) the *primary group*, one that serves as a major social learning force, as exemplified by the family; (2) *formal groups*, organizationally defined groups with finite functions such as task groups or committees, and (3) *informal groups*, those that provide for social interaction or communications purposes, such as the "coffee group" at work. In each type of group, the interaction affects the behavior of individual members. Therefore, groups, especially those that hold high attraction for their members, can be an effective force in individual behavior change. This accounts for the increase in numbers of personal improvement groups such as Overeaters Anonymous, for those who overeat; Parents Anonymous for child abusers, and assertiveness training groups. In these cases, individuals have common needs, interests, or problems, and they recognize that the support of a group will be helpful in promoting the desired change in behavior. A primary group, the family, is in fact, a major force in developing many of the patterns of social behavior in which a person engages.

People *choose* to join a number of the groups in which they participate. They are members of other groups without choice, such as a family; yet even in this "group" the degree of intensity of participation can vary by choice, such as maintaining close and warm relationships or being only a nominal member. In each case, there are two main reasons why one is or remains a group member. The first is *attraction* to the group. The second is *dependency* on the group. Attraction is the primary focus of two theoretical approaches to explaining group formation. The *interaction theory* indicates that the more activities, interaction, and sentiments people share, the more likely they are to form a group. *Balance theory* takes the interaction view into account but stresses that similar attitudes toward relevant objects and goals are a prime force in group formation. *Exchange theory* postulates that rewards must be greater than costs of joining for attraction or affiliation to occur. This would seem to relate to the dependency premise since dependency implies that the individual perceives there are gains to be realized from belonging to the group, and therefore he is attracted to belonging to the group. The gains spoken of in this theoretical approach are not only monetary. They may be the means to meeting a variety of needs not met elsewhere, such as acceptance, shelter, food, love, or freedom.[2]

Groups can be analyzed by considering the *roles* enacted in the group, the *norms* by which members operate, and the *functions* to which their behavior is directed.

[2] Ibid.,p.280.

Functions

The functions of a group's behavior are aimed toward either accomplishing the group's task or maintaining the group. Task-oriented behavior is designed to provide the structure necessary to accomplish work and to clarify the content of thought and action so that group members understand what is being done. Types of actions classified as task-oriented group behaviors are:

- *Initiating*-includes stating objectives, developing an agenda, setting time limits, and other acts designed to "get things moving."
- *Information and opinion seeking.*
- *Information and opinion giving.*
- *Clarifying and elaborating*-restating material for clarity and making additional expanding comments.
- *Summarizing*-reviewing what has been accomplished or stated to this point.
- *Consensus testing*-questioning the group to see if agreement exists on decisions being discussed.

Any of these actions can be taken by any group member since they (the actions) are not strictly a function of the leader.

Group maintenance behavior is aimed toward smooth function among members while doing the group's task. Examples of group maintenance behavior are:

- *Gatekeeping*-assuring that everyone's communications are heard.
- *Encouraging*
- *Harmonizing*
- *Compromising*

These actions are also the responsibility of all group members since without such mutually supportive behaviors, the group will tend to increase in conflict and be less attractive to members.[3]

Norms

Norms are the rules that govern the group's interaction. These norms vary in their extent (how many areas of life are affected), in their explicitness

[3] Irwin Rubin, R. Fry, and M. Plovnik, *Managing Human Resources in Health Care Organizations: An Applied Approach* (Reston, Va.: Reston, 1978,p.152.

(are they stated and agreed upon or just generally known), and in the degree of conformity required of group members.[4] Norms serve the purpose of decreasing ambiguity in relationships, of assuring that the group accomplishes its task, and of creating expectations for some level of group maintenance behavior. Examples of norms are:

New group members keep quiet until they are encouraged to speak by an "old" group member.

The social chatter stops when the group leader arrives and is not acceptable until the day's agenda is completed.

Decisions are made only after each member has spoken her opinion on the issue, but complete unanimity is not required.

The degree to which norms are effective in governing individual behavior is affected by: (1) the relevance of the norm to the individual's reason for being in the group and to the function of the group, and (2) the general cohesiveness of the group.[5] In a rather loosely knit group, a norm that all members wear suits or dresses rather than casual clothes might well be ignored, especially if the group was designed to be a "stop smoking" self-help group where clothing was not a relevant issue. However, in a highly cohesive teenage social group, dressing alike, although not relevant to any purpose of the group, may be a strong norm due to the group's high cohesiveness.

Roles

The concept of *roles* in groups is an outgrowth of the role theory mentioned in Chapter 1. The roles identified as important to group function mirror the task-oriented group behavior categories listed above. That is, there is a role of information giver, information seeker, clarifier, compromiser, etc., each representing a behavior necessary to group function. The fact that some individuals play one role and others choose another is not surprising since different personalities are suited to different types of behavior. In some cases, multiple roles will be assumed by group members. It is the presence or absence of the entire range of roles that defines the group character. For example, without the input of a harmonizer or a compromiser, a group may find itself frequently in conflict. Or without a consensus seeker, there may be difficulty reaching a decision. Clearly, a number of these roles can be taken by a leader, but in an effective group, the responsibility for both task and maintenance is shared.

[4] Edward E. Sampson and M. Marthas, *Group Process for the Health Professions* (New York: John Wiley, 1981),p.68-69.

[5] Ibid.,p.78.

Stages in the Development of a Group

In addition to the norms, roles, and function of a group, theorists have identified various stages in the development of a group. One author identified the following phases: *orientation*-where the issue is"what is the problem", *evaluation*- where the issue is "how we feel about the problem", and *control*- where the question is"what should we do about it".[6] Another researcher called the phases *forming, storming, norming,* and *performing.*[7] The first phase is forming the group. The second or storming phase is one which conflicts or potential conflicts in the group are identified. The norming phase is when the group develops its ground rules, and the performing phases is when it sets to work on the content of the issues at hand. Another author added the *termination* phase. This has its roots in psychoanalytic theory. It is a phase in which acts are performed to signify the end of the group's relationship, such as a final party, good-bye speeches, or exchange of gifts.[8]

As with all such theoretical information, these perspectives offer ways of organizing the observations you will make about groups in which you participate as a professional nurse.

The Leader-A Special Group Role

A key role that can encompass a variety of the other roles mentioned is that of leader. The fact that some people seem well suited to lead and do so frequently has made this a topic of considerable interest to researchers. Early study focused on identifying the traits of leaders, "Great Men" (most of the literature focused on males). The work assumed that if one possessed the traits the research identified, that person would be recognized as a leader by the groups of which he was a part, and he would be expected to bring the group together, to speak for it as advocate to other groups, to be sensitive to the needs of the individual group members so as to provide appropriate support, and to be able to compel the group members to work together to accomplish their function.

6 R. F. Bales, "The Equilibrium Problem in Small Groups," in A. P. Hare, E. F. Borgatta and R. F. Bales, ed., *Small Groups* (New York: Knopf, 1955).

7 B. W. Tuckman, "Developmental Sequence in Small Group," *Psychological Bulletin*,63,(1965),384- 399.

8 W. C. Shutz, *FIRO: A Three-Dimensional Theory of Interpersonal Behavior,* (New York: Holt, Rinehart & Winston, 1960)

More recent research has recognized that interaction plays a major role in determining whether a person becomes a leader. Therefore, leadership has come to be viewed as contingent on a combination of factors in the situation, including other group members' personalities, the nature of the task, and personal characteristics. The fact that, according to current thought, a leader in one group may be a follower in another makes it important to gain skills for either the leader or follower role.

Growing from the research interest in leadership, some rather interesting finer distinctions among concepts have been stated. One of these distinctions is the difference between leadership and "headship." This distinction recognizes that the individual sanctioned from within a group by election or mutual accession by the group members has been granted authority and responsibility from a different source than the head who has been appointed to the position by some external authority. An example is a committee chairperson selected by the committee members versus one appointed by the department administrator. In both situations, functions commonly expected of leaders are part of the expected role performance; but in the case of the appointed head there is accountability to the appointing authority. Accountability of that degree does not exist to the same degree in the case of the elected leader. Their accountability is to those who elect them, but is more global, less direct.

As a professional nurse, if you are responsible for the work of a group of nursing personnel, your management role can be conceived of as both a leadership and headship role. It is one in which you have the organization responsibility for providing supervision, evaluation, and other managerial activities for each individual worker. You also have the opportunity to serve the leadership functions of creating group cohesiveness, advocating for its needs, providing for external communication and buffering, and helping to create group goals. In some other aspects of your work you may also be elected to fill a leadership role by groups of which you are a member. In other words, because you have expert skills in nursing, knowledge of human behavior, and a sense of professional responsibility, you are equipped with a good basis for becoming a leader.

Two additional requirements for leadership are a motivation to lead and practice in doing so. The motivation can be grounded in your recognition that you are capable, that the goals of the group are worthwhile, and that in many cases, "somebody else" will not do it. It just will not be done. Simultaneously, understanding group relationships and leadership responsibilities can be the basis for functioning well as a group member.

The functions and activities of the leadership role in small groups are numerous. These include developing set events (events that create the tone or impetus for the group), serving as arbiter and relieving tension (this requires the ability to be objective and fair, to listen well and encourage others to good humor), and giving needed orders in such a way as to reduce any threats to discipline (this means gauging the way in which direction must be given to gain acceptance and compliance). Leadership functions also include clarifying the group goals, identifying group tasks, promoting cooperation by helping members see where group goals are in their best interest, promoting security and trust, encouraging creative controversy, teaching problem solving to group members, and teaching them to evaluate their group outcomes.[9] It is no small chore to perform all of these activities, and so relatively high energy level is required of the person who leads. Leonard Sayles noted that leaders appear to have the energy and perseverance to keep circulating among their followers and that they must have ability, especially in the task the group is to perform, and credibility with the members of their group and with external "others" to whom they represent their group.[10]

The functions of the leader, mentioned above, can be accomplished in several ways. One type of leader might set the goals for the group and then set out to convince the group that these are the best goals. This same individual could be a vigorous spokesperson externally for the group and also could be respected by group members for her knowledge and ability . The group's tasks are done quickly and with little argument. If there is a problem, the leader settles it. This sort of leader meets the responsibilities of leadership and does so in what is called an *autocratic manner*. Another type of leader might seek the group's thoughts on goals, survey the group for agreement before making a decision, and, in general, share responsibility and decision making with the group while providing structure and support when needed. This leader would be called *democratic*. As with most descriptive categories, these are pure types, not usually found in real life but serve to describe the identifying characteristics of the category.

It would be easy to assume that the democratic style is good and the autocratic is bad. However, there are times when a group can function comfortably and more efficiently with highly directive (autocratic) leadership. Occasions when this is appropriate is when speed is critical to performance, as in a catastrophe or when group members are inexperienced in group functions or in the group's task. On the other hand group-centered

---

9 Carolyn C. Clark, *The Nurse as Group Leader 2nd ed* (New York: Springer, 1987),p.10.
10 Leonard R. Sayles, *Leadership* (New York: McGraw- Hill, 1979),p.33.

or democratic leadership is effective when group members are accustomed to group work, when the task requires problem solving or creativity, or when the group's interaction will continue over a long period of time. The successful leader is one who: (1) has the necessary task abilities, (2) can correctly diagnose the type of leadership needed, and (3) can subsequently perform in that role. All three ingredients are needed. The person who would lead in a variety of situations must be able to vary leadership styles depending on the situational factors mentioned above.

Groups in the Work Setting

Two sorts of work groups will be important when you work in an organized health care agency. The *special task group,* exemplified by the committee, is one type of group and one that frequently falls short of its potential because of poor leadership. The other group of importance is the *primary work group.* Membership and/or leadership in each of these groups can be improved through an understanding of the process and content of each of these types of groups and of some techniques helpful in promoting efficiency and effectiveness in these groups.

The Primary Work Group

In nursing situations, it is common to hear phrases like "working together in giving good patient care" or the "nursing team." Yet on close observation, one finds that most people are working as parallel individuals with a single supervisor. In these situations, one basic element for group formation exists, that is, continuous close proximity. The need for emotional support in stressful patient care situations is another impetus for group formation. Yet, in many situations, the full potential of group formation and of group activity is not realized because there is no leadership exerted to weld the group. Some important reasons for attempting to create group cohesiveness and a sense of group belonging are:(1) tasks may arise that demand some creative input that the group might provide; (2) peer support or pressure might improve the behavior of some member; and (3) the existence of the group as an active entity can be crucial when dealing with some external threat.

Key elements in promoting group formation can be inferred from the information above. Examples of the key elements are listed below.

1. Create a sense of purpose for the group-one can identify both an immediate issue and a set of continuing concerns as the rationale for formalizing group interaction.
2. As an initiator, decide whether you want to suggest electing a leader or to continue to assume that responsibility yourself. Are you the best qualified?
3. Both the immediate task and maintenance skills of the group will need to be dealt with if the group is to become a continuing entity. Can you teach group members how to assure group maintenance through developing skills in the various group maintenance roles?
4. Can you or someone in the group analyze communication patterns and conflict modes well enough to give the group feedback on these important facets of group function?
5. Group development is a slow process. Do not allow enthusiasm for the immediate group task or impatience for "improvement in everything" cloud your judgment or reduce your tolerance and acceptance.
6. If another person emerges as leader, your knowledge of group roles can make you a valuable member. If there is no leadership, your professional concerns should prompt you to assume the role.

Committees

A special task group, the committee, can either be a tremendous waste of time and effort or a valuable source of original, creative thinking. As committee member or committee chairperson, accepting the responsibility to serve implies a willingness to complete the group's task effectively and to perform an appropriate share of the work. In addition to all of the group concerns mentioned above, the formation of a committee involves some additional responsibilities. These are listed in Table 9.1.

TABLE 9.1   List of Committee Responsibilities

1. Estimating cost of the committee's function.
2. Clarifying the group's function and task.
3. Clarifying external resources and assistance available to the group.
4. Assuring the best thinking available.
5. Providing formal channels for the group's recommendation of other output.
6. Terminating the group.

As with other groups, an early orientation activity in the committee will be developing structure and ground rules (norms) for action. An excellent point to make during this phase is the cost in person/time and in salary dollars for each hour of committee work. This emphasizes the importance of efficiency of action. The nature of the group's charge is also an important first concern. Every member should be able to explain in her own words what the comittee's purpose and scope of activity are before task work commences. When committees set to work, it is easy to assume, "This is our job, so we'll do all of it" when, in fact, assistance is available in the form of consultation and staff help with data gathering and report preparation. If these resources are available, committee output can be developed more quickly, so it is to the benefit of both the committee and the organization to provide such assistance as needed.

Andre' Delbecq and A. Vandeven have tested a technique called *nominal group method*, which is one way to assure that the best thinking of the group and group members is applied to the task at hand.[11] This method has group members work for a period of time as only a *nominal* group (a group in name only), not as an interacting group. The rationale is that this change in structure prevents the "falling into a rut" sort of thinking that can occur when a group has developed its own style. In comparing nominal groups with brainstorming by interacting groups, the interacting groups produced a smaller number of problem dimensions, fewer high quality suggestions, and a smaller number of different kinds of solutions than in groups where no interaction existed during the generation of critical problem variables. The nominal group technique very simply stated requires the steps shown in Table 9.2.

TABLE 9.2 Steps in Nominal Group Technique

1. If the group is larger than 9 members, break into smaller groups of 6-9 members.
2. Each individual is instructed to write her own list of problems, solutions, or whatever is the current point of concern without interacting with others.
3. A recorder then lists, without editing, all items produced by each member of the group on a chart or chalkboard.
4. Any new items thought of after this are listed also.
5. The group takes a short break.
6. There is an interacting group discussion of each item, in the order listed, providing clarification, elaboration, or defense of the item. None is condensed or eliminated.
7. The group then votes on its top five items, preferred solutions, problems, or whatever is under discussion.
8. When this is a subset of a larger group, there is a large group discussion of the input from the smaller groups. If not, a decision is reached on the item(s) of choice.

---

[11] Andre' L. Delbecq and A. Vandeven, "A Group Process Model for Problem Identification and Program Planning" in W. Bennis et al., *The Planning of Change*, 3rd ed. (New York: Holt, Rinehart & Winston, 1976),p. 283-296.

When a committee's internal work has been completed, the proper route for transmittal and distribution of its work must be determined in order to be sure the effectiveness of the work is not lost. Forwarding committee minutes to the nurse executive or making a report at a meeting may be only a part of the process. The committee should request formal action in response to its efforts. Formal action may mean a vote for or against actions or recommendations, or acceptance of the report with no other action. In any case, this should be initiated by a specific request from the committee chairperson who serves the leadership function of communicating with other groups. Depending on the structure of the organization and the issue at hand, the committee may also find that a definite person-to-person communications effort in addition to the formal report may be needed to assure understanding and acceptance of the committee's action. Perhaps each member of the group can be assigned specific individuals to contact. As long as a "lobbying" effort like this is conducted openly, with no manipulative secrecy, there is nothing unethical or improper in attempting to promote understanding and acceptance of the committee's work. Aside from assuring that notice is taken of the group's work, this action helps created a sense of closure for the group and prompts some comfort in termination of the committee or in its moving to its next charge or responsibility.

SUMMARY

Information on interaction common to all groups was supplemented in this chapter by specific suggestions for improving primary work group and committee functions. As a professional nurse you will have many opportunities to be group leader or member, so understanding of the process of groups will be a valuable asset.

Additional Reading

Crain,Sharon,"What Kind of Leader Are You?",*Management Accounting*,(Sept.,1985)24-28.

Hein,Eleanor C. and M.J. Nicholson,(Eds)*Contemporary Leadership Behavior:Selected Readings*,2nd Edition,Boston: Little,Brown and Company,1986.

Jay,Antony,"How to Run a Meeting",*Journal of Nursing Administration*,(January,1982)22-28,.

"The Meeting Chairperson: Master or Servant?",*Journal of Nursing Administration*,(May,1981)30-32

Lancaster,Jeanette,"Making the Most of Meetings",*Journal of Nursing Administration*(October,1981)15-19.

Mullen, B. and G. Goethals (Eds) *Theories of Group Behavior*.New York: Springer-Verlag, 1987

Schmeiding,Norma J.,"Face-to-Face Contacts: Exploring Their Meaning",*Nursing Management*,18:11(Nov.,1987)82-86.

Snook,I. Donald,"Advantages and Disadvantages of Committees",*The Health Care Supervisor*(April,1984)39- 49.

Zaleznik,Abraham,"Managers and Leaders: Are They Different?",*Journal of Nursing Administration*,(July,1981)25-31.

PART II

Managing Nursing Care: Processes and Practical Matters

- The Nursing Process

  Chapter 10 deals with the primary process for which the professional nurse is responsible. Although clinical course work and experience will have produced detailed knowledge of this process, this chapter reviews the nursing process and places it in the context of other processes, such as teaching and decision making, important in managing nursing care.

- The Management Process

  The next five chapters address each of the phases of the management process as they are applied in the management of nursing care. Chapter 11 presents an overview of management as a systematic process. Chapters 12 to 15 focus in turn on each of the steps in that process. Both the abstract operations of the management process and some specific techniques and applications are considered.

- The Process for Improving Nursing and Nursing Care

  Chapters 16 and 17 focus on staff development and planned change as two key processes in the improvement of nursing care and nursing as a profession. Also discussed are the abstract phases of each process and specific techniques and activities.

Chapter 10

The nursing process

The idea that nursing can be viewed as a process has found wide acceptance in our field. The concept is seen as one of the organizing strands in many nursing school curricula. It is the basis for the present approach to standards for care. Its usefulness is found in the fact that a process approach:

1. Implies continuity.
2. Specifies systematic progress of action.
3. Provides a structure for utilization of facts.
4. Presents a consistent structure for evaluation.
5. Provides for a deliberative rather than a reactive approach to practice.

Authors vary in their definition of the phases of nursing process, (see comparison in Table 10.1) . Some use nouns to identify the phases, implying products of the action. Others use verb forms, implying that the action constitutes the process. The descriptions that the authors provide also vary in depth of detail and in the extent to which the focus is on the thinking of the nurse as contrasted with a focus on a combination of thinking, interacting, and physical ministration.

The concept of *process* as a systematic way of operation is used to characterize other activities such as teaching, managing, and decision making. Since these activities are directly relevant to professional nursing functions, we need to see what connections among them can be identified. It is not the purpose of this text to develop an in-depth treatment of the phases of nursing. Facility in using this approach can best be developed through consistent guided clinical practice. However, skill in using the process with individual patients/clients does not necessarily mean that the nurse can translate that process to incorporate the increased number of variables introduced when several patients and other personnel become her responsibility. For that reason, subsequent chapters demonstrate relationships between the nursing process and other related processes with detailed emphasis on the management process.

TABLE 10.1 Phases Identified in the Nursing Process by Several Authors

Yura and Walsh	Zeigler, et al	Yurick, et al	Redland and Leonard
Assessing	Assessing	Assessing	Initial encounter*
Planning	Planning	Planning	Negotiating contract*
Implementing	Implementing	Intervening	Data gathering and assessing
Evaluating	Evaluating	Evaluating	Planning and programming nursing action
			Implementing nursing action
			Evaluating nursing process
			*Premonitory steps

Helen Yura and Mary B. Walsh, *The Nursing Process* , 5th edition. (New York: Appleton-Century-Crofts, 1988) p. 106

Shirley Zeigler, B. Vaughn-Wrobel, J. Erlen, *Nursing Process, Nursing Diagnosis, Nursing Knowledge.*(East Norwalk, CT: Appleton-Lange, 1986) p. 32

Ann G. Yurick, et al, *The Aged Person and the Nursing Process,*3rd edition. (East Norwalk, CT: Appleton-Lange, 1988) p. 5

Beverly G. Leonard and A. Redland, *Process in Clinical Nursing.*(Englewood Cliffs, NJ: Prentice-Hall, Inc., 1981) p.

Differentiating Responsibilities

The fondness that has developed in nursing for the nursing process framework has led to some lack of discrimination regarding its use. The attitude seems to be, "If it's good for one nurse, it is good for all."

It is of interest that few authors seem to make any distinction regarding the different levels of responsibility needed in nursing based on educational preparation or competence as they describe the nursing process. Rather, there is either the implicit assumption that people will sort themselves out or that there is no need for such distinctions. Analysis of the preparation of various nursing personnel, even among registered nurses prepared in different types of programs, shows that the second assumption is shaky. There also is no reason to have faith in the quality of individual choices at "sorting out" since these choices are made with varying levels of information. Therefore, it seems important to consider who should be doing what, using the nursing process framework.

It is an admittedly risky business to make assumptions about the capabilities of individuals based solely on their education. But, given a knowledge of general levels of preparation of the nurse's aid, technical nurse, and professional nurse (see definitions below), I propose guidelines as shown in Table 10.2 for job expectations as they are related to the nursing process phases.

Nurse's aid or assistant: One prepared in an on-the-job or brief (4-6 weeks) preservice program to give basic nursing care in a particular setting, usually in hospitals, long- term care, or home health care. These individuals are not licensed but may be certified in certain functions such as "medication aid" or "nursing home aid" where required by state or federal regulations. They are to work under supervision.

Technical nurse: One prepared in a program designed to develop nurses for basic nursing care, usually in hospitals or long-term care. This person is licensed to practice and may function without supervision or with limited supervision in the settings for which she is prepared. Depth of preparation in theoretical concepts basic to nursing is less than that for a professional nurse.

Professional nurse: One prepared in a program that develops nurses for entry level (professional nursing) positions in any health care setting. In addition to depth in theoretical basis and practice of nursing, this person has exposure to theory and practice both in collaborating with other health professionals and in providing supervision to other nursing personnel. This nurse is licensed and can work without supervision. Nurses with additional educational preparation past the basic level such as the Doctor of Nursing (N.D.)and the Master's, Ph.D.,or Doctor of Nursing Science (D.N.S.) degrees are also considered part of the category.

These are future oriented definitions in that they speak to two levels of licensed nurse, one technical, the other professional, without specifying what title, licensure, designation, or degree they hold. At this time, there is much debate about how this goal actually will be achieved. At present *licensure* in most states would indicate that R.N. equals professional and

L.V.N. equals technical. Debate within nursing, particularly among those who are Registered Nurses has persisted since 1965 regarding appropriate education licensure and titling for the two levels of basic nursing practice, technical and professional. At this time, only one state (North Dakota) has made legal changes which make the Bachelor's degree the necessary education for entry into professional nursing. More recently, there has been a shift in the emphasis from titling and licensure changes to distinguishing between appropriate practice roles based on educational experience. The term Differentiated Practice has been used to describe the efforts to establish differences in practice roles, particularly at the staff nurse level, based on education and experience, with the professional level being consistent with most current Baccalaureates degree nursing education and the technical level based on Associate Degree preparation. Some of the projects are developing new practice roles and new models of nursing care delivery rather than simply splitting existing roles.

Conceptually, this is an effort to clarify respnsibility for nursing process phases and or element of phases. Table 10.2 displays a graphic view of nursing process and performance. Consistent with the current work on differentiation of practice, this table shows how the professional nurse is responsible and accountable for the entire nursing process for the patient/clients in her care. Also, it indicates that she may appropriately perform any phase of the process but that there are others who may also perform certain steps competently. This is the basis for some of the decisions that will be considered in more detail as the professional nurse's role of manager is explained more fully.

There is value to trying to help other nursing personnel understand the idea of the nursing process even though they are not responsible for the entire cycle of activity. A description like that shown in Table 10.2 showing different functions helps others to see the professional nurse's responsibility for some activities that are "not visible," such as planning. Further, it gives a framework in which individual nurses' actions can be viewed as a part of a larger whole, important to the patient or client's well-being.

TABLE 10.2 Guidelines for Expectations in Nursing Process Performance

Nursing Process Phase	Description	Appropriate Personnel to Perform This Phase		
		Nurse's Aid	Technical Nurse	Professional Nurse
1.Initial encounter	Nurse and person meet and there is an expression or identification of need for nursing assistance.			x
2. Negotiating contract	Person and nurse agree on terms of relationship.			x
3. Data gathering (a) and assessing (b)	(a)Specific information about health status is collected and	Parts*	Parts	x
	(b) compared with norms and/or desired conditions to identify need, problems, or diagnoses		Parts	x
4. Planning and programming nursing actions	Objectives or goals of nursing activity are generated; specific nursing action or series of actions are sequenced for purposes of meeting goals.		With supervision	x
5. Implementing nursing action	Performing the planned activities	Appropriate to ability and legal limits	x	x
6. Evaluating nursing process	Collect data about structures,process, and product of nursing to compare with standards and specific objectives for this patient/client	Assist in data collection	With supervision	x

*Certain parts of the step described can be performed by this person, with or without supervision as appropriate.

Comparing Processes

The similarity that exists among all activities characterized as "processes" is present in the relationship that exists between nursing and decision making.[1] The decision making process can also be viewed as existing in its entirety in each phase of the nursing process (see Fig. 10.1).

There are a number of discussions of decision making in the literature. Some are essentially descriptive; that is, they list the activities involved in decision making as these occur in some natural or research situations. Another approach is that of the normative discussion. This is one that identifies the way in which decision making *should* be done. The "minimax" approach that arises from the work of economists who have studied decision making is one such normative approach. That description focuses on a purely rational approach that takes into account the probability of occurrence of each possible outcome of each option and the value of each of these outcomes. The decision is made by identifying the choice that minimizes loss and maximizes gain. Figure 10.1 represents a blend between the descriptive and normative approaches. Notice that the figure demonstrates that decision making occurs in each phase of the nursing process. This hybrid, which is intended to reflect a realistic yet rational method for making decisions, is discussed in greater detail in Chapter 12.

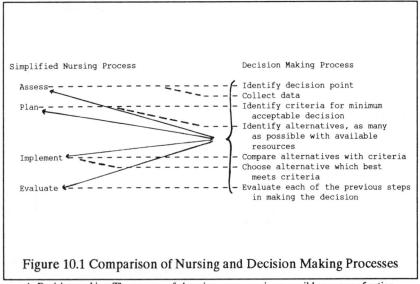

Figure 10.1 Comparison of Nursing and Decision Making Processes

1 *Decision making:* The process of choosing among various possible courses of action.

Another process that is of great importance to the professional nurse as manager or one who is being managed is the process of planned change. It is discussed in detail in Chapter 17.

Teaching is an activity that can also be viewed as a process, one that is extremely important for the professional nurse. Figure 10.2 indicates that teaching can be viewed as a particular type of nursing intervention. In attempts to promote health and prevent disease, teaching patients, families, or clients may well be the main nursing tactic used. Of course, teaching can also be viewed simply as a separate process that has similar properties to nursing and other systematic functions. In Figure 10.2 the connecting line indicate both the similarities between the processes (dashed line) and the "process within a process" nature of teaching in nursing (solid line).

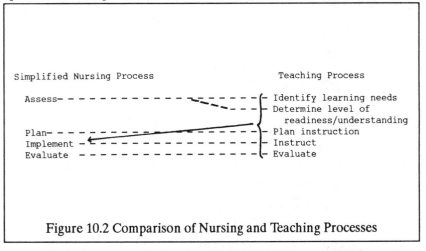

Figure 10.2 Comparison of Nursing and Teaching Processes

This brief overview of processes is intended to demonstrate that professional nursing is a systematic function, that it is similar in some ways to other related processes that are employed *in* nursing, and that principles learned in the use of each systematic process can be useful in understanding and using the other processes.

Additional Reading

American Nurses' Association,*The Scope of Nursing Practice*,Kansas City, Mo.: American Nurses' Association, 1987.

Brill, Esther L. and D. Kilts,*Foundations for Nursing*,2nd Ed.,Norwalk, Connecticut: Appleton-Century- Crofts,1986,p.15-50.

Carpenito, Lynda J.,*Nursing Diagnosis Application to Clinical Practice*,Philadelphia: J.B. Lippincott Company, 1983.

Langford,Teddy,"Establishing a Nursing Contract,"*Nursing Outlook*,26,No.6(June 1978),386.

Rotkovitch,Rachel and C. Smith,"ICON I - The Future Model, ICON II - The Transition Model",*Nursing Management*,18,No.11(November, 1987)p.91-96.

Chapter 11

A view of the management process

The view of management as a process is certainly not a new idea. Writers in the field have implied for some time that a systematic approach for accomplishing work is helpful to those who are responsible for the completion of the work. The nurse who understands the process approach in nursing is well on the way to understanding this same type of approach to management.

The nurse, by virtue of tradition, the centrality of her function in the health care agency, and the constancy of her presence, has often had to assume the role of general manager in acute care settings. She has frequently been the one responsible for housekeeping, supplies, on-unit record keeping, relief pharmacy, admissions, and many other functions not directly involved in providing nursing care. It is the expectation of her providing this sort of management that has become the target for change by nurses in recent years.

The 1960s marked the beginning of a trend toward the use of unit managers and unit clerks for nonnursing functions. The result is that the use of such personnel frees the nurse to deal with the business of giving care. The unit manager is a person who is responsible for the nonnursing management function in inpatient settings. This responsibility generally includes supervision of supplies, arrangements for repairs, housecleaning, liaison with other departments, and other related duties. In many agencies, the unit manager is responsible to the hospital administration. In other agencies, the nursing department retains overall control of the functions of this person. The rationale for this latter placement is usually that the functions are very closely allied to the support of the nursing staff's function and that it is therefore useful to have the accountability for both functions directed by a single department head. These managers are typically responsible for several related units that are geographically near to one another.

In contrast, unit clerks or ward secretaries assist with the nondirect care aspects of care, aspects that relate to maintenance of records and communication on a unit. In most agencies these persons work under the supervision of the nurse in charge or have dual responsibility to the nurse and to the unit manager. The unit clerk is usually present on each shift or at least on the day and evening shifts. Typical responsibilities include noting physician orders, ordering medications and diets, greeting visitors, routine charting, answering telephones, and "directing traffic."

Why then is there reason to be concerned with developing skill in managing if there are others qualified to see that the agency and its units run smoothly? The answer lies in the fact that the *work of nursing*, the high-quality implementation of the phases of the nursing process *requires management skills* when multiple patients are being cared for. Also, the involvement of multiple personnel requires that the responsible person, the professional nurse, be adept in the management of human resources.

The view of the management process utilized for this book is depicted in Fig. 11.1. There are numerous other approaches that include more steps or give different names for the phases. However, they all bear similarity to the one chosen for use here. As you can see, there is a marked resemblance between this process and the nursing process. That is, there are similar steps; there is a planning phase, an organizing phase, an implementing phase, and an evaluation or control phase. A major difference is that although the purpose of the nursing process is to produce nursing care for an individual, the management process produces the structure and coordination necessary to get any type of work done, generally with and through the efforts of more than one person. Subsequent chapters focus, in depth, on activities that comprise these four phases of the management process.

• Plan
• Organize
• Implement
• Evaluate
Fig. 11.1 A View of the Management Process

At this point, the following general description of the phases will serve as an overview.

Plan: To determine, in advance, the objectives to be accomplished and the means by which these objectives are to be attained.

Organize: To put together into an orderly whole by setting up a structure to bring necessary resources into action to carry out plans.

Implement: To perform the activities planned to meet the objectives. In management, to provide the ongoing direction necessary to the completion of those activities.

Evaluate: To determine the degree of quality of the work and in that process to examine any and all factors that may affect that quality.

A great deal of what is suggested as background knowledge and specific methods for management is the same no matter what sort of work is being performed. However, it is debatable whether this is entirely true in the case of nursing, given the differences among types of work and types of workers. Still, it is easy to see that there are many facets of work and workers that are the same from situation to situation. In presenting the management process, as in the nursing process, the intent is to focus on a systematic way of viewing the functions of managing. This framework can serve, then, as a base to which specific knowledge and various techniques relevant to managing nursing can be connected.

There is a large body of management literature, some research- based, some experiential, some theoretical, some purely conjectural, and some diametrically opposed to others. It is tempting to simply choose what suits this author best and present it as "the best way." However, as a professional with a responsibility for lifelong continued education, you will need to gain skill in deciding for yourself what is useful. Figure 11.2 depicts a flow of decisions that can aid in sorting among the numerous theories and opinions in present and future management literature.

Using the chart in Fig. 11.2 requires that you first examine your view of the work situation as objectively as possible. Some of the elements to be examined include the workers, their personal attributes, competence, and performance; the work itself and the quality level at which it is being accomplished; and the organization in which the work is being performed, its philosophy, structure, and environment. If in doing this, you find that you can gain no corroboration for your view of the situation (the "no" branch), there are several possible choices. Self-examination may result in an understanding that your view is clouded by other factors in your life. Perhaps you have some difficulty in dealing with authority figures. As a result, you may perceive the situation as highly directive and stifling to creativity, whereas other coworkers may not sense overbearing authoritarianism at all.]

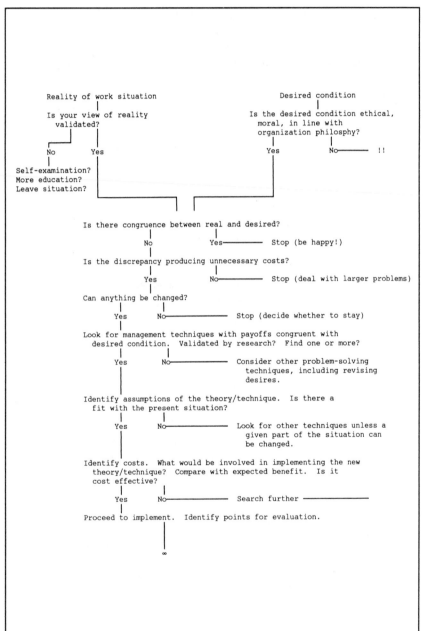

Figure 11.2 Decision Diagram-Using Management Knowledge

Another possibility is that with further education your understanding of the situation may be clarified. Still another possibility is that you may need to leave the situation if you find that (a) you perceive the need for changes in certain management techniques *and* (b) others in the situation find no cause for concern.

The right side of the chart in Fig. 11.2 indicates that the desired condition must be identified in order that a comparison may be made with the real situation. Certainly this definition of the "desired condition" is a difficult task. Frequently, we can say that we want *something* to be different but cannot specify what. It is likely that the first definition of desired states will be rather global, e.g., high morale, good quality of care, or lower turnover. In this phase, also, the nurse may recongnize that it is useful to "bump into" the ideas of others in the same work situation. The result of that collision can be increased clarity of definition. No doubt you are beginning to think that this is more a description of a change process than a method for determining management techniques. The reason for the similarity is that new management techniques are frequently superimposed on top of existing practice. Or the implementation of a new style or new approach is inserted into an already existing work setting. We seldom have the opportunity to begin with an entirely new staff and new work setting. As a result, employing the new management style or technique becomes, in itself, a form of change.

Proceeding through the decision diagram (in Fig. 11.2) the next question of substance is whether a discrepancy between "real" and "desired" is producing unnecessary costs. The concept of cost is most readily viewed in monetary terms. Is money being lost or excesses being spent due to personnel turnover or absenteeism? Is the result of low quality a decrease in customers (patients)? Is the structure or climate of the organization affecting personnel or work adversely? Other factors can be viewed as costs as well. For example, does the attitude of personnnel result in negative public relations, even though work output is satisfactory and turnover and absenteeism are low?

The question of whether unnecessary costs, monetary or less tangible, are being incurred is a key one. The fact that the management style or techniques in a work situation are not new is not sufficient in itself to merit drastic changes if the new technique or style or the process of making the changes will incur additional costs. (These comments are not intended to discourage innovation or a continuing search for useful techniques in managing. Rather, they are intended to encourage critical analysis instead of faddism.)

Assuming that some unnecessary costs are identified with the discrepancy between real and desired conditions, the next question is whether anything *can* be changed. Seldom is any organization so rigid that a new technique or style cannot be tolerated. But it is worthwhile to test the possibility of an innovation's being tolerated before committing yourself to large- scale changes. Ask questions about the past. Have supervisors ever held evaluation conferences with each employee? Has there been a policy that prevents using a team method for providing care in the community health districts? Is there a strong sentiment against professional nurses' giving total patient care on your unit? Also consider the present. Are you in a position to help implement any new activities?

If you find that there is little hope of change in a situation that you and others agree is significantly less than desirable, it is important to consider the possibility of leaving the situation. Hope is a precious commodity, and the conclusion that there is no real hope that change can occur to produce improvement should not be reached precipitiously. But if this is your conclusion, based on solid evidence, it is in your best interest to consider what, if any, important benefits exist in staying in your present position. Perhaps this is a surprising suggestion. It seems, though, that inducing guilt with rhetoric about the need to persist in such circumstances can only contribute to the displeasure some nurses find in their practice.

If, on the other hand, the "Can anything be changed" question nets a "yes" answer, as it usually will, the stage is set to make decisions about what new management theories or techniques are applicable. The first level of decisions must be based on consideration of the particular theory or technique itself. You must read either the original work of the author of the theory or a reliable review in order to make judgments about the validity of the conclusion. It is important that you as a professional cultivate the habit of reading original work as well as text material designed to provide an overview. Numerous insights can be gained by consulting the original work. For example, the comment by Abraham Maslow that his hierarchy of needs theory did not necessarily hold for deprived classes is important.[1]. Yet, most text treatments of his work imply a very broad applicability.

In addition to considering the soundness of the research or the logic of a theory, it is also important at this stage to identify the anticipated outcomes of any new methods under consideration. For example, if personnel turnover is a problem, a method that purports to help personnel become more adept at interpersonal relations may not be particularly useful in dealing with turnovers.

---

[1] Abraham Maslow,*Motivation and Personality*(New York: Harper & Row,1954)

When one or more theories or techniques are found that seem to have applicable payoffs, still further examination must occur. It is important to identify to what conditions the ideas are addressed, what assumptions they are built upon. Cost again becomes a concern at this decision point. In this case, the cost of implementing the new theory or techniques is the concern. Again, the most obvious costs are those that are directly monetary. Other costs such as those of time involved in planning must also be considered. What about extra effort (not more hours, just more attention)? That, too, has its costs. If the benefits do *not* outweigh the costs of implementing your choice of theories or techniques, you will want to think carefully before proceeding. When the reverse is true and a new technique is chosen, the final step (see Fig. 11.2), which in actuality is the beginning step of implementation, includes the identification of points or criteria for evaluation of the new technique or theory.

SUMMARY

This chapter's information has been presented to provide a framework for the material in the next four chapters. Each of these chapters focuses on a phase of the process of management. As you consider this material, keep in mind the process suggested here for selecting new techniques for use in practice.

Additional Reading

Koontz, Harold,"The Management Theory Jungle Revisited" *Academy of Management Review*,5,No.2 (1980)p.175-187.

Chapter 12

Planning

Planning is a sort of catchall term. A plan can be anything from a short list hurriedly written on a napkin to an elaborate document resulting from months of community development activity. It can include a variety of statements on such things as objectives, policies, procedures, rules, budgets, or programs. Planning, when done well, is systematic and contributes to the total operation. In the management of nursing care, planning is essential both for the manager and the managed, and for individual action or group efforts. This chapter describes a general planning framework and gives specific applications of that process along with a related activity - decision making. The specific applications begin with developing daily plans for your own work each day, through planning assignments for other personnel, participating in unit or department planning, and understanding budgeting as a planning activity.

Planning Defined- A Process

Planning can be defined as the process of determining in advance the objectives to be accomplished and the means by which these objectives are to be attained. A rational, systematic series of steps for planning is described in Fig. 12.1. The set of steps shown in Fig. 12.1 can be used as a framework for understanding all types of planning, from small to large-scale efforts.

1.Identifying objectives, including criteria for evaluation.

2.Determining priorities among objectives.

3.Identifying various possible means/actions for accomplishing objectives.

4.Choosing means/actions to accomplish objectives.

5.Developing sequence of activities.

FIGURE 12.1 Planning Process

Plans may vary in their content from situation to situation, but there are general criteria that may be used to evaluate any plan. In their text for nursing administration Clara Arndt and Loucine Huckaby list several criteria for a good plan.[1] They include:

1.The plan is based on clearly defined objectives.
2.The plan is clear and simple.
3.The plan provides stability and flexibility.
4.The plan is economical and realistic in terms of resources needed to implement it.
5.The plan provides for a thorough analysis and classification of activities and for determination of the evaluation criteria.
6.The plan anticipates and forecasts the future.
7.The plan is purposeful, rational, and justifiable in terms of organizational and individual objectives.
8.The plan allows for the unique sociopolitical environment of the organization.
9.The plan specifies the dimension for which it applies.

Identifying Objectives

The first phase, identifying objectives, involves determining as specifically as possible, exactly what is to be accomplished. Delineating criteria for evaluation at this same time will make final evaluation, when the project is finished, a simpler task. There are numerous sources that describe at length just how to develop objectives. The emphasis is on assuring that the objectives are written, are stated in clear terms, and that they are as explicit

[1] Clara Arndt and Loucine M. Huckaby, *Nursing Administration*, 2nd Ed (St. Louis, Mo.: C.V. Mosby, 1980), p.72.

as possible in describing what the planner wishes to accomplish. Ideally, an objective should be stated as shown in Fig. 12.2. It should include a statement of the behavior to be accomplished (a verb and an object), the condition or circumstance under which it is to be accomplished, and the criterion level (the amount or degree of accomplishment).This objective (as shown in Fig. 12.2), when elaborated upon by defining "total nursing care," can serve as the basis for evaluating the plan when it is completed.

Behavior	=	Provide total nursing care
Condition and/or circumstance	=	During the 7 A.M. to 3 P.M. period
Criterion level	=	Any three patients on 3 West

12.2 Example of Nursing Care Objective.

Many authors have addressed the topic of objectives, describing varying levels of behavior; varying foci, including process, structure, and outcome; and various perspectives, including that of manager, of the one who is managed, and of the "product" (patient care). Although these are interesting and potentially useful discussions, it is possible that undue concerns with such matters can inhibit planners, especially those who are less experienced. Therefore, I recommend that primary concern be directed to:(1)*deciding what is to be accomplished;* (2)*considering it from differing perspectives,* specifically the perspectives of the agency, service, or unit (depending on the scope of the plan), the person(s) who will perform the action implementing the plan, and the recipient of service (where the plan involves patients or clients); and (3)*writing the objectives* in words that communicate as clearly as possible to those concerned with the plan.

Of course, deciding what is to be accomplished is no simple task. It becomes increasingly complex as the number of persons and agencies involved increases. For example, it is relatively simple to make a plan for your own day when you are to be alone all day. However, as you begin to involve others, you must also consider their values, priorities, objectives, and abilities. And if you are in an agency, you must consider the constraints or directions implied by existing organizational philosophy, objectives, policy, and procedures.

Another important concern in the first phase is limiting the scope of the plan to a series of potentially accomplishable goals. This demands that the planner have background knowledge of:

1.The nature and extent of human resources available.
2.The nature and extent of material resources.
3.The potential for drastic changes in either of the above.
4.The organization, philosophy, mission, and operating policy of the group or agency. Also important is the degree to which these elements reflect the values of the community served by the agency.
5.Predominant personal and cultural values of those who will implement the plan.

A new employee in an agency may find that even the simplest plan development can fail if the background data are not available as listed above. This information serves as a filter for screening objectives as well as reviewing other elements of the plan as these are developed. For example, from the universe of possible goals for a particular community health agency's care of patients with hypertension, a goal that states that there will be weekly monitoring by nursing personnel of blood pressure on all hypertensive patients may be laudable. However, if there are limited personnel who cannot possibly visit each patient weekly, or cannot even hold sufficient clinics to provide the service, perhaps another objective must be chosen. A revised statement might reduce the frequency of the blood pressure checks. Or possibly the goal may be directed toward involving others such as client or family in performing the monitoring on an intermittent basis.

Take another example. An objective that states, "To provide birth control counseling to all sexually active adolescents in the clinic population" may have agency acceptance, yet be currently impractical if the clinic personnel have personal religious or cultural values that preclude the practice of birth control.

Sources and methods for collecting the necessary background information are numerous. These include: knowledge of staffing patterns and related position descriptions; information on supply inventories; information on current budget and the degree of flexibility of the budget; understanding of the philosophy, goals, mission statements, and master plan of the agency; knowledge of the individual agency personnel; and knowledge of the predominant cultural values of the community. Some of this information is readily available and is presented during orientation to the agency. To gain other data, you may need to ask questions and seek access to source documents or request explanations from administrative personnel. Are you thinking, "I couldn't ask to see a budget," or, "What would they think if I ask a lot of questions about the agency's master plan?" Possibly, such behavior might be novel. Yet, if the reason for the request is stated clearly and honestly, without insinuated negativism, it is likely to meet with acceptance. Role-playing the asking of such questions is one way to rehearse so that your anxiety about such assertive behavior will be reduced.

Another element that must be considered in choosing objectives is the duration for which the plan is to be developed. Are you planning for this week or this year? Logically, the objectives for daily plans will be consistent with longer range plans. But the objectives for short-term plans would be such that they can be accomplished in the allotted time.

Determining Priorities among Objectives

The next phase in planning is to determine priorities among objectives. This implies that some objectives are more important or more urgent in nature than others. Furthermore, there may be a number of objectives that are essentially equal in priority. Therefore, instead of wasting a great deal of time deciding between which objective is ranked fifth and which sixth, it is helpful to use a three-category sorting system, which is viewed as having a variable number of "slots" in each category. The three categories are: Most Important, Very Important, Important. Most Important is reserved for those objectives that are the *life* of the planned activity. In the case of patient care, "life" may in fact be an accurate measure of what is most important. Maintaining basic vital functions in all patients in the coronary care unit (CCU) is an objective that would fit in this category. Or presenting an on-the-job orientation in the use of a new piece of equipment may be a Very Important objective if that equipment is to be used frequently, particularly if improper use could injure patients or personnnel or could damage the equipment. The Important category can be reserved for those objectives that are valuable but which can be deferred until a subsequent planning period.

Do you suppose that if you and I were each given a list of objectives to assign priorites to we would both sort them out in the same way? It is very likely that there would be a high degree of agreement on some objectives, especially those that will obviously maintain life and promote safety. But there might be wide variance in our choice of priorities for many other objectives. This is because some values are widely held by very diverse groups of people, whereas other values are less universal. Given that rather ambiguous and characteristically human state, how can one set priorities among objectives with any hope of acceptance of those objectives by others who may help in the implementation? The answer to that question is found in returning to the information mentioned above as useful background data. That information can provide insight into values that predominate in an organization.

Fay Bower suggests some criteria for choosing priorities among needs of patients.

Criteria of hierarchy should include the consideration of those problems or needs that (1)threaten life, dignity, and integrity of the individual, family, or community; (2)threaten to destructively change the individual, family, or community; and (3)affect the normal developmental growth of the individual, family, or community.[2]

The values implicit here are that (1) the continuation and preservation of quality of life is of great importance; (2) the integrity of the social units of family and community are of high value; (3)as the degree of immediate threat increases, the greater the priority. She also notes that when one begins to deal with groups of patients/clients, additional criteria for priority become relevant. These include safety, efficiency, cost in money and energy, and receptivity, noting that dealing first with the most receptive may free time to use with the less receptive.[3]

It is difficult to draw a direct analogy between these suggestions regarding patient care objectives and the choices required in setting objectives for plans less directly related to specific patient needs. There are some implications to be examined, though. First, the various levels of threat to the accomplishment of *organizational* functions could be used as criteria for establishing priorities, just as levels of threat to life affect priorities with patients. A possible corollary to the "deal with the most receptive first" idea is that some objectives are relatively easily accomplished and can be given high priority simply because they are readily accomplished. For example, "to develop a list of all audiovisual materials owned by the agency that are suitable for patient education " may be an Important objective according to other criteria. But it can be accomplished easily as the shelves in the audio-visual room are cleaned by a volunteer. Thus there is no reason to wait until all higher priority objectives are completed first.

Another issue in choosing objectives and priorities among objectives is attempting to identify a *minimum* expectation. This is particularly important in nursing care because our education encourages that we strive to provide the best possible care. Yet, in situations where personnel are few, best possible care may not be possible. Or, viewed another way, when staffing shortages are acute, the best that is possible may not be good enough to provide for safety. For these reasons, the professional nurse must develop a

[2] Fay Louise Bower,*The Process of Planning Nursing Care*,3rd ed.(St. Louis, Mo.: C.V. Mosby, 1982),p.22.

[3] Ibid.,p.24.

knowledge of what are minimum safe standards of care so that plans can be checked against these. The best circumstance is that the agency as a whole develop such standards so that clear guidelines are available for planning. Choosing priorities is most effective when a "priority re-sort" is performed after actions are developed for all objectives. In the second consideration of objectives, the effort is made to decide which actions can be performed simultaneously. This may increase the opportunity to accomplish all objectives, or greater numbers of them, since low priority activities do not then have to be deferred until high priority activities are completed.

Identifying Various Possible Means/Actions for Accomplishing Objectives

The choice of means, specific actions, to accomplish the objectives is the next step in the planning process. The first activity is to generate descriptions of various possible actions that will accomplish the objectives. It may well be that you can only think of one course of action to meet an objective simply because the activity that comes to mind is feasible, quick, and would pose no problems at all to implement. Certainly, in that case, it would be a waste of time to search for alternatives. However, situations are seldom that clear-cut. Most planning can benefit from creative attempts to develop more than one possible way of meeting objectives. When the series of possible actions has been developed, decisions must be made in order to choose the action to be implemented.

Decisions in this context can be made using a rational approach tinged with reality. This means that the approach is *not* one of complete rationality,(one that assumes that one can know all the possible consequences of every act). Nor is it the "satisficing" approach that merely assumes that any course of action that will accomplish the objective is satisfactory. Rather, the decision combines useful elements of both approaches. From the first approach, the purely rational one, we keep the systematic and objective elements and discard the need to know all possible alternatives and their consequences. From the "satisficing" approach we eliminate the "too ready to accept anything" element but maintain that the decision maker is human and has a limited realm of knowledge.

The phase of identifying alternative means of accomplishing objectives is critical to making a good plan. It is at this point that creativity and the use of sources of information in addition to the planner become important. If you are making a long- or short-range plan for yourelf, you can consult colleagues for suggestions, or you can refer to the literature in your field. When others are involved in the execution of a plan, you may want to include them in the planning. At this point, it is possible to assemble an even larger range of possible alternative methods based on wider participation. Of course, this requires more time. Therefore, the time involved should be weighed against the value of the input, not only in terms of the specific value of the suggestions, but also as it produces greater commitment to the plan. The alternatives should be identified first, without screening them. The thinking encouraged here, free of evaluation, is sometimes referred to as *brainstorming.*

Choosing Actions/Means to Accomplish Objectives

After the series of alternatives for each objective is developed, the next step is to choose the actions that will provide the greatest benefit as compared to any disadvantages. You can ask the following types of questions to help identify the best course of action.

1. Is this feasible, given the available staff, material, and environment? Answering this requires knowledge of the human and material resources available, an important part of any planning effort.
2. Is this efficient in use of time, effort, and materials?
3. Will the action *effectively* accomplish the objective at the level desired?
4. Is this action likely to be acceptable to the persons who will implement it?

When a choice has been made, it is useful to view it in connection with all the others chosen for the rest of the objectives in the plan. You are likely to find that some action will contribute to the accomplishment of more than one objective. Table 12.1 demonstrates that some specific actions, such as that labeled (1), may be directed toward meeting several different objectives. In this example, objectives 1,2, and 4 can all be advanced by the specific action labeled (1). Specific action (1) then is a part of three different courses of action-A,B, and D. A course of action is then a series of specific actions directed toward meeting an objective. Any single specific action can be a part of several different courses of action. This information will be useful in the next step in the planning process.

Developing Sequence of Activities

Generally, the approach in the final phase of planning is simply one of deciding what will be done in what order. Factors to be considered include

TABLE 12.1 Relationship of Actions to Objectives

Objective	Course of action	Specific actions
1	A	(1) (3) (2) (4)
2	B	(5) (1) (6) (3)
3	C	(7) (4) (8) (5)
4	D	(9) (1) (10)
5	E	(11)(3)

priority of objectives, efforts that must be cumulative, and activities that can be simultaneous.

The process as described above (and as shown in Fig. 12.1) is applicable as a general framework for individual or group, long- or short-term plans. It is, however, somewhat abstract until it is applied to a real situation. Examples are presented in later sections of this chapter as specific techniques that can be used in the various phases of planning.

Types of Organizational Plans

The process of planning results in a variety of products, that is, different types of plans. These will differ in their length of use, number of persons affected, and degree of specificity, according to purpose. Harold Koontz and Heinz Weihrich list eight types of organizational plans.[4]

1. *Purpose or Mission:* Basic functions or tasks.
2. *Objectives:* Statements of the end to which activity is directed.
3. *Strategy:* An overall plan for direction, general coupling of objectives with resources.
4. *Policies:* Guides for thinking and solving recurring problems, consistent with objectives.
5. *Procedures:* Plans that establish a required method for actions in commonly occurring situations.

[4] Harold Koontz and Heinz Weirich, *Management 9th ed.* (New York:McGraw-Hill,1988),p.61-69.

6.*Rules:* Standards for action in all occurrences of a particular sort, allowing no discretion.

7.*Budget:* A statement of plans for a given period of time stated in fiscal terms.

8.*Program:* Groups of plans developed to accomplish an overall direction or series of related goals.

You can see that these categories refer to various types of plans for an organization. As an individual you may also want to create a plan, using your own budget, your own objectives, and perhaps a program or strategies. It is likely that you will make daily plans as well as some long-range plans for your own professional activities. Before moving to individual planning, we will consider in more detail two types of planning that occur at the organizational level, strategic planning and budgeting.

Strategic Planning

The term strategic planning has come into use in health care as the level of sophistication of managers has risen and increasing use of the corporate structure has come into vogue. This concept emphasizes that overall strategy or decision about intent and direction of an enterprise must rest on systematically analyzed information about the environment in which the organization functions. With its origin in the military, strategic planning is not different in its general process from other planning, but is different in that is relies on a strong element of data analysis about the external environment and projections about the potential effect of that environment on the target organization. At the direct care level, strategic planning for the facility in which you work may be remote. You may have little input, since decision about strategy - general direction and overall method - are appropriately made at the level of the Board of Directors, Chief Executive and Chief Operating Officers,and executive level administrators. Those decisions do affect the unit level and should be conveyed to the managers at that level so that they can be the basis for planning at the unit level. The strategic decision becomes a "given", the direction for organizational objectives. The strategic plan should be logically consistent with the organization's purpose and philosophy.

How should the strategic plan be communicated? Is there a proper format ? How would you, as a new professional nurse, recognize the plan? The answers to these questions are not definite. No one format is required, no particular method of presentation. Some facilities publish an annual plan, others publish a multi-year document with annual updates. Some provide a document to each new employee. Others discuss the material at employee meetings. As with much planning activity, the nature of the actual plan is only as important as the process of planning. The written plan serves as a way to confirm and communicate the result of a process, which in the case of strategic planning, relies on information about the environment as a major factor.

Budgeting as a Planning Method

The word *budget* frequently draws a rather negative response from those who view themselves as givers of care. Concern with money seems somehow crass when such things as saving lives and preventing family disruption are where your heart is. However, to continue to be unaware of how and by whom budgeting is done and to fail to influence that process will mean losing an important opportunity. Since the facilities and personnel necessary to give care must be funded, there is a direct connection between the budget and the equipment and personnel you have available to give such care. For that matter, whether *you* have a position depends on budget decisions!

What is a budget, the very mention of which brings negative reactions? A budget is the expression, in monetary terms, of the plans for an organization for a particular period of time. It provides the basis for the evaluation of financial performance in relation to those plans. Although philosophy, goals, and objectives may abound, it is in the budget that one can see what will actually be done. There are certain budget techniques that make very clear what funds are spent for what programs, and there are other budget forms that are less specific. Specificity frequently increases with the decrease in the size of the unit (department, project, etc.) that is budgeted for.

This section presents some information about various types of budget elements, their purpose, and the kinds of input you as *managed*, might wish to supply, or as *manager*, may need to collect.

Types of Budgets

The most common type of budget in hospitals is a *forecast budget*-one that is based on estimates for the coming year. In many organizations there is some degree of flexibility in the forecast budget so that there can be adjustments from category to category or from year to year to account for certain variations in income and expenditures.

The components of the forecast budget are the operating budget, the capital expenditures budget, and the cash budget. The nursing department is most directly concerned with the first two components. The operating budget contains the statements of expenses such as salaries and wages, supplies (expendables), other expenses such as insurance premiums, dues, etc., and the expected revenues. The capital expenditures budget indicates the plans for spending for equipment purchases and physical plant changes requiring more than some set amount of money. For example, any item over $100 is considered a capital expenditure in many agencies. The cash budget is an estimate of the cash flow from revenues and direct expenditures.

Where the agency is funded by some source other than direct revenue, such as in hospitals or health departments sponsored by governmental authorities, the forecast budget is submitted and subsequent approval results in an *appropriations budget*. The primary difference between the forecast budget and the appropriations budget is that the appropriations budget is less flexible because the legal limit by category and by year are defined within rigid restrictions for the transfer of funds from category to category ("line to line") or from one year to the next. Once the appropriations are set, there is little, if any, leeway for changes based on new needs or opportunities.

The process by which budgets are determined at the level of the total organization in health care has been influenced in a major way by changes in a source of revenue since 1983. That year, the Congress of the United States passed legislation that changed the method of payment to hospitals for the care of Medicare recipients. Prior to that time a cost based reimbursement system had been in use. With that method a hospital developed charges that were negotiated as reasonable, based on its demonstrated costs of providing services. No incentive was built in to this method to encourage agencies to hold down costs and charges. In fact, the opposite was true since costs were the basis for charges and in turn for reimbursements. In an effort to hold down increases in Federal funds spent on health care, and possibly to model similar changes for private third party payors, a new system was developed. The concept behind the system, prospective payment, is that given sufficient data it is possible to determine typical requirements of medical care and hospitalization for the major categories of illness. Based on wide scale data collection, a system which categorizes illnesses by Diagnosis Related Group (DRG) was developed and costs of providing care were correlated to these groups. Based on these costs along with typical services rendered, a standard length of stay and related cost per hospitalization was determined for each group. These costs were then the basis for a standard payment for that illness, or combination of conditions, regardless of the actual costs incurred by the real patient's hospitalization. The incentive exists in this system for hospitals to reduce length of stay because the payment is fixed, regardless of length of stay. Therefore, if the stay is shorter, and actual costs of providing care are reduced by that shortened stay, the hospital has "made a profit" on the case.

Strategic planning for this environmental change challenges all health care even now since the system of prospective payments is expected to be adapted for all Federally paid care (nursing home, outpatient, psychiatric) and by private third party payors across the country. The *transition* to a wholly prospective paid system is probably the most difficult aspect of the change rather than the eventual changed status. That is because strategy for dealing with a reimbursement based retrospective method simultaneously with a prospective system is difficult to develop and implement. As a result of this change in a revenue source, budgeting in health care facilities has changed, in some cases dramatically. The transition has been one of much uncertainty. Reduced census in hospitals was accompanied by increased patient acuity. One medical outcome of these changes has been an awareness that the degree of specificity afforded by costs and charges aggregated at the "Room Rate" level is probably not sufficient to be responsive to this new fiscal environment. There is now a trend toward developing more sensitive measures of resource utilization at the individual patient level in order to plan for nursing care provision consistent with those needs. This is associated with an interest in charging separately for nursing care rather than as a part of the room rate.[5] [6]

What does all of this mean to the nurse at the patient care level? Perhaps the greatest meaning is that you will be expected to function as efficiently as possible to reduce length of stay, particularly for Medicare patients in hospitals. And, you will have the opportunity to participate in development of new roles to complement these changes. Beyond that, you can expect to be a part of regular data collection about work effort, time allocation for nursing care, and acuity of patient need, much of which may require computer input. I encourage you to participate actively because the decisions which result will affect staffing, pay and benefits for personnel as well as care for patients.

[5] Phyllis Ethridge." The Case for Billing by Patient Acuity"*Nursing Management*16,no. 6 (August, 1985) p.38- 41.

[6] Leah Curtin. "Determining Costs of Nursing Service per DRG"*Nursing Management* 14, no.4 (April, 1983) p16- 20

Another budget system currently in use in some agencies is the *program budget*. Using this system, each program or functional area is budgeted separately rather than being only a portion of a department budget. For example, psychiatric outpatient services may be budgeted as a separate element. Under many hospital systems, several departments might have items that are part of the psychiatric outpatient service, many of which could be difficult to identify as relating to that service. Under the program method, the costs of that program are already identifiable. When program evaluation is performed, then the costs are available to be considered in relation to the benefits of the program.

Process of Budget Development

Perhaps you are wondering just how you might have an influence on budgeting since you do not make decisions about new equipment or numbers of personnel or the salary they receive. The following information describes a typical process of budget development. As you read, you can identify from your own experience how a staff nurse could be involved in this process.

The first step in the budget process is begun when the fiscal officer of the agency, whose title may be controller, accountant, budget manager, or other, sets the budget calendar. This calendar defines the deadlines for the completion of each of the elements of the budget. This calendar is sent to each department head or person responsible for a budget division. When the nurse executive receives this calendar and the budget manual or detailed instructions for preparation, she or he must begin to collect information for decision making. In a nursing service that uses participative management activities, the groundwork will have been done to encourage staff participation in budgeting.

There is no requirement that the nurse executive seek consultation from other staff levels. Certainly there are situations where the budget is only mentioned to staff-level personnel as a reason for being unable to fund some activity or furnish more staff. But where the nurse executive wants to have nursing staff involved in the decisions affecting their work, she will make use of the budget as a planning tool and as a means for comparing plans with actual performance. In order to accomplish this, the next step would be to request the head nurses and supervisors (or the equivalent in that agency) to seek direct suggestions from unit staff and other data to produce the budget recommendations for their units. The major types of information needed are listed in Table 12.2.

TABLE 12.2 Important Budget Considerations

Suggestions regarding new or improved equipment and discussion of rationale for the request.

Requests for remodeling or other alterations or additions to physical plant.

Suggestions about amount of travel and registration needed for staff development off site.

Suggestions for unit, division, or agency-wide consultants.

Data on patient needs related to staffing and any requests for changes.

Obviously the professional staff nurses and other personnel can provide only a portion of the necessary budget information. However, the input from this level can be invaluable. Further, the opportunity to have information about the budget process can be motivating for personnel who enjoy a feeling of involvement in the organization. This is particularly true when the nursing staff then receives in sequence: (1)a summary of the request submitted by the head nurse; (2)information on the budget as it affects the unit when the budget is approved; and finally, (3)monthly or quarterly feedback on operating expenses as compared to the budget projection so that personnel can see the effects of their use of materials and other purchases. This sort of feedback can be furnished only if there is an accounting system that can develop such information.

Importance of Budgeting Data for the Professional

Of what value is knowing about the budget to someone in a beginning professional postion? First, it can help you to understand the ways in which the objectives of the agency are being met. For example, if there is an objective that states that the needs for employees' inservice education will be met on an individualized basis, you would expect to find expenditures supporting individualized needs assessment, times for orientation, staffing ratios permitting "at-work" learning experiences, and materials or funds for rental of materials for learning activity. If no such expenditures are approved, it is clear that this objective has a low priority or that there has been little examination of the fit between objective and budget.

Another possible value in having budget process information available to you is that once you understand the process, you will have a greater possibility of effectively influencing it. Suppose that the preparation of the budget is not something in which the nursing staff is involved, perhaps not even the head nurse (or equivalent) is involved, how can you get information about the process? There is no guarantee that you can, but if you are to learn as much as possible, you must ask questions. You should start with the person in charge of your unit or division. If you find that the head nurse or supervisor is unable to supply the information you seek, you should feel free to proceed to other levels in the nursing service. Questions like those listed in Table 12.3 should gain much useful information.

TABLE 12.3 Useful Questions on Budget Formation

Would you please describe the process by which the agency budget is developed?

In what way do different level of nursing personnel participate in budget process?

What are the factors that cause difficulty for nursing either in the preparation of the budget or in the approval process?

Information such as that shown in Table 12.2 can be very helpful to you in attempting to identify how and at what time requests for additional funds or for funds for proposed activities will be best received and in what terms they are best described to get fullest consideration. There is no reason to assume that such requests should be generated only by head nurses or assistant directors. As a professional nurse, you have knowledge of the needs of your patients and of what equipment and assistance you need to provide for those needs. Therefore you also need some knowledge of how you can effectively influence the process that supplies funds.

If you decide to become better acquainted with facts about budget in your agency, you may well discover that the nursing department is viewed as a drain on resources. This is because the nursing service generally accounts for the majority of personnel employed. Furthermore, there is usually no income credited to the department. Now it is obvious that nursing does provide a service that the patient (or his insurance) is purchasing. Why, then, is the nursing service not considered an income-producing department? The answer is not clear. Probably the strength of tradition influences the accounting system; that is, nurses *give* service, not sell it. Another possible reason is that, until recently, few nurses aside from some visionary nurse executives, have pushed for a change in the system. The status quo seemed satisfactory because it does not demand the greater professional accountability that separate visible charges would require. But, this is changing as the number of professionally oriented nurses increases.

Individual Planning

The most important type of planning ability, from you perspective as a professional nurse, is that of making individual plans for your own activity. Without that, your days become reaction and routine. As manager and managed, you have a responsiblity to initiate and implement plans in several ways.

Daily Planning

The most basic plan is the daily plan. It is tempting to simply "make it" through a day, and certainly now and then even the best organized person does just that. But to accept that mode is certainly less than is expected of a true professional.

The first concern in making a daily work plan is to estimate the amount of time that will be devoted to the day's work. You should include preparation time and finish-up time as well as the actual "contact" time. The time estimate can then be related to the objective, in this case, what is to be accomplished during that day. A list, which is the result of your "choice of action and sequence of actions" phases of planning, is your starting point. Suppose you have a list of 14 items you want to accomplish by the end of the day. This list will reflect goals you set for yourself, your assignment for the day, and any plans of the unit or agency of which you are a part. A sample list for a nurse assigned to a hospital medical-surgical unit as staff nurse might contain the list of activities as shown in Fig. 12.3

---

1. Make a.m. rounds
2. Update care plans for Smith, 201; Riley, 202; Green, 204a
3. Initial assessment on expected admissions 210, 212
4. Complete care for Green in 204a
5. Prepare final notes for class for day after tomorrow
6. Supervise Colson, L.V.N. giving meds
7. Make assignment sheets for this shift
8. Chart early a.m., noon, and close of shift for patients 200- 210
9. Talk with Dr. Adams re: teaching plan for J. Olson, 205
10. Call Public Health Nurse, referral Carson, 208
11. Make complete rounds at least twoce more
12. Prepare tape recorded end-of-shift report.
13. Respond to patient needs/requests as needed.
14. Supervise Mrs. Keynes, N.A. during at least one a.m. care period.

FIGURE 12.3   Sample of Today's List.

It is important to recognize that in daily planning, as in other activities, you are not entirely independent of plans made by others. Also, in most nursing positions, there is the ever-present possibility that emergencies or other nonplanned events will occur. Bearing these possibilities in mind, you can develop a time plan for the day's activities. A chart similar to the one in Fig. 12.4 may be a useful tool until you become accustomed to organizing your time. Assume that you allot 10.5 hours to professional work activity on the particular day for which the list in Fig 12.3 was made. Notice that this plan (Fig. 12.4) allots time to activities in segments of 15 or more minutes. This is done recognizing the fact that this may be an over-estimate that will leave some slack time. Slack time is useful since the "respond to needs" category can easily expand when a patient's condition changes or when crises arise. There is also sufficient open time to include a meal break and to plan adequate communication about all activities.

The time-line chart will probably become unneccessary as you gain skill in estimating what you can accomplish in a day, but list making is a practice that will continue to be helpful. Most busy people find it very helpful to have a reminder of the elements of the day's plan. There is a certain satisfaction in crossing off items as they are completed. It is very important to remember that the work-related plan should be complemented by an effort to do something purely for personal enjoyment each day. Hopefully, you will find that you can remember to take time for yourself without a plan to do so. If you find that you can not recall "having a good time" or doing something non work-related purely for your own enjoyment lately, perhaps you need to plan for that!

A simple technique that is quite effective in relation to your plan is the "follow-up file". In reality, the file may be a notebook, a series of labeled folders, or a calendar with writing space by each date. The choice of collection method will depend on the number of items you will need to follow up on. The idea is that when you have an issue to which you expect a response, or an activity begun that requires further action at a later time, or several plans operating simultaneously, you will write a brief note to remind you when to deal with each item. This method allows you to parcel these activities evenly over a number of days, rather than greeting each day with a continuing stack of "things to do." The same principle can be applied to the ongoing update of your daily plan. For example, when you visit Mr. Burton at 7:30 a.m., you find that he mentions a desire to learn to care for his leg cast. Since you had not anticipated this readiness, you have several other things to do at the moment. You check your plan and see that you have some "slack" built in at 1:45 p.m. Therefore, you make a follow-up note and assure Mr. Burton that you will be back to spend 20 minutes with him then.

The same principle applies to following up on any sort of plan. You may have a file each month when you are dealing with several long-range plans. You may use a file for each day to keep up with a series of ongoing daily plans. The point is that even the best memory is unreliable at times, and a systematic method for keeping abreast of activities is needed.

Perhaps your agency uses some form of assignment sheet for personnel. This is quite common in hospitals and nursing homes. Two types that may be used are shown in Figs. 12.5 and 12.6. The first example, Fig. 12.5, lists all patients and indicates the various elements of care for each. The professional nurse responsible for the group of patients usually completes and/or reviews the sheet and notes on it the name of the individual assigned to care for the various patients. There is usually some space for indicating other assigned duties for each person.

The second form, Fig. 12.6, is an individual sheet for each of the personnel who are working with the patients. It may be used to list patients and elements of care as well as other activities for which the person is responsible. Ideally the source of information for this assignment aid is the plan of care for the patient. But in many cases the care plan is either inadequate, nonexistent, or kept in a holder from which it is not to be removed. It is for that reason that a secondary source of specific up-to-date information, some sort of assignment sheet, is used each day for each shift. From a logical point of view, this may seem wasteful of time and effort. However, in many agencies, this is still the practice, especially when the level of educational preparation of the nursing staff varies.

The use of the "individual worker" sheets also has the advantage of giving each person her own copy of the details of the assignment and a place to record activities and responses. This may pose a difficulty for the nurse responsible for the group of patients if she is accustomed to a form such as in Fig. 12.5, which serves as a summary of activities and observations. Such a summary can be combined with a routine of hourly "mark offs" to provide a current quick overview of the progress of the care of the total group of patients. Notice that this example (Fig. 12.5) includes a section for care planning and teaching to be noted. It is rare to find such notations on forms of this type.

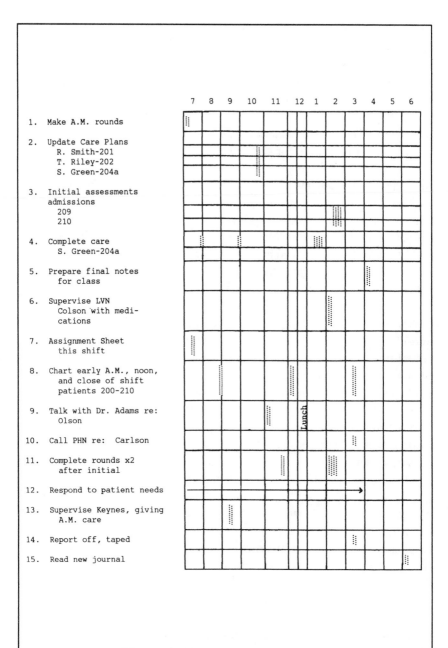

Figure 12.4 Sample Time-Line Chart

Nurse	Room	Patient	Vital Signs	Bath	Postop Exercise—Turning	Treatments	Elim.	I&O F.F.	Activity	Meals Assist	Observations	Care Planning or Teaching	Comments
E	301a	Ms. Albert	7 12	Complete	T-q 2h 8-10-12-2	P.T. @ 9	Check for impaction		In chair 30 min.	Assist	Check for pressure areas	McD - update	Encourage self-hygienic measures
E	301b	Ms. Bailey											
E	302	Mr. Carson											
McD	303	Ms. Allen											
E	304a	Mr. Jackson											
E	304b	Mr. Halston											
E	305	Admission 1 o'clock											
C	306a	Ms. Powell											
C	306b	Ms. Denton											
C	307	Ms. Hladek											
C	308	Vacant											
C	309	*Complete Isolation* Mr. Banks											
C	310	Ms. Williams											

Lunch 11:30 ———— 12:00 ———— 12:30 ————

Figure 12.5 Assignment Summary

Name_____   Interregional General Hospital   Date_____

Room/Patient	Bath	Ambulate	Meals	Elimination	I & O	Vital Signs	Postop Exercises	Special Treatments	Notes
307 Ms. Aleorn	Self	Ad lib	Reg. self		–	8	–	Soak rt hand 15 min 10 and 2	Observe hand lesion for amt. redness

Figure 12.6 Individual Assignment

Where primary nursing is the method for organizing, the need for aids such as these is eliminated since each nurse should be prepared to do her own planning and can do so directly from the patient's chart or care plan. A similar situation exists in community health agencies. The use of secondary information sources, outlining data in primary records, increases as the level of preparation of staff decreases.

Making assignments is a form of planning for individuals. From your perspective as planner it is a series of interlocking activities that requires careful consideration of the available resources in determining courses of action. In this case, the human resources are the important concern. The information about the job description, educational preparation, and personal characteristics of the personnel are entered in to your planning as key elements. You ask yourself such questions as: Who is *qualified* to care for the patient who requires teaching before surgery? Who *prefers* to care for elderly persons? Are there union contract elements that prescribe type and amount of assigned activities? Other important concerns relate to the usual activities on the unit or in the assigned area. For example: Do personnel usually assist one another? Are assignments usually grouped geographically? Are there norms regarding what makes "equal" assignments?

The answers to these questions are related to the knowledge you have about the objectives of care for the day and the routine activities that must be performed in order for you to choose a series of actions. These actions are, of course, the day's assignments. This sounds like a very complicated explanation of what looks rather routine-making assignments for a day's work. However, the difference between a simply routine act of filling in spaces on a sheet and making a useful plan is the thought that goes into it. That is where the planning process becomes a useful tool.

A technique that has useful results is for the professional nurse to write her assignment along with those of other personnel, even after the need for time-line charts is long past. Why? When there are other nursing personnel for whom you are responsible, it is very easy for their perspective of your functions to be quite different from yours. If you doubt that, go to a clinical unit and ask a nursing assistant or practical nurse to tell you what a professional nurse does that is different from what she does. Typically, the response is, "She can give some medications that I am not allowed to, pass tubes for patients, and be in charge." If you probe for more information, like what does "be in charge" mean, you may be surprised to know that this means "take doctor's orders, sign requests, and check on things." Hopefully, this is a limited view of what professional nurses actually do. But the only way to change that perception of others is to have them see that you have specific plans for you actions, just as they do. It is doubly important that you take the opportunity to make your plan *visible* as a written assignment or list since many of the most important activities you perform are not, in themselves, visible. For example, the preparation for teaching a patient or family may involve a period of *thinking* (not visible, except as staring into space), or some time reading, writing, and assembling materials.

Participating in Management by Objectives (MBO)

In addition to daily planning, you may be making plans for some extended period. Six months or a year is long enough to accomplish some major project yet still provide feedback for reimbursement. Using the process outlined earlier, you can develop a plan that will help you move toward objectives that pertain to long-range plans.

A management technique called *management by objectives* (MBO) has been used to provide structure for this type of planning. Its techniques make it possible to incorporate the unique plan of the individual into the performance evaluation. MBO was originally developed to encourage improved performance among managers. Its originator, Peter Drucker, was directing his suggestions to business and industry when he devised this method.[7] He proposed that each manager should be expected to set objectives for his performance in managing his section, store, or division, within company goals. The goals were to be discussed with his organizational superiors. When agreement was reached, the subsequent responsibility for accomplishment was the manager's. The underlying principle is that participation in developing one's own goals encourages investment in them. Also, evaluation based on these goals is expected to be meaningful and provide a reinforcing feeling of accomplishment.

While Drucker was not focusing on health care in recommending MBO, variations on his method have been applied with a relatively high degree of popularity in some nursing services. The expected value of the use of the method is based primarily on the expectation that the condition described above (investment and reinforcement) will result, viewing the nurse as the equivalent of the manager. Effective use of MBO requires that both the manager and the managed participate. The manager will probably need to interpret the goals of those at other levels in the organization, so that the objective developed will be consistent with and contribute to the overall goals for the agency. She may need to teach the "managed" how to state goals clearly. She may also need to provide some supervisory counseling in order that the nurse with whom she works can develop realistic

7 Peter Drucker,*The Practice of Management*(New York & Row,1954),pp.121-136.

objectives that are possible to accomplish during the evaluation period. The technique for MBO could well proceed as shown in Table 12.4.

TABLE 12.4 MBO Procedures

Supervisor notifies professional nurse of the intent to use MBO.

Supervisor solicits feedback from nurse regarding the concept.

Supervisor furnishes more information, both in discussion and as handout material on MBO.

Further discussion is held to clarify the procedure and the purpose. Nursing service goals and supervision objectives are discussed.

Nurse prepares objectives and time limits for each.

Nurse and supervisor discuss the objectives and alternative methods for meeting them. They also identify any objectives that may be unrealistic and possible additional areas for objectives.

Nurse pursues activities to meet objectives during the set time period.

Supervisor provides intermittent feedback on positive movement toward objectives (based on earlier discussion of objectives).

Review session is held at six months or one year (as determined previously) to discuss accomplishments and plan for new objectives.

What are the primary problems with MBO? More importantly, why may you find that it is *not* used in the agency where you work? Probably the most direct answer is that this technique takes time. It requires that both supervisee and supervisor spend time developing, discussing, and evaluating the goals. Another problem frequently encountered is lack of administrative support. Although MBO can be used at any level, it works best when modeling of the activity occurs at each successive managerial level. In addition, administrative support may well mean the difference in whether the objective can be related to the performance appraisal and to organizational rewards. Consider how much more important a series of self-generated goals could be if their accomplishment were related to merit salary increases or to promotion. Attempts to relate incentives to the objectives of MBO prove difficult when personnnel are represented by collective bargaining agents or by a highly structured personnel system. Such a system tends to focus on very explicit, objective standards being applied to the placement of personnel on salary and rank schedules. This was not problematic for the original MBO scheme since managers were its target population.

But, by definition, managers are not represented by collective bargaining agents.

Perhaps you can see from this discussion that, at the very least, there is a useful kernel in the MBO technique. If your agency or supervisor does not make use of formal MBO, you might still wish to initiate your own long-range planning and discuss the plan with your supervisor. Speculate about the possible outcomes! Or you might instigate some similar activity on a limited basis among those for whose work you are responsible. If you do make this attempt, be prepared for a period of adjustment as well as the possibility that there may be some staff who will not participate voluntarily. Earlier material on motivation (Chapter 1) may help you to understand the reasons for this lack of cooperation if it occurs.

Group Planning

Many of the situations in which you will work as a professional nurse will cause you to be responsible for making plans for groups or for seeing that plans for a group are generated. Managing that sort of responsibility requires an understanding of the behavior of individuals in groups as well as some techniques for moving groups to accomplish tasks. The content in Chapter 9 describes useful information about relationships in groups.

Therefore, the following material focuses on some practical concerns relevant to you both as a person responsible for a group's planning and as a member in groups for which you do not bear sole responsibility.

Conferences-A Method for Group Planning Activities.

"Let's all go to the treatment room, we're going to have a conference." This statement, frequently made by an RN, with the best of intentions, is just as frequently met with sighs, eyes rolled heavenward, and other less than enthusiastic gestures by personnel. There are a number of reasons why this potentially useful activity is not a favorite for many health care workers. Several of these reasons are:

1.Conferences take time away from the "important" work.
2.Conferences are a ritual; nothing real is accomplished.
3.People are expected to contribute, but they are not educationally prepared to do so.

4.People are expected to contribute, but they are not emotionally prepared to do so.

5.There is no reward for holding or participating in conferences.

These statements address the problem of resistance to conferences in general, since many persons make no distinctions among the various types of group meetings.

There are a number of reasons for assembling a group of nursing personnel or an interdisciplinary group of health care providers. For example, conferences can be categorized according to general purpose as follows:

1.Providing information, educational activities.

2.Developing group plans, making decisions.

3.Business meeting of a group, conducted to manage the ongoing activity of an organized group.

4.Team development.

5.Combination of two or more of the above purposes.

As the purpose of the group meeting varies, so also may the techniques necessary to produce a successful meeting. So the list of objections to conferences may be more pertinent to some types of conferences than others. Using conferences for purposes other than planning or group decision making was discussed in Chapter 9. The following paragraphs focus on techniques that can be used in group planning and decision making and that may overcome the objections listed earlier.

Preparing for the Conference

An important decision that you, as a professional nurse, will make is *whether* a conference should be held to involve a group in planning. The notion that a conference should be held simply in order to say it has been held probably accounts for the charge that "conferences are a ritual." Since the advent of team nursing, literature on team leading and leadership and management in nursing has emphasized the team planning conferences as a key element in success in organized nursing services. However, little evidence supports the assertion that daily conferences are a "must." In fact, when conferences are conducted ineptly, the usual result is a break in the regular series of nursing care activities, probably accounting for the "conferences take time away from the important work" objection. This is not intended to discourage you from using conferences. Definitely not. Rather, it is intended as a warning that when group conferences are used, the conditions as listed in Table 12.5 should be observed.

TABLE 12.5 Conditions for Using a Group Conference

1. There should be identifiable potential benefit from group involvement in the planning effort. There is nothing quite so destructive to group morale as the negative reaction that results from pseudo-participation. This type of reaction is likely to occur when the plans developed by a group are not used, either because they are of poor quality or are incomplete. A negative reaction may also occur when the actual intent of the conference is other than announced. For example, when the conference is announced as a care-planning conference but is used only as a time for transmitting information from administration, participants quickly realize that their unput is not desired.

It is almost certain that all nursing or health care personnel who are familiar with a patient can contribute information useful in planning. This is because each will have information about the patient or about possible approaches to care gained from his or her own perspective. Therefore, the condition for potential benefit from group involvement is usually met in health care setting.

The potential benefit should be weighed against the time and effort required to hold the conference. If you, acting alone as the professional responsible for nursing care, can develop a nursing care plan that will result in high-quality care and you have other means for involving personnel for motivation purposes, perhaps you should limit the number of care planning conferences to an absolute minimum. The time spent in planning might be better used for team development activity or for educational conferences.

2. It should be feasible for the group to develop the plan (or make the decision) with the information and skills available to it. If you ask a group to develop a plan of care, it is important that you recognize what each member is able to contribute so that individuals are not placed in the position of being expected to perform in ways or at knowledge levels for which they are not equipped. For example, a person with little experience as a home health aid should not be asked questions regarding which technique is best for home colostomy irrigation. However, this person might well provide competent information about which family member is most interested in learning to assist the patient. This will obviate the "lack of education" complaint mentioned above.

As a professional educated in techniques of planning and decision making, it is likely that one of your main contributions will be to assure that the plan or decision is arrived at through a sound process. You will model the sort of questioning and other structuring activities needed to ensure the quality of the planning or decision-making process. As you do this, you can expect that it may serve as a learning experience for other group members. This, along with other staff development activities, can contribute to the development of a cohesive, competent group. It will also be your responsibility, whether group leader or participant, to contribute factual information regarding health, disease states, and nursing techniques. This information should be from a continuously growing knowledge base that you assemble through your own professional continuing education activities.

3. Participants in planning or decision-making activities should receive feedback on the implementation of the plan or the outcome of the decision. This condition is designed to provide some of the reward element so often lacking in conference participation. If participation in group planning is viewed as a basic part of each worker's responsibility rather than as an "if there is time" addition, then competent participation can become relevant in the performance appraisal.

Providing feedback may also prove to be a motivator for those individuals for whom job enrichment is important.

4. If you are the person responsible for deciding whether and/or when to hold a planning conference, you should hold the conference only after(a) you are convinced that the conference will have one or more of the benefits mentioned above, and (b) you have prepared to provide the structure, content, and continuity necessary for a successful group conference. The confidence and enthusiasm you will feel then this condition is met will help set the emotional tone important to encouraging the group.

Certainly, as you read, you will note that much of what is stated about planning conferences holds true for other types of group meetings. Keep these ideas in mind as you consider conferences held for other purposes.

When the decision has been made that a conference for planning or decision making will be held, the person responsible for conducting it must make preparation. Some of the simpler elements of preparation involve place and time. Choose a room that provides seating for all attending. It is difficult to promote group discussion when some people are seated on windowsills, others are standing, and still others are in comfortable chairs. It may be no small chore to arrange for such a meeting place. This is especially problematic if you are working in a hospital where space is frequently at a premium. The space for the conference should be private so that the meeting can proceed without interruption from other personnel, patients, or visitors.

The time chosen should be at other than peak hours. In a hospital, this may mean choosing a time when most patients are having visitors or are sleeping. You may find it useful to set a regular "meeting time" on certain days of the week. The period can then be used for any necessary group meetings, not just those for planning. The advantage of this sort of arrangement is that the meeting period is then viewed as a regularly scheduled activity, not one that occurs only "when there's time." The length of time for a conference will depend on the purpose, frequency, and pressure of other required activities. For example, a group that has interdisciplinary staff conferences for planning care and meets once every two weeks may need an hour or longer to do its work; whereas a group of nursing personnel working on a hospital unit, meeting twice weekly, may only need 30 minutes to develop care plans for three patients. The important point is to decide on the length of time needed and notify the group at the beginning of the meeting. As the group becomes familiar with its work and functions with open communication, as either leader or participant you may find it productive to ask the group to set its own time limits. This is but one of several sorts of "group function" decisions that the group should be able to assume as it becomes less leader-centered in its activities. (See Chapter 9 for discussion of changing group relationships.)

When you are a group leader, you will find it useful to have "walked through" the conference in your mind. The purpose is to identify the way in which you will structure the conference, the information people will need in order to participate, the preparation that you might request from various group members, behavior you desire and/or expect from individuals (recognizing that each has a different level of entering ability and experience), and how you will respond to any resistance or lack of participation. As you do this thinking, keep in mind that you have two purposes: (1) accomplishing the task set for the meeting and (2) helping the group do so in an efficient and effective fashion. When you identify preparation or contribution needed from individuals, take the time prior to the conference to speak directly to the person concerning the request, indicating why the contribution is important. Again, it is important to keep in mind the individual differences mentioned earlier. Providing opportunities for group members to participate successfully requires beginning where the person's present ability allows him to function.

The time, location, and purpose of the conference should also be announced to the group by some written and/or verbal means. A note can be posted on a unit bulletin board (if anyone ever looks at it), individual assignment sheets can have a notice written on them, or other similar means can be used. When the conference is an interdisciplinary group meeting with members who have office or work space away from your unit or clinic, it is useful to send a memorandum and/or contact the person by telephone at least one day before the meeting. This simple bit of advance activity can make the difference between a successful meeting or no meeting at all.

As you are mentally rehearsing the conference, the structure of the meeting is an important concern. Specifically, you should consider the suggestions for conducting the conference as listed in Table 12.6.

When you have prepared for and mentally rehearsed the conference, you will be well on the way to success. If you still find yourself a bit shaky, you could ask a couple of friends to role-play the situation. This gives you an opportunity to get feedback on your tactics in a relatively low-threat situation.

Tools for Planning

A new professional nurse can adapt to personal time management/planning activities with relatively little equipment or formal techniques other than the simple forms, lists, and follow up files discussed earlier. But, as you become a more experienced member of the nursing profession and begin to participate in larger scale planning, additional tools and techniques will assist. The next section gives a brief review of some of these aids to planning which you may encounter or may seek to improve your skills in planning.

TABLE 12.6   Conducting a Conference

1. *Setting the right mood at the beginning of the conference.* The leader sets the pace and the mood by beginning with a statement of what is to be accomplished in terms that are as clear and specific as possible. For example: "We are going to use the next 30 minutes to develop a plan of care for Mrs. Smith. When we finish, we should have agreement on the method we will be using to give her care. I have talked with the patient about some goals for her care, and after we are through, I will tell her about our plans. If she has no objections, we will proceed with the plan as we have developed it."

I feel compelled to state that my personal belief is that the professional nurse should work directly with the patient or family to develop the plan for nursing care, that other levels of nursing personnel should be involved in collection of information to update the plan, and that collaboration in conferences for planning should be for interdisciplinary coordination. I recognize, however, that many agencies/nursing services will expect you to function according to the prescription of team nursing. Since you must first succeed in an agency before you can help to change its practice, the items in this table allude to care planning with group participation as well as other planning. The principles are the same for group planning and group conferences, no matter what the purpose.

A chalkboard or newprint pad can be used to write key phrases throughout the meeting. This serves to focus thought on the topic at hand as well as to record the decisions that are made.

Your manner as leader can influence the group. If you are relaxed but businesslike rather than anxious and distracted, the group is more likely to respond favorably to your leadership.

2. *Moving the conference to complete its task.* Your concern with encouraging participation and reducing irrelevant conversation will be a model for the group. When talk seems to be straying toward the trivial, a series of statements can be used to help move everyone back to the work at hand. The first "off-track" comment by an individual can usually be ignored. Make no remark, no nod of the head, no response at all. (This is a hard thing to do, especially when much that you have learned about listening to patients requires either verbal or nonverbal responses to their utterances.) Usually, ignoring the remark is sufficient to return the individual's attention to the mainstream. When a second unrelated comment comes from that same individual, you can ask, "How does that relate to what Mr. B just said? I'm not sure I understand." Perhaps, to her there is a connection between her idea and the main discussion. If so, she can explain. If not, you can smile as you say, "Since we have limited time, it is important to stay on the main point." This last comment or something similar can be used if there is continuing distraction. If there is one person who continues this behavior, you can speak to her privately after the conference about ways in which she can make a better contribution, indicating why her behavior is unacceptable and the consequences of continuing it.

When you are a new group leader, it is easy to feel somewhat affronted by persons who "don't play the game," and therefore it may take extra effort to avoid being defensive until you feel confident with the group.

Questions and continuity statements will also help lead the group through the planning process. For example, "Now, what activities could we use to accomplish this goal?" Or, "So, now we have some ideas about things we can do to meet our objectives." Or, "Number one. Let's talk about a timetable for doing them and who will do what." The steps in planning discussed earlier furnish the cues for these structuring statements.

Suggesting amounts of time to allot to various elements of the group's task is helpful if there is a tendency to bog down on some phase. As the group works together more, you may want to request that it consider if scheduling of time is needed. If it is agreed that such action is necessary, then you might well ask the group to suggest the time periods.

Finally, liberal praise for useful participation and feedback on results are useful in encouraging continued participation.

3. *Bringing the conference to a successful conclusion.* Many a good conference ends with a fizzle, not a bang, because the group leader fails to bring closure. A sense of having completed something

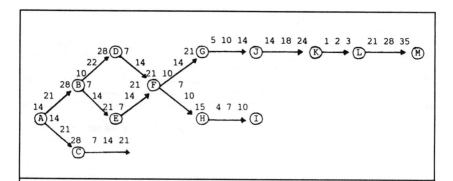

Event Symbol	Event
A	Plan begins.
B	Analysis of present methods completed with identification of problems
C	Completed review of literature.
D	Consultation completed-other hospitals
E	Consultation completed-Communicable Disease Center.
F	First draft of procedure revision.
G	Complete pilot test of new procedures.
H	Data collected on effects of procedures on other departments.
I	Review of procedure completed by other departments.
J	Final adjustments of new procedures completed.
K	New procedure reviewed with all nursing personnel for implementation.
L	New procedure implemented.
M	Period of supervision of initial implementation is completed.

FIGURE 12.7 Simplified PERT Network. The circled letters represent the completed activities or events described in the accompanying table. The arrows flow from left to right and indicate the action required to complete an event. The three numbers accompanying each arrow represent, in this order, the most optimistic time, the most likely time, and the longest time alloted for completion of the action.

is very important, especially when group members place high value on their time. To finish the conference, begin winding up with a comment like, "It's five minutes until our stopping time; let's finish on this part of the plan and then summarize." Then in a couple of minutes, "Now, let's summarize the decisions we've made and the assignments for next time." After you or a group member summarizes, you can then ask, "Did I cover the main points or are there other things we need to add?" This summary can serve as a meeting record if it is recorded when the meeting is going on, is used for the closing remarks, and then is corrected and signed by the person who did the recording. Of course, it is not necessary that all meetings be formally recorded unless there is to be some use made of the record.

As the group becomes well-acquainted and is ready to move to less leader-centered functioning, you can begin to help the group evaluate its process of action at the end of the meeting. The concern should be first with having the group identify how it should be functioning. Certainly you may make recommendations, but there should be *group* attention to aspects such as quantity and quality of participation, ways in which decisions are reached, consideration of others, and quality of decisions. When there are statements developed regarding how the group wishes to function, there can then be a brief evaluation of this at the end of the meeting. One group member (a different person each time) can be requested before each meeting to observe and comment on the process. An alternate method is to have the topic of evaluation be a point of discussion for the entire group. This is not particularly fruitful if done *each* meeting, but it is useful as an intermittent feature of the conference.

PERT

The acronym PERT represents Program Evaluation Review Technique, a method for phasing and sequencing actions chosen in a plan. The technique was developed by Navy researchers in 1958 at about the same time that DuPont scientists developed the Critical Path Method, a very similar technique. The visible result of PERT is a network, a graphic representation of the events and activities that are planned. The PERT chart typically contains a series of circles and arrows. It may also contain a series of three numbers along each arrow representing time elements. The network in Fig. 12.7 is an example of a PERT chart that describes the plan to develop an improved isolation procedure for a medical unit.

Notice that the chart in Fig. 12.7 reads from left to right, showing events or completed activities in the circles. The arrows represent the activity necessary to produce the event. The numbers along the arrows are three estimates of the time needed to complete the activity. The first is the optimistic time, the least possible time required. The second is the most likely time, and the third the pessimistic estimate or the longest time allotted. In many cases, these estimates are arrived at arbitrarily, by guess. In other situations, past experience will provide the basis for sound estimates.

Sarah Archer describes a method for arriving at a time estimate for completion of an activity that takes into account the three usual estimates and weighs them according to the probability of their occurrence.[8] The formula is:

$$Te = \frac{(O+4m+p)}{6}$$

Te is time estimate, *O* is the optimistic time, *m* is the most likely time, and *p* is the pessimistic estimate. Using this formula, the weight of the most likely time is greatest, but the two extreme estimates also influence the result. When several arrows exit from a particular event, this indicates that several activities can be accomplished simultaneously, with no one activity prerequisite to the others being completed at the same time. IN Fig. 12.7, event interval *A - B* has an optimistic estimate of 14 days, 21 days the most likely, and 28 days the pessimistic estimate. Using Archer's method, the *time estimate* for this event is:

$$Te = \frac{14+4(21)+28}{6} = \frac{126}{6} = 21 \text{ days}$$

This is a case where the *Te* is the same as the optimistic estimate. However, this is not always the case. Consider event interval *G - J*, where

$$Te = \frac{5+4(10)+14}{6} = \frac{59}{6} = 9.8 \text{ days}$$

There is no one right way to develop such a chart. If the chart is extensive, events may best be identified by numbers rather than by letters. You may find it useful to include descriptions of the activity along an event path in addition to the completed event. The key is to include the information that will make the network display useful as a reinforcement and evaluation device.

8 Sarah E. Archer,"P.E.R.T.: A Tool for Nurse Administrators,"*Journal of Nursing Administration (September-October 1974),p.18.*

The path through the longest series of activities is often called the *critical path*. It identifies the series of steps that will define the length of the project. The critical path through the procedure development leads from events *A - B - C - D - E - F - G - J - K - L - M. The resulting time, using any of the series* of estimates-optimistic, most likely, or pessimistic-is the time required to complete the project.

The PERT method can be used to display simply the series of activities already identified in a planning process, or the development of the chart can parallel the decisions regarding activities. In this latter method, the planners can begin with the last event and work backward, identifying each preceding event in a logical process. Using the PERT method can thus serve as either a stimulus for, or a reinforcement of, the activity sequencing phase of a planning process. When you are using PERT in planning with a group, there are some important points to recall (see Table 12.7).

When the chart has been developed, it can then serve as a guide for evaluation. As events are completed, the chart can be used to provide a visual summary of accomplishment. The actual time can be compared to estimated time. Some advantages of the use of this technique mentioned by Koontz and Weirich are: (1) it forces one to plan and to plan "down the line," (2) it concentrates attention on the critical elements of a project, and (3) it facilitates contact.[9]

At the same time, there are some disadvantages noted by those authors. For example, PERT is difficult to use when the project is a nebulous one. Also, a major fault is that the technique does not deal with costs.[10] It is, however, quite useful, especially when helping a group to plan. You can certainly make use of this tool as a leader and may well suggest it when you are group participant.

TABLE 12.7 Important Points to Remember in Using PERT with a Group

---

1. Orient the group to the use of the chart, explaining it as a visual display of the thinking the group will do.
2. Use material that can be erased and/or disposed of inexpensively when the group is still considering possibilities.
3. Transfer the final network to a more permanent form for continuing use during implementation.
4. Use the network development *only* as an adjunct to the planning process; making a chart does not necessarily mean that deliberative planning has been done.

---

9 Koontz and Weirich,*Management*,pp.574-577.
10 Ibid.,pp.576-577.

Computers

The development of the microcomputer and its widespread availability at relatively low cost has affected us all in countless ways. From entertaining games to learning tutorials, from pre-school to advanced education and from merchandising to space exploration, the computer is our current version of pen, pencil, and slide rule. As a new professional nurse, it is likely that you have used computers in your education, for word processing, for tutorials, and for simulation. You may even have been fortunate enough to have used computers for clinical record keeping and data analysis. Since you are probably "Computer-Friendly", the use of computers as an aid to planning will be natural to you. Without ever needing to learn programming, you can use applications software, which uses English language commands and which prompts the user through the required input (menu-driven). Following are brief descriptions of three types of software which can aid in planning. Proprietary names are not mentioned since any list becomes rapidly obsolete. A visit to a local software vendor or a consultation with a nearby university will bring you up-to-date choices.

Database Programs

Database programs are the computer analogy of an excellent cross indexed file cabinet. Unlike a file cabinet, however, the database can also manipulate the information in the files, given the commands to develop specified reports. Therefore, if staff data on absences have been "filed" in the database, with certain information noted in each file, such as type of absence, length of absence, next day off, age of nurses, number of children - etc, the database program can "go through the file folders" and develop a report to answer the questions you might need answered. For example, suppose a benefits committee is planning a proposal related to on-site child care. This database could report on the number of absences related to nurses with children ages 0 -12 years.

The program does not do anything a human could not. But, the fact that the database is kept, is orderly, and is readily retrievable for reports make it possible to have information for planning which would likely be unavailable if we were to depend on human effort.

Spreadsheets

A spreadsheet is a way of displaying a series of figures and the relationships to one another so that the results of changes in one element can be seen across all other elements simultaneously. This is a technique that has long been used (manually) in accounting. But, computerizing the calculations and automatically updating the displayed material make asking "what if" an easily answerable question. Such a program can be made to identify the progressive costs of changes in salaries, the estimates of required personnel related to changes in patient acuity, or any number of types of information which are relevant in planning in nursing. These are particularly useful in budgeting and related analysis. The calculations can be performed automatically by the program as long as the user can input the relationship among the elements in each segment of the spreadsheet. Knowledge of simple algebraic statements is the basic requirement for use of most of these commercially available packages.

Modified PERT

The value of a project planning device that supplies a graphic as well as verbal display of project steps was discussed earlier in the section on PERT. Computer based project planning packages can now prompt a user to input the steps in a plan and can then produce the graphics including calculated time estimates. While the software does not perform the planning, it does prompt the systematic thinking, automate calculations, and produce a well organized display. Several such project planning packages are available.

SUMMARY

This chapter has presented planning as a process which is important at the individual and at the organizational level. Individual planning emphasized efficient use of time through use of planning aids such as forms and lists. Organizational plans considered included strategic plans and budgets.

Used to its optimum, the budget can serve as a unique sort of plan. For a beginning professional nurse, involvement with its development can provide a challenge. Other aspects of planning for groups included a systematic approach and the use of such techniques as PERT and planning conferences.

Additional Reading

American Nurses' Association,*DRGs and Nursing Care*,Kansas City, Mo:American Nurses' Association,1985.

Bell, Mary L.,"Management by Objectives",*Journal of Nursing Administration* (May,1980)19-26.

Brewer, Carol,"Variable Billing: Is it Viable?",*Nursing Outlook*,32:1(Jan./Feb.,1984)38-41.

Cerne, F.,"External Data Can Improve Strategic Planning",*Hospitals*,62 No.8(April 20,1988)p.85-86.

Charns, Martin and M.J. Schaefer,*Health Care Organization, A Model for Management*,Englewood Cliffs,N.J.:Prentice-Hall,Inc. 1983,p.63-77.

Cox, Helen, B. Harsanyi, and L. Dean,*Computers and Nursing*,Norwalk,Connecticut:Appleton and Lange,1987.

Curtin, Leah,"Determining Costs of Nursing Services per DRG",*Nursing Management*14:4(April,1983)16-20.

Daubert, E.,"Strategic Planning in Home Care",*American Journal of Nursing*,87 No.9(September,1987)p.1161-1163.

Drucker,P.,*The Practice of Management*,New York:Harper & Row,1954.

Ethridge, Phyllis,"The Case for Billing by Patient Acuity ",*Nursing Management*,16:8 (August,1988)38-41.

Grimaldi, Paul L.,"Case-Mix Reimbursement for Nursing Home Patients",*Nursing Management* 17:3(March,1986)64- 66.

Odiorne, G.,*Management by Objectives*,New York:Pitman,1965.

Sovie, Margaret and Toni C. Smith,"Pricing the Nursing Product : Charging for Nursing Care"*Nursing Economics*,4:5(Sept.-Oct.,1986)216-226.

Sweeney, Mary Anne,*The Nurse's Guide to Computers*,New York:Macmillian Publishing Co.,1985.

Trofino, Joan,"A Reality Based System for Pricing Nursing Service"*Nursing Management*,17:1(January,1986)19-24.

Walker, Duane D.,"The Cost of Nursing Care in Hospitals",*Journal of Nursing Administration*,(March,1983)13-18.

Chapter 13

Organizing

As a phase in the management process, organizing might well be defined as in the dictionary, "To pull together into an orderly, functional, structured whole."[1] Stephen Robbins elaborates in the following way, "Organizing is the establishment of relationships between the activities to be performed, the personnel to perform them, and the physical factors that are needed."[2] You, as a manager of nursing care, may wonder just how you can establish such relationships when you have relatively little discretionary power in the organization. Perhaps you wonder if you can actually organize anything, given your position. Possibly you think organizing is a function of administrative positions only. Actually, given the broad definition of organizing and the importance of such activity in any enterprise, it is extremely important that you, as both manager and managed, share an understanding of and responsibility for elements of organizing. This section describes various levels of organizing activity in a nursing service and suggests techniques for your participation in a number of these activities.

Organizing at the Agency Level

Even if you have never directed much thought to the topic, you are probably aware that the various organizations of which you are a part differ in their structure and in the ways in which responsibility and relationships are defined. The League of Women Voters, the Church of which you are a member, the Civil Air Patrol, and the City Hospital in which you work may

1 *The American Heritage Dictionary of English Language* (Boston: Houghton-Mifflin, 1976), p. 926.
2 Stephen T. Robbins, *The Administrative Process* (Englewood Cliffs, N.J.: Prentice-Hall, 1976), p. 17.

all be organizations in which you participate. Yet each of these is organized differently, and your behavior in each organization differs according to its structure and your position in it.

Organizational Chart

The overall framework or structure of an organization is commonly represented by an organizational chart. This is a graphic representation of the functional relationships among persons in the enterprise. The chart can indicate lines of responsibility, accountability, and communication. Conventionally, unbroken lines between positions represent lines of communication and authority. The relative placement of the hospital administrator at the top of the page indicates that he has the top level of responsibility and accountability for the hospital. This position carries various titles, such as chief administrative officer, administrator, president, and executive director. Successively lower positions on the chart indicate decreasing scope of responsibility. The vertical unbroken lines indicate both flow of communication and delegation of elements of responsibility and authority. However, the complete picture of relationships cannot be determined without the opportunity to read position descriptions that clarify the scope and nature of responsibility for each position.

Horizontal unbroken lines represent communication flow between positions of similar levels with separate spheres of responsibility. The positions linked by these unbroken lines are referred to as *"line positions."* The responsiblities of these individuals are the actual daily operation and long-range operation of the agency.

In contrast to line positions, there are certain positions that are called *staff positions.* These appear on the charts linked to one or more other positions by a dotted or broken line. This sort of position has primary responsibility for an advisory or consultative function or some activity other than direct operations. For example, in Fig. 13.1, the Assistant Administrator in Nursing for Special Studies serves a staff function. All reasearch studies are coordinated through her office as is the planning for demonstration projects in nursing. When a plan becomes operational and is incorporated into routine, it becomes the province of the line personnel. Until that time, the activities are an adjunct to, rather than an operational part of, the daily activity of the nursing service.

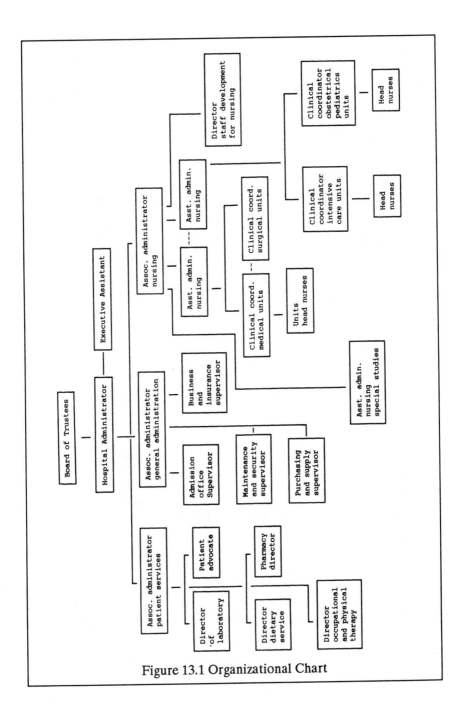

Figure 13.1 Organizational Chart

It has become popular to draw organizational charts in a variety of shapes for the purpose of demonstrating some particular concept. For example, the nursing service has been represented by a circular design with the patient in the center. Although this serves to demonstrate the concept of the centrality of the patient to the concern of all the staff, it fails to inform the viewer of the relationships among personnel defined by traditional structural chart methods.

Types of Organizational Structure

Understanding the method of describing the organization is useful only if it is clear how the method is related to the decisions about the nature of the structure itself. Decisions about what responsibilities will be combined and vested in which positions, which positions will be related in what ways, what staff functions are necessary, and what degree of autonomy various positions will have - all are the stuff of which an organizational structure is made.

A major consideration in developing an organizational structure is the type and extent of decision-making authority that will be expected (or permitted) at each level in the organization. That answer will, to some extent, predict the number of levels necessary in the organizational hierarchy. The resulting decision-making and authority/responsibility structure can be described according to the *centralization-decentralization* concept. This refers to the degree to which decisions are made at the central or top level in the organization.

You may hear a nursing organization referred to as "a centralized service" or a "decentralized unit." It is difficult to know specifically what is meant by these terms since the concept cannot be realistically dichotomized in that way. It might be more useful to think of these terms as end points on a continuum that can be called the "Locus of Decision-Making Continuum." As in Fig. 13.2, an organization or its elements can be conceived of as existing at some point on this continuum. Identifying the locus of decision making may seem to be an academic exercise. However, you may find that it becomes increasingly important to you as you become more confident of your professional ability. For example, a person who is equipped with knowledge to make decisions regarding the care of patients may be uncomfortable in a situation where the supervisor makes any and all decisions for which there are no standing hospital procedures or routines.

Extremely Decentralized (most major decisions are made at the point of implementation)	Extremely Centralized (most major decisions are made at top administrative level)

FIGURE 13.2   Locus Of Decision-Making Continuum.

Some modes of organizing to deliver nursing care are conducive to a wide latitude in professional judgement by the nurse dealing directly with the patient. Other modes of organizing depend on established routines and strong supervision to deal with decision making. These two general modes of organizing will be discussed in detail later in this chapter.

When an organization is designed to move important decisions toward the top, as size increases, the number of levels of personnel increases. Many of the levels, as a result, function mainly by supervising successive levels. When a chart is drawn to depict such an enterprise, it is shaped like a pyramid. This is frequently described as a "tall organizational structure." The form typifies the bureaucratic structure, a common one in many large organizations. This structure was formally described by Max Weber early in the 1900s as a part of his work on the sociological theory of organization.[3] This theory focused on the efficient, impersonal utilization of individuals to accomplish the work of the organization. According to Weber, the main attributes of the bureaucracy are: (1) clear job descriptions with job activities routinized and well defined, (2) clearly defined formal relationships, (3) reliance on objective impersonal treatment of personnel, and (4) a system of formal policies and procedures.

It is clear that the term *bureaucracy* presently carries a negative connotation. Possibly the reason for this is the ponderous rate at which nonroutine action can be taken. Robbins notes, however, that contrary to that belief, the bureaucracies "have proved to be the most efficient manner in which to structure certain types of complex activities."[4] Perhaps this organizational form persists because it is efficient for certain types of enterprises. Keep in mind that this description refers to the pure form of bureaucracy. That pure form would be at the extreme right of the continuum in Fig. 13.2.

The "flat organizational structure" reflects an effort to move decision making downward from the upper levels toward the point of implementation. There are few administrative levels as a result. The resulting structure

---

3 Max Weber,*The Theory of Social and Economic Organization*, trans. by A.M. Henderson and Talcott Parsons,(New York: Oxford University Press,1947)pp.329- 341.

4 Robbins,*The Administrative Process*,p.260.

is characterized as decentralized, or the end point opposite the bureaucracy on the continuum mentioned above. Advocates of the move toward this structure reason that it promotes more democratic participation, increases information flow, and decreases distortion of communication among levels. Along with these anticipated advantages, certain potential problems are recognized. These include the possibility that the ability of personnel will not be equal to the decision-making requirement and that the efforts of various units will not be coordinated.

Many decisions regarding structure seem to reflect a choice based on the alleged merits of one of the two structural forms discussed above. The general tone of much literature suggests that the flat structure is the only one that the rational person in a democratic society would choose. This is because the increased individual decision making is seen as growth-promoting for the employee, aiding in self-actualization.

Another line of reasoning is presented by Paul Lawrence and Jay Lorsch.[5] In one of the earliest expositions of what has come to be known as "contingency theories," they make the point that there is no one best way to organize. These authors claim that many of the studies that support one particular structure or another are *not* multivariate. Yet life is, in fact, highly multivariate. Therefore, study of the organizational structure should take this into account. Major areas (variables) of concern are differentiation, integration, nature of the task to be performed, individual motivation, and environment. *Differentiation* is viewed as a condition existing along a continuum, with high differentiation reflecting a large number of special functions to be served and resulting in multiple specialties operating in the organization. *Integration* is the state of collaboration that exists among departments that are required to achieve unity of effort.[6] The higher the degree of differentiation, the greater the efforts (in terms of communication , policies creating linking structures, etc.) required to accomplish integration. Neither differentiation nor integration is a specific function of organizational size., but rather of complexity.

In their work, Lawrence and Lorsch found that successful organizations were not necessarily similar in structure. Rather, success seemed to be related to how well the structure facilitated integration and differentiation.[7] These findings must be applied to the nursing service cautiously since the

    [5] Paul R. Lawrence and Jay W. Lorsch,*Organization and Environment*(Homewood, Ill.:Richard D. Irwin,1969).

    [6] Ibid.,p.11.

    [7] Ibid.,pp.185-245

unit of analysis for Lawrence and Lorsch was the manager in the organization or the work of the manager. Perhaps the health care agency is analogous; perhaps not. But simple observation of the wide variation in effectiveness among health agencies utilizing similar structures does seem to substantiate the conclusion that organizational structure should *not* be based purely on the democratic ideology. Rather, each organization should be structured in a fashion that takes into account all of the variables of its own individual needs. There is no one best structure.

The choice of structure is frequently viewed as a static decision. This would be true only if all the factors that caused the decision remain constant. Have personnel changed? Has the environment changed? Are the goals the same as three years ago? These questions should be considered at regular intervals to determine whether structural changes should be introduced.

In the past several years, a second generation of organizational structures has emerged that do not necessarily lend themselves to description on the tall versus flat dimension of earlier organizations. One of these forms is an example of how decisions about structure can reflect the variables mentioned above. The form is called *project organization*. The project organization is one in which the structure reflects teams or groups organized to complete a particular job. The teams are generally composed of specialists of different types, each having a contribution to the project. As new projects are added, new teams are formed from existing groups that are disbanding or from the outside. The structure is extremely fluid. As a result, there is a high degree of ambiguity, and there is potential for conflict due to problems of communication among groups. This form is not well suited to tasks that are routine or well defined or are continuing in nature such as assembly or production. It is better suited to research and development activity where continuing production is not a major concern.

You may question to what extent nursing is similar to either the research and development activity or the production function. The answer to this question is certainly affected by one's approach to nursing. For some, nursing has become routine. This is more true in some settings than in others due to length of patient stay and number and type of patient problems. However, even in the most stable settings, the view of nursing as nonroutine and creative, especially the practice of the professional, can be supported if the approach is focused on the patient or client as a unique individual. On the other hand, when tasks alone are the focus, the picture of nursing in practically any setting becomes much more routine.

In any health care agency, there are certainly a number of ongoing functions that do not lend themselves to a project structure. Examples are maintenance, purchasing, and supply. But a project to develop a new oncology service might well be managed as a single project within an otherwise traditional organization pattern. Here again, the distinction is one of degree. The critical difference is between a total project structure and the use of the form when it is appropriate, based on function, personnel, and all the other factors, such as task and environment, mentioned earlier.

One other structure discussed in current literature is the *matrix*. This is formed when a project structure is combined with the basic elements of a hierarchy. The individual worker is at once a part of a department and a member of one or more program staffs. This means that the program administrator is responsible for the individual's work in relation to program objectives and that the department administrator deals with ongoing concerns such as evaluation of competence, salary, and initial assignment to programs. The matrix structure offers the accountability of one program manager for each program area and the potential for greater responsiveness to needs within programs. Problems that tend to arise are caused by conflict between program and department managers and the increase in numbers of administrative positions. Also, the multiple authorities to which the individual worker responds can prove problematic for some personnel. This problem is reduced when there are few status distinctions between the personnel and the manager such as in the situation where all personnel are professionals.

Each of these last two structures - the project organization and the matrix - demands managers who are willing to be open to continuous change and who communicate well.

Shared Governance, A Professional Concern - Implication for Organizing

The concept of shared governance emphasizes creating organizational structures and process that emphasize professional accountability and involvement in decision making by all members of its professional nursing staff. The organizational changes proposed consistent with this concept include a professional staff organization for nurses paralled with the medical staff organization, with direct input at the highest level of nursing decision making. This organizational element is typically charged with the responsibility for peer review and for a credentialing process.

Peer review processes are included in a shared governance operation as a mechanism for providing colleague input into performance. The form that the processes take vary with the organization. For example, peer review may be the mode for all performance evaluation; it may be used for recommendation for merit salary increases; it may be used for review of disciplinary situations, it may be used for some combination of these. As with all organizational processes, it is desirable that the method and extent of decision responsibility and authority be in writing. This is often an element of a bylaws document for the staff nurse organization. Participation in peer review demands a strong sense of professional accountability and a commitment to maintaining appropriate confidentiality regarding actions related to individual nurses. Because decision by such a group affect a nurse's practice, the written documents (e.g. Bylaws) empowering the group should have legal review to reduce threat of individual liability for professionals who participate. Structures for peer review in the nursing service usually place the structure parallel with and reporting recommendations to the chief nurse executive. In this way, actions from the peer review process are enacted through the organizational *line*.

Credentialing processes involve review of the qualifications of nurses seeking appointment to the nursing staff. The result of the review is a decision about practice privileges. That is, under what position description may this nurse practice? What is the scope and authority? What are the expectations? With this type of process in place, all nurses who practice in the agency, either regularly or intermittently, as paid employees, consultants, or as part of the roles such as faculty, are reviewed for privileges. Categories or descriptions of scope of practice and responsibilities correlated with experience and education guide the decision in this process.

Participation in decision making, the key element of the shared governance concept can be facilitated by certain structured arrangements, such as committees as part of a professional staff organization. But, alone, structure is insufficient to produce shared governance. These must be an organizational commitment to the validity of staff participation in decision making and a related commitment by staff to participation. If both do not exist, form and ritual are substituted for involvement and impact. Reintegrated professional practice, with its emphasis on service beyond the immediate confines of the job as an integral element, is consistent to the type of service involvement that shared governance requires. A line structure which tends toward decentralization facilitates shared clinical decision making and fosters colleagiality. In this atmosphere shared decisions about policy and procedure for practice standards could flourish more readily.

The potential benefits of a shared governance arrangement (whatever form might be developed) include increased job satisfaction related to increased involvement and increased retention of staff related to professional recognition. The possible hazards include disruption in existing decision processes resulting in some inefficiency for a period of time and frustration among staff due to lack of experience with participative professional behavior. Disruption may be aggravated by perceived loss of authority and control by some personnel in nursing administration roles. For these reasons, change to create shared governance by developing organizational structure and processes consistent with it should be initiated only when a core of administrative *and* direct care staff are favorable to its development. A services concern must be the varying educational preparation of nurses in staff roles. Many will have little, if any, preparation to participate effectively in professional practice decisions. Another issue will be individual motivation to participate. Without a professional horizon which extends beyond the end of the shift and payday, a nurse has little reason to seek broader involvement. Fortunately for nursing, there are many nurses who are motivated to the highest level of function. It is these whose motivation and enthusiasm must become contagious if broad adoption of shared governance is to occur.

Use of Committees

The use of a series of committees is a structuring technique designed to encourage participative management and to promote inter-and intradepartmental coordination. Committees are compatible with any of the structures discussed earlier. The committees may be composed of administrative personnel from the same level across several departments. An example of this type of committee is one composed of all department heads in an agency. This is a particularly useful group for developing suggestions for widely applicable problem solutions. The degree to which the input of this or of any committee is used depends on (1) the defined authority of the committee and (2) the willingness of the administrative personnel to accept the input provided by the committee.

Another type of committee is a staff group composed of personnel from a variety of staff levels. A personnel benefits committee could profit from such a composition.

Within the nursing department, both types of committees - administrative and staff - may be generated. For example, the nursing service executive committee might be an administrative committee composed of the nurse executive and all associate and assistant directors. This group could make recommendations to the nurse executive regarding policy and planning as well as on daily operation. The procedures committee might be a staff committee and have a membership of staff nurses, a head nurse, and a staff development nurse.

Some committees may be *standing* committees with a membership defined by positions and/or representing specific groups in the nursing service. A standing committee is one that has a continuing function in contrast to the *ad hoc* or *special* committee. As its name suggests, this latter type is charged to accomplish a particular purpose and is then disbanded. Another distinction to be made is between the ad hoc committee and the use of project groups or an organizational structural unit. The ad hoc committee is usually expected to make its recommendations to some administrative officer who makes the final decision about implementation. The project team, by contrast, has responsibility for all phases of its project, with its own manager being responsible.

The likelihood of success of the committee mechanism can be increased by attention to the techniques mentioned earlier for conferences. When you accept committee membership, it is important to plan time for adequate preparation for the meetings. Participating in committee activity is one very good way to gain a better knowledge of the agency in which you work. It is also an important way to influence the policies and procedures that affect the care given to your patients or clients. Your broad background preparation and your acquaintance with the use of libraries and other sources of information will give you a good basis for performing effectively as a committee member or chairperson.

Informal Organization

The structures mentioned above are those designed intentionally for the purpose of accomplishing the work of an enterprise. In health care agencies as in all other forms of group endeavor, relationships other than those depicted on the charts will develop. The informal patterns of communication and influence that are formed are sometimes referred to as the *informal organization*. Chapters 5 and 9 have discussed these types of relationships. This information can help you to analyze your organization and particularly your nursing service and functional unit. In this way, you can gain the information necessary to function efficiently. It is certain that such relationships will exist and that, in some way, you will be affected by the resulting influences. For that reason, it is crucial that you not operate from the naive belief that all communication and influence proceeds through official channels.

Modes for Organizing Patient Care

The previous discussion has focused on organizing at the level of the total enterprise and the nursing service as a whole. The next level of concern is with the modes by which care actually will be given. Several methods have been developed over the years for organizing at this level. These methods, described below, have each been in vogue at some time in modern nursing. In the following discussion, the elements that influenced the development of the method will be identified. In addition, each mode will be examined for compatibility with overall organizational structure. The methods are case assignment, functional method, team nursing, primary nursing, and case management.

Case Assignment

Early in this century, nursing was practiced in homes and in hospitals. The care in hospitals was largely for those patients without the resources to be cared for at home. At that time medicine had relatively little to offer in terms of care that could not be effected in the home. Therefore, many nurses worked in the homes of their patients. The average nurse worked a 12- hour shift, six or seven days a week. The "case" was her total assignment for the time she worked.

The nursing student, in preparation for such practice, was assigned "cases" in the hospital where she trained. These hospitals were staffed almost entirely by students. The head nurses and the director or superintendent of nurses were frequently the only graduate nurses who were staff members. The student nurse assumed responsibility for the total care of the patient while she was on duty.

It would seem that this method would be quite compatible with a very decentralized structure allowing for much decision making at the operational level. It is also easy to see that this method was quite feasible given the condition of the times. All those in the work force worked long hours. Nurses were among the groups whose motivation was expected to be primarily altruistic, if not religious. There was little technology and relatively little medical or nursing science upon which to base activities of care. Nurses provided for the patient's basic needs of hygiene, ventilation, elimination, comfort, and activities of daily living. The responsibilities also included preparing and serving the patient's food and cleaning the room in which the patient stayed. As a result, nursing was less complicated, with little in the way of specialized medication, machinery, or knowledge and no ancillary personnel to teach and supervise.

Marjorie Beyers and Carole Phillips reported that the Depression resulted in nurses' being unable to find work in homes, and as a result they returned to hospitals to work in order to earn room and board.[8]. The number of students was reduced, and the "case" method of care by graduate nurses in hospitals became the mode. The method of assigning a *caseload* is frequently used in community health agencies. The number of individuals or families in a caseload varies, but it is certainly more that one *case* due to the fact that the nurse is providing assistance for selected problems rather than total care. The case method continues to be used for private duty nursing in the home, though such care is not nearly as commonly provided by registered nurses as in the past. Probably due largely to cost and low availibilty of nurses, care in the home tends to be more specific, with interim care between visits by the nurses provided by family or a nursing assistant. However, the nurse providing the home care will have case assignments, and have responsibility for the provision of the care which has been contracted for and/or approved by the insuror for the patient.

The term "total patient care" is also used to describe this type of assignment as it is used in some hospitals. The main difference between this and earlier case methods is that the cases are assigned for the shift, not for the entire hospital stay. The nurse will have a group of cases, one to several patients, depending on the acuity of their condition. And the nurse may have the same or different cases on subsequent days.

Functional Method

The impact of World War II on the fields of nursing and medicine in the United States was dramatic and extensive. Many of the nurses who were living and working in hospitals in the States went into the armed forces to care for the wounded. At the same time the techniques of medical science were improving rapidly, resulting in increasing demands upon nurses both for assistance with medical routine and for new techniques of nursing care. As a result of the increased demands for such activity and the relative dearth of graduate nurses, other levels of personnel including volunteers, nurse's aids, and practical nurses became part of the delivery of nursing care. Because these new personnel were not graduate nurses, they were unable to provide total care for most patients. Therefore, a method was evolved that assigned responsibility for specific tasks to each worker, depending on

[8] Marjorie Beyers and Carole Phillips,*Nursing Management for Patient Care* (Boston:Little,Brown,1971)

training and personal ability. This is known as the *functional method*. The nurse's aids were responsible for housekeeping chores and delivering meals and, in some cases, feeding patients. Practical nurses performed activities such as bathing patients, some treatments, and comfort measures. The registered nurse staff provided the other nursing care and supervised all care. This division of labor seemed quite logical in view of classical management principles. It fits quite nicely with the typically pyramid-shaped organization structure. The new chain of command placed the graduate nurse in a position of responsibility for supervising the actions of other workers.

This functional method offers each individual worker the opportunity to perform in a highly efficient manner in completing relatively few tasks for a relatively large number of patients. Some personnel are satisfied with this sort of arrangement, and it is found in use in some agencies today, especially on evening and night shifts in hospitals. The condition that is likely to prompt use of this method is a high ratio of unlicensed staff to professional nurses. Using this method reduces the complexity of supervision of large numbers of such personnel.

There are two factors that tend to discourage the use of the functional method for giving care. The foremost is the resulting fragmentation of the care received by each patient. The fact that several workers are providing small bits of care increases the possibility that problems of omission of activities, lack of coordination, and poor communication will arise. From the viewpoint of the personnel, some may feel that they are not being used to their full potential. For example, the licensed practical nurse (LPN) who spends her work time performing only treatments for a larger group of patients may wish to give total care to patients whose needs her education has prepared her to meet. The work of Frederick Herzberg, Bernard Mausner, and Barbara Snyderman regarding job satisfaction would prompt careful consideration of the possibility that for many nursing personnel, a functional assignment is not satisfying.[9]

How do we explain, at the same time, that there are some personnel who are not only content but are actually pleased with a functional assignment? The work of Morse and Lorsch mentioned earlier, offers some explanation.[10] For such personnnel, the need for a sense of competence may best be met by a well-defined predictable routine in their jobs.

[9] Frederick Herzberg, Bernard Mausner, and Barbara B. Snyderman,*The Motivation to Work*,2nd ed.New York:John Wiley,(1959).

[10] John J. Morse, and Jay W. Lorsch,"Beyond Theory Y,"*Harvard Business Review*, Vol.48,No.3,(May-June 1970),pp.61-68.

Team Nursing

The team method of organizing to provide care was developed to correct problems of the functional method while at the same time allowing use of nurse's aids and practical nurses. Understanding the two key concepts upon which the team nursing method is based is important in ensuring its success. These two concepts are (1) that professional nurse should provide leadership for the team and (2) that good open communication among team members is essential to the method.

In team nursing, the group of personnel includes individuals with different levels of preparation such as nurse's aids, LPNs, and RNs. These persons are assigned as a team to provide care for a group of patients. The method was developed for use primarily in inpatient settings. The basic idea is that each team member is assigned the total care of patients to the extent that it is within his/her capability. The assistance necessary to complete care required for patients assigned to an aid or LPN is provided by the professional nurse, and since the group works as a team, each member will assist the others as needed. The idea is that the professional nurse will provide leadership and that the team as a total group will be responsible for its group of patients.

The proper functioning of this method depends on group planning to develop and update a nursing care plan for each patient. In order to develop such plans capably, the professional nurse needs conference leadership skills (mentioned earlier in Chapter 12) as well as knowledge of appropriate nursing care measures. The importance of the professional nurse as the team leader cannot be understated because it is her use of her educational preparation in leadership and group management that makes it possible for the team to function as more than a collection of individuals with various levels of skills. The main advantage of the use of team nursing (when practiced at its best) for personnel is that mixed levels of personnel can be employed without the problems of boredom with routine that may result when a strictly functional system is used. The potential benefits for patients lie in the probability that fewer persons will be providing care per patient than in a functional assignment, resulting in less fragmentation, and that all team members should be well acquainted with the plan of care.

Sadly, the communication required to assure that team nursing works is the thing that is most often lowest among priorities. Also, since the leadership of the group and the nursing care planning and communication elements are largely "invisible," the team leader is often thought of as being responsible only for medications, treatments, and for keeping up with new orders. Since most of these activities are within the scope of the LPN's ability, the reasoning goes that the team leader's job can then be done by this level of nurse. Although this may be viewed as happening only occasionally, the notion that team leadership can be assigned to the LPN at any time implies that the professional nurse's skill is not actually required. Although some who wish to justify such assignments speak of job enrichment for the LPN, this is actually reducing the nursing function of the team leader to a series of isolated activities, thereby losing the essence of the method. Lest the reader believe that these statements represent a dislike for the practical nurse, I would hasten to note that these statements are based on differences in educational background, not on individual differences. There are always some persons who are exceptionally good and poor in ever field, but decisions of principle about assignments must be based first upon education and licensure.

If team nursing is practiced in your agency, it will be your responsibility as either a team member or team leader to make every effort to function according to your best ability as a professional to provide the patient with comprehensive nursing care.

Primary Nursing

The primary nursing method was designed to provide the patient with comprehensive, nonfragmented, planned nursing care and to increase the accountability of the professional nurse. In primary nursing, the patient is assigned upon admission to a primary nurse. That nurse is responsibile for the care the patient receives during his entire hospitalization and for planning for smooth transition to follow-up care by family or by other nurses if needed after discharge.

In order to reconcile the needs for round-the-clock nursing care with the "my nurse" arrangement, nurses on shifts other than that of the primary nurse are assigned as associate nurses. These associate nurses are responsible for implementing the plan developed by the primary nurse. This is done essentially by the case method with the associate providing complete care for her own primary patients, if assigned any, as well as for those for whom she is associate. The intent is that all care will be planned, implemented, and evaluated by a professional nurse. In some agencies, this has been altered to include LPNs acting as associate nurses. In agencies that use this method, the nurse's aids perform very little direct nursing care and are involved in messenger and transportation activities.Recently, with a shortage of Registered Nurses, the role of the aid as a partner in care has been examined as a way of extending the scope of the R.N.'s effect.

There may be a number of difficulties involved in beginning to use this method since most agencies are staffed with a combination of staff levels suitable for functional or team nursing. For this reason, a change to primary nursing must necessarily be gradual, requiring phasing in as attrition helps reduce the number of aids and LPNs. The only alternatives to a gradual phase-in of this sort are reassignment to nonprimary units or termination of personnel. There are some areas, especially rural areas, where the number of professional nurses is so limited that this method of organizing is unrealistic. However, the notion that a shortage of nurses exists in a particular place should not be accepted too readily. Aggressive recruitment coupled with the development of incentives can be effective but is unlikely to occur unless there is some greater benefit anticipated than can be achieved from the current pattern of staffing.

Karen Ciske has noted that it is important to anticipate that a change to this method of delivering care will cause some insecurity among those nurses who have not been accustomed to the degree of accountability required.[11] The primary nursing method places an emphasis on the nurse's ability to manage the care of a group of patients rather than on management of personnel as in team nursing. The primary nurse-associate nurse relationship is one in which each nurse may participate in each role. The result is a requirement that the nurse function as a peer and that the interaction be collaborative rather than superior-subordinate.

A frequently mentioned concern related to primary nursing is the necessity for more personnel hours and/or more expensive hours. One author commented that more personnel hours would be required in a hospital changing to this method than in other methods of assignments only if available personnel hours were inadequate in the present delivery method currently in use.[12]

Case Management

Not so much a delivery method, or assignment pattern as an adjunct to routine assignments, case management is the name used for a variety of arrangements which have in common an intent to move a patient or client effectively and efficiently through elements of the health care system. Some case management is performed by non-nurses, often social workers. In these arrangements, the case manager's role, particularly in relation to the hospital nurse or other institution-based nurse, is to gather information necessary

---

[11] Karen Ciske,"Primary Nursing: An Organization That Promotes Professional Practice,"*Journal of Nursing Administration*,4,No.1(January-February 1974),30.

[12] Ibid.,p.31.

to make referals and provide guidance as the patient moves from one health care setting to another (e.g. hospital to nursing home). In these case management arrangements, the emphasis is on effective synthesis of information to assure effective, cost conscious use of services. Each health care professional is continuing to perform his or her function in the usual way, with communication to and from the case manager. Many insurors or government sponsored health programs employ this type of case management with cost containment as a primary concern.

Two other general models of case management are prominent in current nursing development. The first was developed by Zander and her associates at New England Medical Center. This system builds on a primary nursing assignment method and has "four essential components:Achievement of clinical outcomes within a prescribed timeframe; The care giver as case manager; Episode- based RN-MD group practices that transcend units; and Active participation by patients/families in goal setting and evaluation."[13] In this system, patients are admitted to a group practice comprised of a group nursing staff and an attending physician. One nurse is designated as case manager. That nurse will be the primary nurse when the patient is on her/his geographic unit, but the case manager's responsibility is not limited to a unit. It goes across units, along with the physician's role.

Initial findings show that use of the method, which relies on Critical Paths and Case Management Plans as guides to expected outcomes, results in better quality and/or lower cost care. Critical Paths are short versions of the Case Management Plans. These Plans are detailed protocols for care, nursing and medical, which are jointly developed to reflect the typical course of an illness, its most desirable treatment, and the activities of care needed to accomplish designated outcomes. These plans reflect effort to move a patient through a hospitalization in a period equal to or shorter than the usual time designated for the DRG. Subsequent focus in outpatient care is on preventing unnecessary readmission.

Zander emphasizes the professional accountability fostered by the type of practice which demands collaboration. While, at present, the case management extends only to certain diagnostic categories, expansion is intended.

While the advantages of the method are readily evident - reduced costs, high accountability - some disadvantages must be considered. First, a strong motivation to collaborate must be present and the part of both physician and nurse, at least as long as the Case Management Plans continue

---

13 Karen Zander,"Nursing Case Management: Strategic Management of Cost and Quality Outcomes" *Journal of Nursing Administration*,18,No.5 (May,1988)p.23.

under development. This may require some behavior change. Second, since creating the Case Management Plans subjects medical practice to a certain degree of regimentation, there may be resistance to this scrutiny. If other agencies were to develop the New England Medical Center model, it would be neceassary to either revalidate at the local site the New England CMPs or to use them as a prototype to develop locally acceptable CMPs.

Case Management is also the name for a nursing function which is in use at St. Mary's in Tucson. This model is based on a nursing practice philosophy which emphasizes holism. Case managers may have a variety of other assignments in the hospital. They have in common the role of manager for the care of clients which become a part of their caseload when they are admitted to the hospital. The person continues in the caseload until discharge by the nurse. Case managers base their action on nursing diagnoses which require resolution, in contrast to identified outcomes and activities as in the New England model. The St. Mary's Case Manager's activity also goes beyond a particular unit and relies on collaboration and referrals specific to the case. This method, sponsored by the hospital, has a case manager role which combines the best of a community health practice with access to participation in hospital care activities. Initial reports demonstrate cost savings under the DRG system attributable to the case manager's function.[14] Similar concerns about individual motivation are relevant in considering this case management model as in the Zander model.

Selection of Mode of Delivering Patient Care

The selection of one of the various methods of delivering nursing care is frequently dictated by convenience, tradition, or fad. This is an extremely important decision, one that should be reached in a rational fashion and that may result in different answers for different nursing services. The notion that nursing services are affected by many variables that combine to produce differing optimal staffing is borne out by the study by Harry Levine and Phillip Joseph.[15] Their work takes the position that there is no single optimum staffing level or ratio in hospitals; but rather the optimum is relative to the purpose and philosophy of the hospital, the desired level and type of care provided, and a series of other factors related to personnel. The

[14] Phyllis Ethridge and Dr. Kathy Michaels, St. Mary's, Tucson personal communication,1988.

[15] Harry Levine and Phillip Joseph,*Factors Affecting Staffing Levels and Patterns of Nursing Personnel* (Washington,D.C.: U.S. Department of Health, Education and Welfare,1975)

same is true for choice of method for delivering care. Of course, the delivery method choice, in turn, affects staffing, although in some cases the relationship has been reversed, with staffing determining the method of organizing at the unit level.

The following are concerns that must be addressed in determining the choice of method of care delivery at the direct patient level:

1. What is the objective of the agency and how does that reflect the philosophy of the agency's governing body?
2. What types and quality of care *should* be involved in order to meet the objectives of the agency?
3. Does the budget reflect commitment to the objectives?
4. If the budget is not adequate to meet objectives, which objectives assume priority, or what change in level of care is realistic?
5. What educational levels and performance abilities are evident in the present staff?
6. What is the availability of various personnel for recruitment?
7. Are there attributes of the environment that affect the ways in which care can be provided efficiently? (For example, are there particular architectural characteristics of the hospital or nursing home that make communication activities difficult? Are there geographic aspects of the location that hamper supervision of home health aids in the community health agency?)
8. Are there labor contracts that would affect the assignments of various workers and/or changes in staff composition?
9. What is the quality of care presently being provided? In the case of a new unit or service, the question would be, What does research literature indicate is the expected type and quality of care rendered using this method?
10. Are the nursing personnel satisfied with the quality of care they are providing and with the way in which it is organized? Do personnel generally seem interested in and happy with their work?

Based on the combined answers to these questions, a decision can be reached regarding which mode of nursing care best suits the purpose of the agency. As a professional nurse in the agency, you could provide critical information to answer these questions. In fact, you might well prompt consideration of the above questions if they are not being asked as change is being contemplated. Possible avenues for participating are: (1) by directing written suggestions following verbal discussion through the appropriate administrative lines; (2) by participating as a member of an ongoing committee concerned with quality of care (The names of such committees vary as do the specific committee charges, depending on the agency; but, in general, the focus is on determining quality of nursing care and identifying methods for improving quality.); (3) by suggesting the formation of an ad hoc committee to develop information and/or make recommendations regarding method of organizing and related topics and by volunteering to serve on the committee. As a manager of the care of patients, you have an investment in assuring that the care is provided in the most efficient manner possible. As a member of the staff you are a participant in the method chosen, and it will affect the way in which you can function as a professional nurse. For these reasons it is important that you seek to be involved in providing information for decisions about the way that nursing care is organized in your agency.

Staffing and Scheduling as Elements of Organizing

The plan for organizing to give nursing care is made operational through staffing and scheduling. Since you are directly affected by these activities, it is useful to learn the kind of information regarding different approaches to developing staffing plans and schedules.

The American Nurses Association issued a publication entitled *Nursing Staff Requirements for In-Patient Health Care Services.*[16] In the introduction to the booklet, the Commission on Nursing Service noted that no single formula, ratio, or numerical concept should be viewed as *the* approach for all inpatient facilities. Instead, it recommended that the nursing service administrator develop individualized staffing patterns for each department.

That same publication describes the essential elements of a staffing plan for an inpatient agency. Although you may not be in a position to develop the overall plan, it is still useful for you to be aware of these components since you will see that you are an important participant in gaining portions of the necessary information and in implementing the plan. The elements are:

1. A written statement of purpose, philosophy, and objectives of the nursing program.

[16] American Nurses Association,*Nursing Staff Requirements for In-Patient Health Care Services* Kansas City,Mo: ANA,(1977).

2.A statement of the purpose, philosophy, and objectives of staffing.
3.An indication of the data base.
4.A statement of rationale for the staffing method used.
5.A set of personnel policies and procedures related to scheduling and a plan for implementation.
6.A basic staffing pattern for each unit.
7.A set of performance standards.
8.A plan for supplementing staff at times of illness, emergency, etc., and for reducing staff when prolonged low load occurs.
9.A quality assurance program.
10.A plan for evaluating the staffing program.[17]

Four Approaches to Determine Staffing

Statement number 4 above may be a puzzle to you unless you are aware that there are various approaches to developing staffing for nursing services. These approaches can be categorized into four groups: (1) descriptive, (2) industrial engineering, (3) management engineering - including the Medicus system, and (4) operation research. Each of these is described briefly below.

The least precise methodology is the *descriptive* one. This method essentially focuses on using the experience and judgement of the administrative personnel who make the staffing decisions. Although several variables are included in making decisions about staffing, their use is generally imprecise. Variables considered may include census, occupancy rate, personnel training, and personnel policies. Some simple ratios or other formulas may be used in this method, but their use is generally not based on research.

The *industrial engineering* methodology focuses on deriving staffing needs from studying nursing work at the unit level. The tools used are work measurement, time studies, physical work layout studies, and analysis of work distribution. The underlying assumption is that nursing can be viewed as a series of discrete and visible activities that can be rearranged to form the most efficient method for performance. The "rearrangement" of activities then predicts the needs for staff. The assumption is certainly open to criticism since planning and other mental acts are seldom considered in developing the required time to accomplish work. As a result, the industrial engineering method is frequently viewed as an incomplete basis for staffing for nursing.

17 Ibid.,p.3

Management-engineering methods combine the techniques of industrial engineering with systems analysis. This approach is based on the installation of a continuing system that monitors the staffing functions in relation to performance standards. The use of this approach requires the assistance of consultants and special training for agency personnel to function in the quality-control activities. You may have encountered the use of such a system when you participate in the daily classification of patients into standard care categories. This is probably the most commonly used formalized approach to staffing. The patient categories represent standard needs for nursing hours as based on previous industrial engineering studies. These standard hours result from averages of times needed to perform typical nursing activities for patients in these categories. The number of patients in each category is multiplied by the standard number of hours per patient, according to an equation that varies somewhat from method to method. The result is the number of nursing hours needed by patients in that category. The category totals are then summed to determine the number of nursing hours needed for the shift. (The standard hours per category vary by shift in most of these methods, with the day shift usually requiring the greatest number of hours.)

The number of these hours to be provided by each level of personnel is defined by a ratio that is usually determined by the agency. The total number of hours per level of personnel is then divided by a standard number of hours worked per person to identify the numbers of personnel needed for the shift. The "hours worked" number will vary with the formula or method being used. However, each method recognizes that some standby or idle time is to be expected as is some allowance for nondirect patient care activities. In some methods, the nondirect care activity is built into the patient care categories; in others, it is considered at the point of determining hours of care needed by multiplying the direct care time by a given factor for nondirect activity. In still other methods, the nondirect care activity is estimated as that portion of each individual worker's time that is unavailable for direct care, thus reducing the "hours worked" figure to correspond.

Figure 13.3 indicates the factors usually considered in calculating staffing needs through a management-engineering approach. There are a number of these methods that are described in the literature or are provided by consulting firms, so this figure is only a general description. You will notice that the calculation depicted results in a statement of personnel need for one shift. By using these daily figures to derive averages, a plan for daily unit staffing needs is derived. The daily needs are then multiplied by a factor that compensates for off-duty time and any personnel benefits that result in nonworked days. The result of that calculation defines the overall staffing pattern, that is, how many personnel must be employed to provide care. You can see that this method assumes that the type of care given at the standard

---

1. Patients are classified by activity or need level. Result is number of patients per category.	2. Number of patients per category is multiplied by standard nursing care hours per patient per category.	3. Total hours needed per category are summed. Result is total hours nursing needed for group of patients on this shift.
4. Nursing hours needed is divided by hours worked per individual worker per shift. Result is number of persons needed.	5. Predetermined ratio of various levels of personnel is used to identify number of personnel by level.	

FIGURE 13.3 General Method of Staffing Determination: Management-Engineering Approach.

---

times mentioned is of the quality desired. It also assumes that the standard times and categories are valid. These assumptions are critical and should be checked for the particular nursing service before the rest of the method is employed.

A more informal descriptive method than the calculation system shown in Fig. 13.3 is in use in a large number of agencies. This is a variation on the management-engineering method in that it uses the calculation techniques only on an intermittent basis to adjust estimates of staffing pattern needs. For example, a one- month data collection period will be used to identify the average needs for personnel by unit. The staffing pattern is then based on these estimates, and the daily collection of data on patient categories is eliminated until the next estimate period. This is commonly done to support budget requests for changes in the personnel budget.

A management engineering approach is used by some consulting firms. An example is the *Medicus system*.[18],[19],[20] This approach differs from other management engineering approaches in that it focuses on the difficulty of assignment and the assignment to staff of clusters of activities rather than simply on classification of patients. It also uses the individual

[18] Ronald B. Norby and Lewis E. Freund,"A Model for Nurse Staffing and Organizational Analysis,"*Nursing Administration Quarterly, Vol.1,No.4(Summer 1977),1.*

[19] Carol A. Smith,"Adequate Staffing: It's More than a Game of Numbers,"*Nursing Administration Quarterly,*Vol. 1,No.4(Summer 1977),15

[20] Ronald B. Norby, Lewis E. Freund, and Barry Wagner,"A Nurse Staffing System Based upon Assignment Difficulty,"*Journal of Nursing Administration, Vol.3, No.9 (November 1977),2.*

institution's data as the basis for determining the relative difficulty of various clumps of activities. Although this is very time-consuming, it allows for the particular characteristics of the institution and its personnel and standards to influence the equation used to determine staffing levels. Before wholeheartedly endorsing this approach as superior to others, one would need to see comparative studies between this and the other management engineering methods, including a cost- benefit analysis of each.

The *operation research* methodology uses computer simulation techniques to derive solutions to real-life problems. For this reason, extensive use of consultants is a part of this methodology as is the use of computer facilities. The related costs make this a less frequent choice of method for determining and monitoring staffing than those mentioned previously. However, as a research methodology, this holds much promise for use in analyzing new methods of delivery of care as they are developed.

Choice of Staffing Methodology

The staffing methodology used by an agency must be intimately related to its personnel policies. For example, the number and frequency of weekends off will affect availability of personnel and/or the need to use supplementary part-time personnel. The length of vacations and number of holidays will likewise affect availability of personnel, and the staffing pattern must reflect these factors. Another important factor related to the staffing pattern is scheduling, that is, the way in which personnel are designated to be on or off duty and to work various shifts. Decisions about scheduling should reflect written policy and should be applied fairly to personnel. Generally, the decisions about number of weekends off per month, number of consecutive days off and on, rotation of shifts, and frequency of rotation will be somewhat similar from agency to agency in a particular area. The similarity is necessary to ensure that the agencies can remain competitive for personnel. It is very important that you make your choice of position with full knowledge of these policies and practices as well as an understanding of the patterns of staffing and the effect on the care of patients as well as the resulting demands on personnel.

Scheduling-Some Typical Patterns and Problems

The most common schedule for a full-time employee in the United States is the eight-hour, five-day week. That 40-hour week was hard won after the early part of the century when men, women, and even children worked long days every day of the week. The organized labor movement achieved this as one important improvement in conditions for American workers. However, the fact that hospitals and some other health care agencies are in operation 24 hours a day, seven days a week, makes it somewhat difficult to provide all health care personnel with the same Monday through Friday schedule of the office worker. Therefore, careful planning is required to achieve sensible schedules that are workable and predictable for shift work personnel.

A common complaint among shift workers is that rotation of shifts is ill-planned and results in fatigue and disruption of their personal life. Rotation refers to changing from one shift to another. The reason for requiring rotation of personnel is generally to distribute the less desirable shifts among all personnel. In some agencies, this rotation is avoided by recruiting persons to work "straight nights or evenings." These individuals usually have personal preferences for the shift chosen. There may also be a pay incentive offered to those who work permanent evenings or nights, or those who rotate may receive the extra pay when they work other than the day shift. It is relatively common to find that a new employee will be given a choice of either a continuous non-daytime shift or a rotation schedule that includes some day shifts. The need for such a policy is related to the availability of personnel and the practices in other health care agencies in the area.

When shift rotation occurs, the complaints that result are frequently thought to result simply from dislike for changes or from negative reaction to disruption in routine. Some nurses who have "paid their dues" by working all shifts over the years are heard to generalize with such statements as, "These young nurses don't really want to work. They don't care about their patients or they wouldn't complain." It is possible that all of these factors contribute to the complaints of fatigue and other problems, but it is also possible that the way in which the rotations are developed may influence these complaints. The reason for such complaints may well be actual psychological and physiological disruptions caused by lack of synchrony between activity and circadian rhythms. Researchers have studied the variety of body functions that vary cyclically over approximately a 24-hour cycle. The variations are called *circadian* (from Latin "about a day")rhythms. It has been noted that mental efficiency varies directly with body temperature. Further, there is information that body temperature, in the individual on a typical daytime schedule, tends to be low in the morning, rises to its peak in the late afternoon, and then decreases gradually. In addition, several researchers have noted that the body temperature cycle adjusts slowly to changes in the waking activity cycle. As a result, a person who is accustomed to a daytime schedule who suddenly changes to an 11 P.M.-7 A.M. work schedule will be working at the time when her/his body temperature and hence, mental and physical efficiency are at a low ebb. Other research has indicated that irritability, extreme fatigue, and difficulty in concentrating are related to lack of synchrony between circadian rhythms and activity requirements.[21],[22],[23],[24]

Given this evidence, it seems important to have rotating schedules that leave an individual on a particular shift long enough for the circadian rhythms to adjust to the new activity cycle and to allow for off-duty periods for gradual adjustment of routines between shift changes. Although it can not be specified that any single period of time between shift changes is optimal, it is rather easy to determine that changing from a 7 A.M.-3 P.M. shift to an 11 P.M.-7 A.M. shift in a 24-hour space is far too rapid. The ideal would be to move to the next shift (3 P.M.-11 P.M.) and to have two or more days off before the change.

There have been some variations in the usual eight-hour shift routine for hospitals, variations that have been developed in response to a variety of needs. For example, the concern with fatigue and high stress levels in some critical care units has prompted consideration of shorter days and/or shorter work weeks at regular pay rates for these nurses. This is in contrast to the more typical practice of paying a differential in salary for work in these units. Another, more widely accepted variation is use of the "four-forty" work week. There are a number of versions of this schedule, but all have in common the use of a four-day week with ten-hour days. In some agencies, the ten-hour day is used only for the day shift, and the other shifts work the usual eight hours. The two-hour overlap is used to provide for activities that cannot be performed with the usual minimal complement of staff. Such activities include patient and family teaching, discharge follow-through, and consultation with other care givers. Another "four-forty" plan uses two ten-hour shifts per day with a five-hour mid-shift. This is particularly attractive when part-time personnel are available on a regular basis to fill the five-hour shift. The day can be constructed so that the five-hour element can be placed at 8 A.M. to 1 P.M. or 9 A.M. to 2 P.M. to provide a convenient shift for individuals who wish to be home after their childrens' school hours.

[21] W. P. Colquhoun,"Circadian Rhythms, Mental Efficiency and Shift Work,"*Ergonomics,12,No.5 (1970),*558- 60.

[22] W. P. Colquhoun, M. J. F. Blake, and R. S. Edwards, "Experimental Studies of Shift Work I: A Comparison of Rotating and Stabilized Four-Hour Shift Systems," *Ergonomics,*12,No.5 (1969),743-47.

[23] W. R. Colquhoun, M. J. F. Blake, and R. S. Edwards, "Experimental Studies of Shift Work III: Stabilized Twelve-Hour Shift Systems,"*Ergonomics,* 13,No.6 (1969),865- 82.

[24] Geraldine Felton,"Effect of Time-Cycle Changes in Blood Pressure and Temperature in Young Women,"*Nursing Research,*No.1(1970),pp.48-58.

Other arrangements of these hours are possible. Any use of this method would depend on acceptance by personnel and availability of sufficient part-time personnel to make the short shift feasible.

A different arrangement of schedules that is feasible for some nursing settings such as certain community health agencies is called *flex-time*. This arrangement offers the opportunity for workers to choose their own schedule within certain restrictions. The main restriction is that all personnel must be available during "core hours." These are generally the high-volume work hours and are used for communication among personnel, meetings, and similar activities that require availability of all personnel. The individual is then free to choose additional hours that best suit his needs and the needs of his job. The available hours usually begin at 7 or 7:30 A.M. and end at 6 P.M. The result is that personnel can choose a schedule which permits a variety of activities within a day and the agency can still be assured that work can proceed as expected. In the case of the community health nursing agency, this type of schedule might well meet the client's needs better than the usual 8 A.M. to 5 P.M. schedule. Of course, in some agencies, the professional nurse is free to develop her own schedule to meet patients' needs since she is considered a professional employee, exempt from the usual constraints of hourly wage concerns. If, however, this is not the case in your agency, it is to your benefit to understand the basis for staffing and scheduling plans. As you are responsible for other personnel, you will find that such information is helpful in providing explanations and determining scheduling choices with them.

The idea of cyclical scheduling is another one that can be very helpful both to the person responsible for scheduling and to the individual worker. This method does not depend on any particular set of policies but rather simply requires that there is a policy regarding the pattern of days worked, the number of weekends off, and the pattern of staffing designated for the unit. In this case the pattern of staffing refers to the number and type of personnel planned for each day. The schedule is then developed to meet these requirements. The result is a schedule that repeats itself as a cycle over a given period of time, six weeks, for example. The names of personnel are placed in the "slots" on the pattern, and the schedule is then predictable for an extended period. The only necessary changes are for vacations or other nonwork time, which are usually dealt with by use of float or supplementary personnnel or short-staffing.

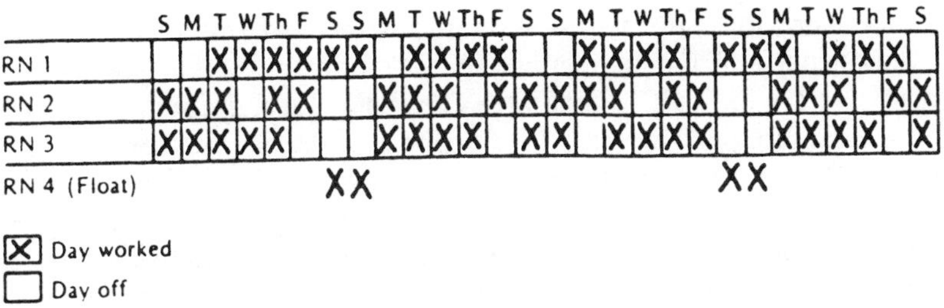

Figure 13.4 Sample Cyclical Schedule: Four Week Rotation: One Shift-Two Weekends Off per Four

Figure 13.4 is an example of a cyclical schedule. Notice that the employee can predict far in advance which days will be available for off-duty activities such as business appointments.

This type of scheduling can be viewed as a rather rigid disadvanatge if one wishes a particular day off "out of pattern." A policy allowing "trades" by persons in the same personnel classification, if proper notification is given, can relieve this complaint. The other method for dealing with this problem is scheduling an annual leave day on the desired day off.

Another feature of this cyclical scheduling plan is that when new personnel replace former employees, they are simply inserted in the available slot in the pattern. For the scheduler, this method is considerably simpler than dealing with special requests and responding to the subsequent distress resulting from perceived lack of fairness. In fact, with this sort of system, scheduling can be the responsibility of a nonnurse, thus freeing the head nurse or supervisor for more nursing-related activities.

The specific arrangements of staffing and scheduling in your health care agency will reflect its particular character, its policies, and the other variables affecting staffing in any setting. The information presented in this section should give you a basic overview of methods and concerns from which you can critically examine the policies and procedures that affect you, the care you give, and those with whom you work.

Organizing at the Level of Your Direct Responsibility

The previous information about the methods and effects of organizing at the agency and nursing service level demonstrates that planning and organizing are difficult to separate. The same is true in organizing at the unit level where the concern is the nursing care that is your direct responsibility and that of the personnel working with you. At the upper administrative levels, concern is with securing and arranging staff and resources to provide for acceptable care, along with creating relationships that will assure that communication regarding work is facilitated. When this concern is addressed at the unit level, your personal level, it is visible as efforts to identify the most efficient methods to accomplish work. Another concern besides the care itself is with creating communication activities that will provide appropriate information about the care. These organizing activities are relevant whether your position is in a hospital, in other inpatient agencies, or in community health agencies.

Making Work Simpler and More Efficient

Industrial engineering has developed a methodology that studies the expenditures of effort in work activities and designs methods and procedures for doing work more efficiently. Obviously, this is an approach applicable to only the physical activities involved in nursing; but since much of nursing involves these physical activities and since it is this work that frequently takes priority over teaching and counseling aspects of nursing, efficiency in the performance of these physical activities is critical. Any savings in time and effort gained from efficient performance can be applied to the other functions of nursing.

Some principles derived from industrial engineering are presented in the following paragraphs in order that you may apply them in organizing your work.

1. *Reduce travel to and from activities.* This principle can apply to any procedure or a series of procedures. For example, if you will stop a moment to think before going to a patient's room, you can decide what equipment you will need and probably can identify multiple activities that can be performed on the same trip. Then you can assemble your materials, picking up all items that are stored together at the same time. Finally, you can make one trip to the room, using a tray or cart, if necessary, to carry equipment. If you work in a community health agency

and give care in the home, such organizing is absolutely essential. If you have need of equipment or materials and leave some at your office, the trip back to retrieve the missing item is time lost.

2. *Group activities for patients who are near one another.* This certainly sounds simple, but it is a frequently overlooked principle in organizing. When no other priority intervenes, you can group the activities you must perform for patients whose beds are in the same room or whose rooms are nearby; or in the community, you can group activities for patients whose homes are in the same vicinity. In making assignments to personnel, you should keep this principle in mind.

3. *Use time estimates to identify activities that can be completed simultaneously or those that must come first.* You probably use this principle if you cook. For example, potatoes must bake for one hour and the squash casserole for 35 minutes. Therefore, you place the potatoes on to cook before putting the casserole together since you want both items completed at the same time. In nursing, you may have one patient who needs a warm moist pack and another who needs assistance to ambulate. Since the pack will stay on for 15 minutes, you can put it on, walk the other patient, and return to remove the pack. However, you would not choose to use the "pack time" to teach a patient how to give insulin because this would take more than the 15 minutes estimated for the moist pack.

4. *Store items together that are used together.* In many hospitals and nursing homes, you may not be able to decide where certain supplies should be stored since architectural features may dictate this. But at the patient's bedside or in the home, you can place all items that are to be used together near to one another. This save steps and motion.

Organizing requires not only that you make a plan but also that when the plan is complete, you stop to think again before actually beginning to work. The "stop to think" period is when you consider ways to put people, activities, and material together to accomplish your plans. It is at that point that the principles just mentioned are used. These principles, although relatively simple, can mean the difference between your being labeled "disorganized" or being viewed as efficient. Although efficiency does not *produce* effectiveness, its absence can *prevent* effectiveness in nursing.

Creating or Improving Unit Communication Methods

A key factor in organizing to provide care in any nursing agency is the choice of methods used for unit communications. As mentioned earlier, the organizational structure with its position descriptions defines the official *lines of communication. However, this does not prescribe methods* for communication. Since the effectiveness of communication can have a direct effect on the care that patients receive, the decisions about methods and techniques for communicating become an important part of organizing to give care.

At the direct care level, decisions must be made about communicating plans for general nursing care, specific directions, general information, day-to-day or shift-to- shift updates, and statistical information. The choice of methods should be made with the following concerns in mind:

1. Will the method reach all who need the information?
2. Will the method be timely in reaching those who need the information?
3. If feedback is necessary for adequate communication, does the method make that possible?
4. Will the method use time and material resources efficiently?
5. Is a permanent record of the communication needed for later use as verification or for follow-up?
6. Are the channels the method employs appropriate for the message?
7. Is the content delivered in a manner that reduces unintended messages in the communication?

The focus of questions 1 and 2 above indicates that you must identify all those for whom a particular communication is intended and estimate the speed with which it must be received. If you wish to communicate the day's assignment, choosing to send typed memos would be a very slow way to do this, although it might assure that each person actually received the message. If, however, the communication is a routine summary of monthly quality of care audit results, which can be received any time within a one-week period after the audit, a typed message might well be appropriate. A typed message is also suitable when the audience may be nurses on several units rather than on a single floor.

Perhaps you wish to communicate a referral to a nutritionist for a family in your community caseload. In this case, a telephone call is a rapid method of reaching the necessary person (see questions 1 and 2.) This method also meets the concerns of question 3 in that the opportunity for feedback is evident. Question 5 is also relevant in this case, since there is a need for a combination of methods of communicating, and a written referral should be developed to confirm the phone discussion. Most agencies have a standard form for this purpose, but in many instances, the use of the form alone may not meet all the concerns. Therefore, a combination approach is frequently needed.

Question 6 is intended to point out that some types of messages are best communicated in writing, whereas others are best communicated orally, that is, either face to face or via the telephone. For example, when the message includes abstract descriptions and/or numbers, most persons are aided by some visual presentation. In cases where the message is relatively straightforward, perhaps routine, an oral communication may be adequate. Where an interchange of ideas or verification of understanding is needed, an oral exchange is usually necessary.

Question 7 regarding unintended messages is extremely important, so much so that even though it is basically a "content " question, it is included here among concerns about the choice of methods of communicating. Consideration must be given to whether a particular method of communication arouses an unintended emotional response. For example, does your receiver view a memorandum as a cold and depersonalizing way of avoiding face-to- face contact on a touchy issue? If so, a written response alone to a request for a change in assignment may carry an unintended message, "I don't want to face you when I say no." Perhaps in this case it would be better to respond face to face and then make a written confirmation if it is needed. Perhaps a formal written communication from a group of personnel describing a concern with working conditions on you unit is presented to you. Simply responding verbally and immediately may imply that their message is not viewed as very important and, therefore, does not require a formal written response.

These questions are useful in making a choice among methods of communication. The following section presents a brief discussion of some specific concerns and techniques for communicating that will provide some alternatives from which you can choose in this aspect of organizing.

Cultural Differences Affecting Oral Communications

The more common aspects of face-to-face oral communication will not be discussed since they do not, in themselves, constitute a discrete method of communicating. You, no doubt, will have spent some time in studying both general and therapeutic communication in other portions of your nursing program. There is one item that bears special mention since it becomes quite relevant when you are responsible for guiding the work of others, and that is to gain information specific to cultural differences in communication among those with whom you work. For example, in some cultures it is not deemed respectful to look directly into the eyes of persons communicating information to you, especially when there is a perceived difference in organizational status. This and other information of a similar nature will aid you in understanding the behavior of those with whom you work and can help you to be alert for the possibility of differences in communication from individual to individual.

End of Shift Report

The end of shift report is a method used in many inpatient agencies to provide a summary of the major events of the past shift for the incoming personnel. It should be a relatively concise resume of the information regarding nursing care, medical treatment, and other pertinent facts so that there will be continuity in the care provided from shift to shift. This report is usually an oral face-to-face report. It should include the following information:

1. For each patient:
   (a) Identification (not just room number).
   (b) Primary nurse or Case Manager if this system is in use.
   (c) Admitting physician.
   (d) Major nursing and medical diagnoses.
   (e) Current condition, including specifics regarding special observation such as fluids and output, neuro checks, etc.
   (f) Any changes in nursing or medical plan of care since last shift.
   (g) Any specific observations or activities related to more general statement of care plan in (c) above.
2. Any new activity, policy, or procedure of which the shift may not have been informed.
3. Any anticipated admissions or dismissals.
4. Any necessary or expected communication with other departments.
5. Any changes in staff for the shift, such as presence of new orientees, float personnel, or absence of personnel.

The report should *not* include unnecessary remarks that might be viewed as gossip about patients or staff. Neither is it necessary to elaborate upon difficulties with physicians or other departments when these factors have no bearing on the functions of the incoming personnel. It is tempting to use this fresh "audience" to ventilate frustrations, but the responsibility of the professional is to deal with these frustrations in a way that will not adversely affect the function of other staff members. Your position carries not only an element of managerial responsibility but also an expectation for leadership through modeling appropriate behavior.

The oral end of shift report may be given to all incoming personnel by one nurse-the charge nurse or head nurse. A variation is to have only the charge nurse and/or staff nurses receive reports. They then transmit the necessary information to personnel on the new shift. When primary nursing is used, each primary nurse may report to the incoming associate, *or* a clinical coordinator (similar to the head nurse) may give an overall unit report.

Variations in reporting are the use of the tape-recorded report and the "walking report." The tape-recorded report is advantageous in that the report can be completed by one or several persons, and it frees the nurse(s) to attend to patients until the new shift has listened to the report and is ready to take over. Since there is no one to chat with, there is less likely to be time spent in making gratuitous remarks than in the usual face-to-face arrangement for report. The disadvantage is that since there is no opportunity for feedback, some important questions may go unasked and unanswered, although offgoing personnel can be available for questions, thus reducing such problems.

The "walking report" moves the site of the report from the conference room or nurses' station to the patient's room. This offers the incoming shift the opportunity to see the patient first-hand, along with the information given to them. It also gives the patient an opportunity to see the new shift's personnel and to mention any concerns. If each patient is actually visited, this activity takes more time than the traditional report. However, this is time well spent, especially in an inpatient unit where your first priority as a shift begins must be to determine each patient's needs and condition. A visit to each patient therefore is a useful way of transmitting the report.

Assignment Conference

The assignment conference is another important method of communication. The activities necessary to structure and facilitate this type of conference are the same as mentioned in relation to the conferences used for planning (Chapter 12). The only difference is in content. The assignment conference calls together all personnel caring for a specified group of patients for a particular shift or other relevant time period. The content relates to the specifics of what work is assigned to each individual and to the group as a whole. In situations where all personnel attend the shift report and *do not* receive combination or team assignments, there is little need for such a conference. In such cases, the person making assignments will meet with each individual worker to discuss her assignment. In any situation, the concern must be with clarity in the assignments and providing an opportunity for feedback to assure that the communication was clear. Any assignment should specify the following:

1. What is to be accomplished.
2. The desired result of the action.
3. Expected timing.
4. Any necessary follow-up.

The degree of specificity necessary in each element of the assignment, listed above, will be determined by your knowledge of the personnel, their experience, and all the same factors that went into your assignment decisions during planning. There is a fine balance between offending the person with too much explanation and supplying sufficient information to assure safe performance. You cannot simply give one type of assignment to all personnel. The amount of information must be chosen to fit the person.

Written Assignment Summaries

Most inpatient agencies use some sort of written summary of assignments. This is most common when either functional or team assignments are used. There is less need for such a summary when the primary nursing approach or case (total patient care) assignment is used, since one person is giving all of the care for any particular patient and assignments do not change from day to day. (Figure 12.5 in Chapter 12 is a sample of a typical written summary sheet.) The primary advantage for its use is that it provides in one place the major information regarding the specific activities to be performed during a particular shift. The need to refer to the medical record is then reduced. Notice that the usual categories of activities are listed so that check marks can be used to complete much of the form. A problem with such forms is that such activities as care planning and teaching are not identified as part of the "work to be done." As a result, much of what the professionl nurse should do as an assignment is not visible to the other staff members.

Many agencies require that some notation be made to indicate that work has been completed. The summary sheet can provide a quick reference on progress of work. A variation on the use of a single sheet for a unit or team is providing a separate smaller sheet for each care giver, regarding her patients. These are small enough to carry in a pocket and, as a result, are a useful personal reference.

Summary Reports

Another important organizing communication is the summary report. The form and content will vary by agency, as will the frequency of completion. For example, in hospitals, there will be census reports and summaries of patient conditions prepared for each shift. In community health agencies, statistical summaries also are completed regularly.

These reports serve a variety of purposes. Some summary reports include staffing levels as well as categories of patient conditions, census, and remarks. Specific data can be accumulated to support requests for changes in staffing. Also, certain facts are required for accreditation and licensure survey. You can see that it it necessary to assure that the information reported is accurate. Generally, much of the standard information can be completed by clerical assistants, but the professional nurse should be concerned with the accuracy of the content.

Other Written Communication

Two other types of written communication you may use are items on the bulletin board and the memorandum. The primary concern with a bulletin board is that one can seldom be sure that all persons will read the material placed there. This is especially true if the board tends to be a collecting area for "dead" material and if much of what is current is inconsequential. If you choose to use a bulletin board for group communications, you should consider these problems and be sure that the board contains only recent pertinent information. In addition, all persons on the unit must be informed that the bulletin board will be a source of certain kinds of communication. The fact that this method does not encourage feedback or clarification should be kept in mind.

Memoranda are less commonly used in communicating among persons at the direct care level than between organizational levels. A memorandum serves at least two purposes. First, it is a means of communicating a message. Second, it can be used as a lasting record of the communication. In a nursing service, this latter purpose is sometimes important for indicating that certain information regarding policies, procedures, or clarification has been communicated. To that end, many units maintain a notebook or file of memos received from the nurse administrator for reference. For your own purposes, you might wish to use a memo for confirming a verbal communication that has occurred or for formalizing a request or suggestion especially when the receiver does not work directly with you daily.

Since any written communication is available, potentially, to other than the intended recipient, it is important to write it with that in mind. If you are referring to another person in your memo, be certain that your reference is factual or clearly indicate that it is your impression, not a fact. When the message is signed by you, it represents *you*. It should do that in the best way possible. In addition to the content of the message, your memo should include the date and the purpose as well as your signature. Of course, you should retain a copy of what you have sent.

If the whole idea of writing memoranda seems unnecessarily formal to you, perhaps you should consider how frequently we forget good ideas that are discussed with us. The details tend to escape. The memo is one method of keeping track of the progress of an activity, recording the fact that communication has followed all appropriate channels, and providing a basis for evaluating the outcome.

SUMMARY

The organizing phase of management can contain many important activities. All of these are designed to assure that there are appropriate personnel, supplies, and lines of communication available to perform the work designed in the planning phase. This chapter has presented a variety of such activities that affect and are affected by you, the professional nurse.

Additional Reading

Allen, David, Joy Calkin, and Marlys Peterson, "Making Shared Governance Work: A Conceptual Model", *Journal of Nursing Administration*,18:1(January,1988)37-43.

Apostoles, Frances E. and Charlotte Naschinski, "Instituting A Clinical Privileging Process for Nurses",*Journal of Nursing Administration*,17:1(January,1987)33-38.

Beecraft, P.,"A Contractual Model for the Department of Nursing",*Journal of Nursing Administration*,18,No.9(September,1988)20-24.

Bolger, Anne, "Shift Reports: Using Nursing Diagnosis",*Nursing Management*,18:10(Oct.,1987)17.

Chavigny, Katherine and Alcinda Lewis, "Team or Primary Nursing Care",*Nursing Outlook*,32:6(Nov/Dec,1984)322-327.

Creighton, Helen,"Understaffing - Part I",*Nursing Management*,17:4(April,1986)26- 28.

Creighton, Helen,"Understaffing - Part II",*Nursing Management*17:5(May,1986)14-16.

Creighton, Helen,"Legal Significance of Charting - Part I",*Nursing Management*,18:9(Sept.,1987)17-22.

Flood, Sandra D. and Donna Diers,"Nurses Staffing, Patient Outcome and Cost",*Nursing Management*,19:5(May,1986)34-43.

Loveridge, C.,S. Cummings, and J. O'Malley,"Developing Case Management in a Primary Nursing System",*Journal of Nursing Administration*,18,No.10(October,1988)36-39.

McLennan, Marianne,"Nursing Care Delivery Systems: What is the Most Effective Means of Assigning Patient for Nursing Care?",*Nursing Leadership*,6:3(Sept.,1983)72-77.

Magargal, Polly,"Modular Nursing: Nurses Rediscover Nursing",*Nursing Management*,18:11(Nov.,1987)96-104.

Manthey, Marie,"Primary Practice Partners (A Nurse Extender System)",*Nursing Management,19:3(March,1988)58- 59.*

Manthey, Marie,"Can Primary Nursing Survive?",*American Journal of Nursing*,88:5(May,1988)644-647.

Manthey Marie,"Myths That Threaten",*Nursing Management*,19:6(June,1988)54-55.

Manthey M.,"A Theoretical Framework for Primary Nursing",*Journal of Nursing Administration*,(June,1980)11-15.

Metcalf, Marion,"The 12-Hour Weekend Plan - Does the Nursing Staff Really Like It?"*Journal of Nursing Administration*(October,1982)16-19.

Nagaprasanna, Bangalore R.,"Patient Classification Systems: Strategies for the 1990s",*Nursing Management*,19:3(March,1988)105-112.

Ortiz, Marlaine E.,Phyllis Gehring, and Margaret D. Sovie,"Moving to Shared Governance",*American Journal of Nursing*,87:7(July,1987)923-926.

Palmer, Mary Ellen, and Edith S. Deck,"Assertiveness: Phone-calls, Memos, and I Messages",*Nursing Management*18:1(January,1987)39-42.

Parasuraman, Saroj, Bruce H. Drake, and Raymond F. Zammuto,"The Effect of Nursing Care Modalities and Shift Assignments on Nurses' Work Experiences and Job Attitudes",*Nursing Research*,31:6(Nov/Dec,1982)364.

Peterson, M.E. and L. Allen,"Shared Governance: A Strategy for Transforming Organizations, Part I",*Journal of Nursing Administration*,16,No.1(January,1984)9-12.

Peterson, M.E. and L. Allen,"Shared Governance: A Strategy for Transforming Organizations, Part 2",*Journal of Nursing Administration*,16,No.2(February,1986)11-16.

Porter-O'Grady, T.,"Credentialing, Privileging, and Nursing By-laws",*Journal of Nursing Administration*,15,No.12(December,1985)23-30.

Price, Elmina M.,"Seven Days On and Seven Days Off",*American Journal of Nursing*,81:6(June,1981)1142- 1143.

Przestryelski, David,"Decentralization: Are Nurses Satisfied?",*Journal of Nursing Administration*,17:11(November,1987)23-28.

Richard, Judith A.,"Congruence Between Intershift Reports and Patients' Actual Conditions",*Image: Journal of Nursing Scholarship*,20:1(Spring,1988)4-6.

Shukla, Ramesh K.,"Primary or Team Nursing? Two Conditions Determine the Choice",*Journal of Nursing Administration*(November,1982)12-15.

Van Servellen, Gwen Marram,"The Concept of Individualized Care in Nursing Practice"*Nursing and Health Care*(November,1982)482-485.

Wolf, G., L. Lesic, and A. Leak,"Primary Nursing, The Impact on Nursing Costs Within DRGs",*Journal of Nursing Administration*,16,No.3(March,1986)p.9-11.

Yano-Fong, D.,"Advantages and Disadvantages of Product-Line Management",*Nursing Management*,19,No.5(May,1988)27-31.

Zander, K.,"Nursing Care Management: Strategic Management of Cost and Quality Outcomes",18,No.5(May,1988)23- 30.

Chapter 14

Implementing

Another important phase in managing the nursing care of patients is the implementation phase. In many management texts this aspect of activity is called *supervision* and *coordination*. The nurse not only supervises and coordinates, she frequently participates directly and regularly. Therefore, the term *implementing*, connoting a direct involvement of the manager, seems appropriate for the title of this chapter.

Guide to Individualized Supervision and Coordination

Information throughout this book's previous pages emphasizes the variety of individual differences in motivation, education, and experiences among nursing personnel. As a manager your challenge is to capitalize on these individual human differences to accomplish high quality care. Hersey[1] has formulated a theoretical perspective which can guide you in this effort. The model is a contingency approach that matches supervisory or managerial strategy to readiness level of the target worker. Each of these concerns, managerial approach and worker readiness is comprised of two major dimensions. Employee readiness level is determined by assessing ability (knowledge, skills, education, and experience) and willingness (confidence, motivation). The result of different combinations of these two factors is characterized as readiness level. Figure 14.1 indicates the readiness level associated with each of four combinations.

The description of readiness of the individual (or group) being considered is in regard to a particular task, function or job aspect. For example,

[1] P.Hersey and K.Blanchard,*Management of Organizational Behavior*, Englewood Cliffs, N.J.Prentice Hall, Inc.1988.

Joe Dixon, R.N., who has just begun a new job in a nursing home in a city to which he has just moved may have general knowledge of providing care in nursing homes, but not of the specific routines of care in this facility. Much of the equipment is different from that with which he is familiar. Competence or ability could be called low to moderate at this time, in regard to many aspects of the job he is to do in this facility. He wants to succeed in this new job, so he could be considered to have high willingness. With these factors in mind, the manager would consider Joe, at least during this initial employment period, to be at readiness level 2 - R2.

Each readiness level is characterized by a different combination of the two factors ability (knowledge, competence, experience) and willingness (confidence, commitment). The readiness level most nearly characteristic of the individual or group in regard to the task(s) or function is the appropriate identification. This will guide choice of manager behavior. Assessing these two factors is relatively easy. Asking specific questions which are open-ended and do not elicit yes-no responses will gain information about past experiences with the task, knowledge of it, and recency of practice. Sensitivity to non-verbal cues and to questions from the worker will help to identify willingness.

If a manager is uncertain about readiness level, there is less risk to patients to err on the side of too low an estimate (R1 instead of R2 for example). This will result in more task behavior by the manager, thus assuring more direct supervision and safety.

Able and Willing or Confident	Able but Unwilling or Insecure	Unable but Willing or Confident	Unable and Unwilling or Insecure
R_4	R_3	R_2	R_1

Figure 14.1 Readiness Levels of Workers from Hersey and Blanchard

Manager strategy is comprised of two primary types of behavior, task behavior and relationship behavior. Task behavior is focused on the task to be performed by the worker and can vary from "high" where frequent over-the-shoulder inspection occurs and much verbal instruction and little inspection is used. Relationship behavior emphasizes a focus on the importance of the person and his/her work to the overall enterprise. This behavior also varies from high to low in amount and intensity.

If these two dimensions were placed on intersecting axes and the extremes identified, then four quadrants could be identified in Figure 14.2. In this figure, "Telling" is the name given the strategy which is high directive and low supportive. High directive and high supportive is called "Selling". "Participating" identifies the high support, low directive quadrant and "Delegating" characterizes the low, low segment.

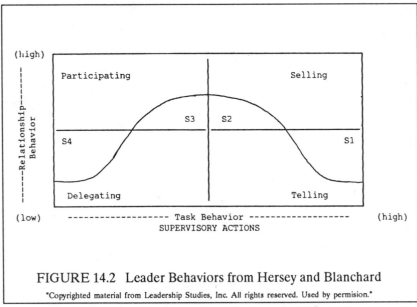

FIGURE 14.2 Leader Behaviors from Hersey and Blanchard

When the readiness level of the worker is associated with manager strategy as in Figure 14.3, the bell shaped line is the guide to which strategy to use. Where a vertical line from developmental level intersects the curve, the managerial strategy named is most desirable. As R1 intersects at "Telling", the manager would choose to give explicit, frequent verbal directions and regular over-the-shoulder supervision. Minimal emphasis is placed on supportive behavior. At R2, supportive behavior, tinged with enthusiasm combines with consistent explicit direction. This worker has some competence, but is ready for support, not to be undirected. "Participating", low direction with high supportive behavior is used for R3 and "Delegating", low direction with low support is used for the highly developed R4.

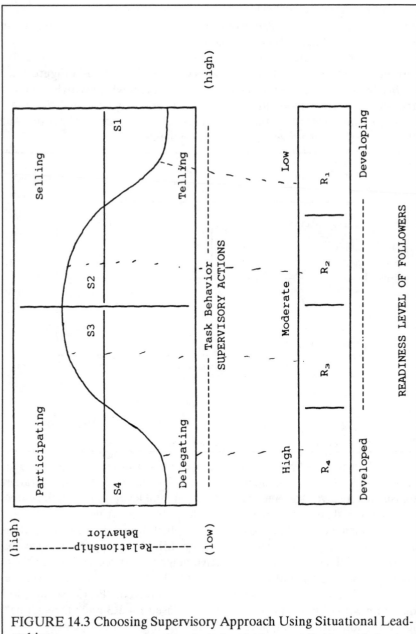

FIGURE 14.3 Choosing Supervisory Approach Using Situational Leadership "Copyrighted material from Leadership Studies, Inc. All rights reserved. Used by permission."

Recall that people change over time. For that reason, readiness estimates must be regularly reassessed as the worker acquires experiences *or* as the job changes. This model focuses the idea of readiness level as a job or task specific assessment. Therefore, any person in a new job, with new tasks and responsibilities will probably be R1 or R2 for at least a short while. Motivation changes too, so a worker's level of willingness may increase or decrease, thus changing the readiness level.

This model is a way of analyzing the overall approach the manager will best use. In any of these strategies, certain information about managerial activities such as in the following pages will be useful. Note that in the following pages, delegation refers to designating authority and responsibility not to the strategy mentioned in this model as a general direction or approach, which characterizes a manager's behavior when it is low in direction and low in supportive behavior.

The fact that some employees are in various stages of learning their jobs (R1 and R2) may mean that you wish to delegate limited authority, such as delegating the authority to make all decisions *except* those involving physician referrals. As long as it is clearly understood between superior and subordinate (1) what the limits of responsibility and authority are, and (2) what the reasons are for any limits, then two prime requirements for good delegation are met. The third requirement is that the subordinate accept the obligation implied by the delegation.

Another distinction that is useful to make in delegating is that between the delegation of a *function*, on a continuing basis, and the delegation of a *task*. The delegation of function, for long periods of time, is quite appropriate when the subordinate is a competent, well-oriented worker. This makes close observation of activities less necessary and can help create a greater sense of autonomy for the worker. On the other hand, the assignment of specific tasks or a series of tasks is appropriate when a worker is being oriented and is developing new skills, or when the superior is not well acquainted with the worker's ability. Obviously, the general level of skill and extent of preparation of the worker are important considerations. These factors of skill and preparation, combined with the general tendency of the individual worker toward more or less independent functioning, and the goals you have for the type of work group you want to create, are basic to delegation decisions. As with other aspects of management activity, the interaction between superior and subordinate and the degree of openness of communication between them are important in producing effective delegation.

Supervisory Observation

In supervisory observation you are doing two things. First, you are observing to determine if patient care is being accomplished on time and in the manner expected. In this way supervision aids in the later phase of evaluation of work. Second, you are collecting observations on the type and quality of work activity of individual workers. These observations are the basis for counseling and evaluation of the work performance of those individuals. In each case, the basic activity is observation of work in progress.

There are several decisions you must make as you prepare for supervisory observation. A critical one is how closely you will observe and how frequently you will check on the progress of work. It is not uncommon that the "new" nurse will create some distress among seasoned personnel when she is given responsibility for supervising their work. The distress results from her efforts to know firsthand what is being done, which conflicts with the worker's perceived need for independent decision making. You will hear comments like, "She doesn't trust anyone." Or, "I am getting tired of being watched; after all, I've been doing this for five years now."

It is not easy to balance your need to know *what* is being done and *how*, against the need to help personnel feel valued and trusted. The problem of your being new to a unit, yet needing to provide supervision, can be dealt with very directly by discussing this problem with the personnel involved. A frank statement that acknowledges that you have a responsibility for seeing that good care is given, that they also wish to give good care, and that you are as unfamilar with their work as they are with yours can encourage cooperation. You could also describe the ways in which you expect to behave in relation to everyone, that no one will be singled out, and that you will discuss with them any changes in you plan for supervision. Emphasizing that your purpose is to assure that the patients receive the best care possible and that the nursing personnel will receive assistance as needed will clarify that the intent is supportive rather than punitive. Of course, this assumes that your basic premises about people at work include a positive view of their motivation to work.

It is also true that simply because the persons with whom you work have been in nursing for a number of years does not guarantee that their performance will always be adequate. For such reasons, it is necessary to plan in advance the way in which you will supervise. Considerations in that plan should include the following:

1. What are the critical elements of work on this day that are non-routine, both overall and for each worker in particular?
2. What information do you need about the typical work of individuals to contribute to their overall evaluation? What part of that information will you plan to collect today?
3. What do you already know about the performance of the individuals that will prompt you to make observations more or less frequently?
4. How can these observations be combined with the other activities you have planned for yourself?

When you have considered these questions, there are some techniques that you can then use to carry out your supervisory activity. One such method is *participant observation*. You can plan to offer assistance to the individual in performing some of her work. In this way you are both assisting and gaining firsthand information on her performance. This is especially useful when some atypical activities are scheduled or when you have little firsthand knowledge of the individual's typical performance. The use of *anecdotal notes* can augment your memory in collecting this type of observation. These notes are written descriptions of observed behavior. They should include an indication of the time, date, and circumstance along with the observation. No evaluation is attached at the time of observation. As these observations are collected, on note cards or in some other sort of file, they can create a picture of overall performance, including both negative and positive aspects.

Another activity you may find helpful is to indicate, at the time assignments are made, when you need a report on the progress of certain activities. For example, "Please let me know at 4:30 P.M. what progress you have made with ambulating the postsurgical patients. I will be in with the new patient, Mr. Fry until then." This does not replace the need for some firsthand observations, but it does reduce this need. You will still need to plan time for direct observations. Some observations can be combined with "making rounds," that is, your routine visits to all the patients for whom you are responsible. You can see the patient and determine his condition *and* observe the personnel at work at the same time. In addition, you can observe the condition of the patient's environment.

A Special Issue - Working Effectively With The Impaired Nurse

Nurses, along with other health care professionals, are among groups in which there is a high rate of substance abuse. Until the relatively recent past, nurses with alcohol or drug abuse problems tended to hide the problem; eventually be discovered, often as a result of work-related errors; lose employment; move on to another job; never seek treatment, and often lose the privilege to practice due to revokation of their license. Guilt and fear surrounded the whole issue of substance abuse and nurses with known substance abuse problems, particularly drug addiction, found seeking treatment risky in regard to subsequent employment.

Recognition of the problem of substance abuse as something amenable to treatment, as an illness, not a moral failure was a major step for health professionals in dealing with their colleagues. With that view, nursing as a profession is actively seeking to aid nurses who are ill in this way and in doing so, to protect patients from harm and reduce the loss of these nurses from the profession.

This text is not the place for information on the incidence of substance abuse nor a discourse on treatment methods. Suffice it to say that specialists continue to be frustrated that, at best, substance abuse/addiction must be considered a lifetime chronic illness, not curable. It is more positive to note that in recognizing this illness model, several states have now created programs for "Impaired Nurses". These programs are designed to confront and supervise treatment and monitoring for nurses as an alternative to revocation of licensure.

One of the usual methods in the programs for impaired nurses is a "back to work contract" designed to provide a structured work setting for the nurse who has received treatment and is returning to work. You may encounter such an arrangement as a colleague or as a manager. You may wonder how best to respond. Following are some guidelines which should help both you and your impaired colleagues:

- Accept that the illness model is the best approach we currently have to help the person who is chemically dependent.
- If you have reservations, talk with your supervisor or with a colleague who works in mental health or substance abuse, to clarify your thoughts.
- If you will supervise the nurse, know the stipulations of the "back-to-work contract" so that you can be consistent with its expectations.
- Do not be afraid to be direct-give performance feedback as with all other employees.
- Keep confidential any knowledge of this person's situation as a result of your supervisory role. Only discuss the situation with those to whom you report or who have a legitimate need to know.

- Know the signs of impending relapse. Notify the nurse (Impaired) and the person who is responsible for the back-to-work contract of your concerns. Signs include:
  — erratic or disorganized behavior
  — unexplained illnesses
  — unkempt or changed appearance
  — questionable clinical decisions
  — poor charting, errors in medications
  — unexplained disappearances from the work area
  — volunteering for or accepting large amounts of overtime, working a second job

You are responsible for the work of each person you supervise, even if that person is licensed. But, you are not responsible for the person. The individual makes his or her own life choices. As a manager, be cautious that you separate your managerial role from your therapeutic role. If you work with an impaired colleague, you can help by creating a postive work environment and by encouraging them to continue with their treatment through appropriate treatment methods. Learn about the Nurse Practice Act in your state or the statutes related to impaired professionals. The program information will help you understand the rationale for the structured environment and the urine screening which are often a part of supervision required for an impaired nurse to maintain licensure.

Based on the above information it is evident that you may encounter a chemically dependent nurse who has not yet identified the illness. It is your professional obligation, and in some states a legal requirement, to report observations which indicate a possible substance abuse problem. The behavior mentioned above under signs of impending relapse are those which serve as indication of the impairment. Learn the reporting route in your agency for such situations so that you will be prepared if, as a supervisor or as a colleague, you observe these behaviors.

Focus of Verbal Interchange

One of the most important changes a nurse makes in becoming manager, at any level, is the change from incidental verbal interchange which may include professional and social topics to a more focused type of interchange which is intended to affect others' work. Making the change may be viewed by others as "you're becoming more thoughtful" or "My, you're all business aren't you?". With practice, you will be able to be pleasant and attentive yet focused on the effects of your interchanges with colleagues/subordinates in the same way as with patients.

Remember, as you interact in a supervisory role, that the main focus of verbal interchange should be the following:

1. State expectations (tasks, functions, reporting expectations, performance standards)
2. Seek information about assigned work or response to it, ideas about performance
3. Give information about assigned work
4. Give feedback on performance

These guidelines are not to suggest that some social or trivial conversation is absolutely inappropriate. Rather, it is to emphasize that the purposeful exchange may be overlooked by the supervisee if it is not a clear, consistent, major part of the conversation. Do you feel uncomfortable about this? Do you recall when you first attempted therapeutic communication with a patient or family? Managerial communication is the workplace equivalent of therapeutic communication. Neither has to be stiff, excessively formal, or unfeeling. Rather, they are both purposeful and genuine.

Value of Feedback

Collecting information by observation is only one part of supervision. You must also put the information to work. One important reason for collecting information is to provide feedback. The value of feedback as a reinforcer is well known. Therefore, when performance is good, you should tell the individual that you have noticed the quality of her work, commenting on the specific observations and indicating not only your approval but also that her performance will influence the care of a patient or patients. The concept of positive feedback is based on two principles. First, there is relatively widespread acceptance of the idea that genuine praise can serve to reinforce the behavior that prompted the praise. The reinforcement will prompt repetition of the behavior. Of course, that is dependent upon whether praise is reinforcing to the particular individual. For some, only compliments from certain persons can have this effect. The second principle is that, according to the contingency view of motivation of work,[2] as well as Abraham Maslow's and Douglas MacGregor's theories,[3] people can be motivated by a need to do important work and to do it competently (see also Chapter 1). Your act of praise and explicit statement of how the work is important should be directed toward capitalizing on these motivating factors to encourage continued good performance.

Feedback regarding poor performance is also an important part of supervision. There are two levels of such feedback. The most basic is the *immediate response* indicating that at this particular moment some action was incorrect or in some way was unacceptable. There is a focus on the specific action, and there is no implication that this represents a pattern. For example: "Mrs. Jones, I just noticed that as you changed the linen on the patient's bed, you placed it on the floor. That can cause an increase in the number of germs already being walked from room to room. It could be dangerous for the patients in other rooms. If you will place it in a bag directly as you remove it, that will be the proper technique."

The second level of such feedback is a *formal counseling* session. This is used when it becomes apparent that a performance problem exists. Such a problem will become evident when you begin to collect daily performance observations. When you see that you have made more than one informal feedback effort of the sort described above for the same reason, or you notice that the same person is frequently the object of such concerns, a formal counseling session is in order. Each agency will have certain specific rules about the form in which such counseling is documented and the consequences of recurrent counseling. You should determine what these procedures are. In any case, though, there should be both verbal discussion and written confirmation of the counseling session.

In the counseling session, it is important to focus on behavior and fact and the relationship of the performance to expected standards. The following aspects should be covered:

1. What has been observed.
2. What is not acceptable in that performance.
3. What the employee's perception of this problem is.
4. What needs to be done to correct the performance.
5. Is the correction something only the employee can do, or does she need inservice training?

---

2 See Chapter 1.p.11

3 Abraham Maslow,*Motivation and Personality*New York: Harper & Row, 1954; and Douglas McGregor,*The Human Side of Enterprise* New York: McGraw-Hill,1960.

6.Agreement on what steps will be taken to correct the performance. (If there is no agreement, the employee may choose to terminate employment.)

7.Agreement on time limits for improvement in performance.

8.Reiteration of expected standards of performance.

9.Consequences of failing to improve performance as indicated.

The words you choose should be as nonemotional as possible and you should think through just what you will say and how the employee may respond. It is helpful to role-play the first time you must do this in order to better judge your own reactions. Remember, you want to help the person maintain her diginity as a person, even though you are describing a problem with her performance.

Frequently, in an effort to spare the person's feelings, the supervisor will minimize the description of the performance problem. This is actually unfair to the individual since without accurate feedback, there is less chance for competent performance. If you surround the problem statement with a mass of anxious words, the impact is lost. Therefore, you can use the role-playing to prepare you to deliver your message in the most effective manner.

From your alternate perspective as employee you should consider whether you are receiving adequate supervision and assistance. In most organizations there will be someone to whom you report, even if the primary nursing method is used and the structure of the nursing service is largely decentralized. Although you are a professional, you do have need of some feedback on your performance. The typical organization in which most nurses work will have at least some defined supervisory lines. Where these lines exist, use the relationship to your advantage to gain feedback for improved performance. If the organizational structure does not define such relationships, you can contract with a colleague to provide this feedback for a period of time. Your agreement could specify the type of feedback you wish, the frequency, and the duration. It is also useful to discuss and "give explicit permission" to your colleague to provide negative feedback as well as positive. It is very likely that this behavior on your part will be viewed as atypical, but this is all right so long as you are ready for the responsibility that such professional behavior demands.

Adjusting Plans

Another important aspect of the implementation phase is making adjustments in plans as conditions change. The flexibility required to make such changes is not simple to cultivate. As the size of the work group increases, rapid changes in group activities become more difficult. Since much nursing care is accomplished by individual action, you may find that many changes implemented must be managed by one-to-one discussion between you and the person assigned to the care or element of care. The adequacy of information regarding what is changed and the implications of the change are crucial. To illustrate, suppose that a patient's physician is notified that the patient's condition has deteriorated, with symptons indicating a possible bowel obstruction. The resulting medical orders include giving nothing by mouth, and giving an antiemetic medication intramuscularly until the physician arrives. If the person responsible for giving medication is unaware of the change, she may take the patient his regular medication, given by mouth; so you must intervene before this happens.

Another possible type of needed adjustment is that resulting from fluctuations in staffing. When you had planned the assignments with one other RN, and LPN, and an aid, and the LPN suddenly must leave due to a family emergency, you must adjust your plans to provide adequate coverage. The considerations that affect how you choose to adjust actions during implementation include the following:

1. What do you observe that indicates a need for adjustment of plans?
2. Is it a change in the condition of a patient? If so, can the person(s) currently assigned to provide care manage the needed activity changes, or will there be a need for a person of a different skill level to provide care?
3. Is the need for adjustment due only to schedule changes, either on the unit or in other departments? If so, is there a domino effect on other scheduled activities? What do you need to do to deal with this problem?
4. If the adjustment is prompted by changes in personnel, do you have adequate personnel overall to provide the necessary care? If not, what is your next level of resources? Can someone on the unit from another group assist, or should you ask for assistance through your direct supervisor?

In order to make necessary adjustments, you must have a well-developed plan to begin with, and you must be familiar with that plan. It is difficult to develop adjustments unless you know both what is planned and approximately what amount of time is necessary for each element. In addition, that information will be incomplete unless you are knowledgeable about the skills of each of the personnel with whom you work.

SUMMARY

The primary activities for the manager in the implementation phase of a management process are supervising work and workers and making any necessary adjustments in the plan of work. The Situational Leadership model provides a framework for choice of managerial behavior strategy. Delegation of authority, supervisory observation, managerial communication, and methods of feedback-including formal counseling, are all discussed.

Additional Reading

Creighton, Helen,"More About Floating"*Nursing Management*,18:8(August,1987)17-18.

Feutz, Sheryl A.,"Nursing Work Assignments: Rights and Responsibilities"*Journal of Nursing Administration*,18:4(April,1988)9-11.

Hersey, Paul and Bonnie Duldt,*Situational Leadership in Nursing* East Norwalk, CT.:Appleton and Lange. 1989

Housley, Charles E. and Nancy Grom Nichols,"The Responsibilities of the Responsible Supervisor",*Health Care Supervisor*,(April,1984)1-15.

Kabb, G.M.,"Chemical Dependency: Helping Your Staff"*Journal of Nursing Administration*,14 No.11(November,1984)18-23.

Loraine, Kaye,"Release with Love",*Nursing Management*,18:11(November,1987)18-20.

Marriner, A.,"Problem Employees ..."*Nursing Management*,17 No.6(June,1986)58-60.

Westphal, Barbara C., Ruth Jenkins and M. Clinton Miller,III,"Charge Nurse: When Staff and Management Meet",*Nursing Management*,17:4(April,1986)56-58.

Wilson, Janet S.,"Finding the Key to Problem Behavior",*Nursing '87*(February,1987)89-90.

Chapter 15

Evaluating

The final phase in the management process presented in this book is evaluation. This step, as the others, does not necessarily begin and end in sequence with the other phases of management. Rather, activities of evaluation can and should occur simultaneously with planning, organizing, and implementing.

Figure 15.1 describes a view of activities involved in evaluation. You will notice that the description is rather general. The steps could easily describe any type of evaluation, whether used in hospital management or in the evaluation of a student's performance in school. The generality is intentional since at least two sorts of evaluation are involved - that is, evaluation of nursing care and evaluation of the performance of those providing the care. A description of each of the steps in Fig. 15.1 is presented below, followed by a discussion of the types of evaluation systems in use today for each purpose, evaluation of care and evaluation of personnel.

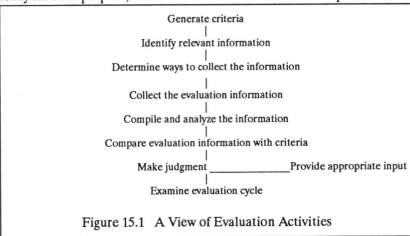

Figure 15.1   A View of Evaluation Activities

Generate Criteria

The generation of criteria for evaluation is a key step. The ultimate judgment of value of what is being appraised is reached only after comparison of the facts about it with the desired standards, the criteria. If the criteria do not address all important aspects of the objects, process, or performance being evaluated, the resulting judgment may be inaccurate or at least incomplete. The criteria should be stated in terms that are as clear as possible.

Ideally, each criterion should specify the desired behavior or visible product, the conditions under which it is to be present, and the degree or amount of the action or product that should be present. For example, a standard might be stated as: "The primary nurse will have completed an initial assessment of each newly admitted patient within six hours of his/her admission to the unit." In this statement the words *initial assessment* describe the product. The condition is clarified as *upon admission* and *within six hours*. The degree or amount is indicated by the words *each newly admitted patient*. In addition to these specifics, it should be noted that this one criterion addresses only one element of nursing care; therefore, it would be only one of many relevant criteria for evaluating care. Furthermore, the term *initial assessment* is clear only if there is a commonly understood definition of what constitutes a complete initial assessment in the hospital. Defining such criteria is no small chore. It requires both careful examination of the desired performance as well as skill in stating the resulting decisions.

The terms *standards* and *criteria* are used interchangeably here. Some authors use these terms to describe different levels of specificity. The words *goals* and *objectives* are also related and are frequently debated. The only importance of such discussion is to clarify the distinction between increasing levels of specificity in statements. There is relatively wide acceptance of the idea that goals, objectives, standards, and criteria describe increasing explicitness, with goals the most global and criteria the most specific statement of intent. It is worthwhile to clarify the general connotation of each of these terms in your agency as you begin to work with the idea in order to reduce miscommunication. One way of thinking about this relationship is depicted in Fig. 15.2. With each level of specificity, the potential number of statements increases. As a result, one goal may be reflected in many criterion statements.

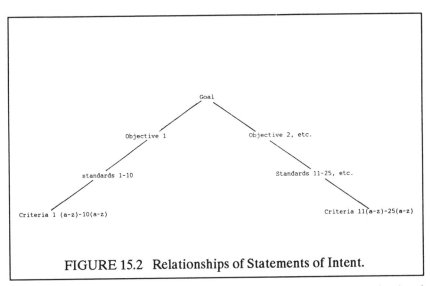

FIGURE 15.2   Relationships of Statements of Intent.

The potential number of statements increases with the increasing level of specificity.

Identify and Collect Relevant Information

The next phase in this general view of evaluation is the determination of what information is relevant for comparison with the criteria. In the case of the criterion mentioned above, necessary information would be whether the nurse has performed the assessment *and* the length of time that had elapsed after admission. Information about administration of medication would not be relevant in regard to that particular criterion. However, as you assemble all of the relevant criteria for evaluating care of patients on a unit, the medication data will very likely be relevant to one or more of the other standards. Therefore, this step may require identifying numerous bits of information that will need to be collected as the evaluation proceeds.

When you have listed all of the data that are necessary for the evaluation, the next step is developing some method for collecting the information. The purpose of this activity is to make some systematic and efficient plan for gaining the maximum amount of information with the minimum amount of effort. Examples of the tools or methods used in this phase are performance rating scales, quality assurance monitoring, and a plan for daily personnel supervision. These tools and methods are *not* the evaluation, although this is frequently how they are thought of. Rather, such tools are *aids* to gaining the information required to perform the evaluation. The distinction is important in order to point out that tools may be changed as criteria change or as more efficient tools are developed. Furthermore, the tools and methods must be chosen to reflect the information needed, not simply because they are in vogue. For example, it would be senseless to adapt an attractive new form for performance appraisal of registered nurses that seeks information on their abilities to supervise nurse assistants if your agency does not employ nurse assistants. Rather, your agency's choice of forms should reflect the current standards for personnel performance expected there.

Only some of the methods you will use for data collection will be forms. In addition to the right form, it is important to develop a systematic plan for making direct observations of care in progress, of personnel performance, or of whatever is being evaluated. It is all too easy to be so busy with your own assigned direct care activities that observing personnel or examining the quality of care becomes a "sometimes" occurrence. Another possibility is that observations may be made, but with no systematic plan. In that case they may address only certain criteria, usually those for which data are most readily available, and important aspects may thus be overlooked or forgotten.

The plan for collecting data may be relatively short-term, as when evaluating care on a unit using a monitoring method that samples the care of some patients monthly in order to make judgments about overall care. Or the plan may be long-term. For example, long-term plans may be developed for evaluating performance of nurse assistants during a six-month probationary employment period. Another possibility is a long-term self-evaluation plan that covers a year of your practice.

The actual collection of data is the next phase in this general view of evaluation. Of course, as with other processes, adjustments may be made during the actual collection of data. Perhaps you will alter your plan for observation of a nurse assistant's performance when you determine rather quickly that she has mastered many of the necessary skills. Maybe you will find that the data collection plan needs some refinement in order to speed up the procedure. As the information is collected and compiled, the next phase is entered. That is when the information about the actual performance or product is compared with the criteria.

Compare Data with Standards

Suppose that you examine the charts of 15 patients admitted during the past week. You are collecting data related to the admission assessment criterion mentioned above. When you complete your review, you have a tally of 10 records with assessment completed in less than 6 hours after admission. Five records show that assessment records were completed in from 8 to 48 hours after admission. Your *compare* that result with your standard and note that the standard is not met and identify the way in which it is not met. This simple act of comparison is repeated with all data and criteria. You now have a measure, although the degree of precision may be crude, of how performance or product reflects standards. It answers the "how," "how much," "how many," and "how often" questions. This does not, however, provide you with an *evaluative* statement. An evaluation of any sort results in a judgment regarding the quality or worth of the item or process under scrutiny, not only the *measurement* of the elements related to criteria.

Judgment Techniques

There are a number of approaches for arriving at a final judgment in evaluation. One is to set predetermined levels that represent adequate, excellent, or less than adequate quality (or quantity). The key point is that the judgment is made *prior* to the actual collection of data rather than after the facts are assembled. The number of scale points and the terms applied will vary. There may be five categories or two, or a percentage, or a raw score may be identified as being equal to "excellent" or"satisfactory". Any number of methods can be used as long as there is a clear understanding that the measurement does not automatically represent the judgment. There could be predetermined cut-off points related to the measurements that represent the evaluative judgments. When a predetermined judgment is used with the statement, "All newly admitted patients must have a complete initial assessment within 6 hours," the result might be any of the following, depending on your judgment:

1. Only 100 percent of standard will be adequate. Less that 100 percent is unsatisfactory.

2. 100 percent of standard is excellent, 90 percent is satisfactory, 80 percent is unsatisfactory.
3. All completed in less that 6 hours is excellent; all completed in 6-10 hours is satisfactory; less than all completed in any time period is unsatisfactory.

The possible combinations are numerous, but in each case, the evaluative judgment has been made *prior* to the collection of the data. As a result, situational problems are not likely to influence the decision, nor are problems of a "halo" or favorable bias likely to occur. This technique lends itself well to evaluations that will be repeated so that overall performance from one period to another can be compared.

When the evaluation is specific to the care of a particular patient, predetermined judgments may be less useful since no matter what judgment might be reached, other areas for improvement might still exist. So rather than pronounce a "satisfactory" and leave it at that, you might wish to make a specific *situational* evaluative judgment. This contrasts with the predetermined judgment in that factors other than simply the measured facts compared with the criteria are considered in making the judgment. For example, you may have reckoned that since a particular patient's emotional state is very depressed, his request to skip a bath and to go to the day room immediately after breakfast represents some improvement. If hygiene measures were being evaluated, that patient's care might well be substandard by a prejudgment method. Yet, using a situational decision, you might conclude that the overall care is good since it meets his individual needs that day.

As you can see, the two approaches-predetermined and situational-are similar in process but different in specific activity. This is appropriate since the specific purposes differ. Yet, in each case the steps in the evaluation are the same.

Analyze the Evaluation

A phase that is frequently overlooked is that of analyzing the evaluation as a whole. The purpose is to determine if the judgment reached was appropriate and complete. Critical questions to ask are the following:

1. Were the criteria sufficiently explicit and complete? Perhaps the evaluation overlooked important activities or outcomes because the criteria were not complete.

2. Were the correct data collected in the most efficient and effective manner? Maybe a judgment was reached with insufficient evidence, or possibly excessive amounts of time and money were spent in gaining information that was irrelevant.
3. Was the comparison of data with criteria performed objectively?
4. Is the evaluative judgment consistent with the previous phase?

It is not necessary that this analysis be performed each time an evaluation is done, but it should be frequent enough to provide a quality check on the evaluation activity.

Provide Appropriate Input

The phase represented by the input branch at the bottom of Fig. 15.1 is the action that determines whether evaluation of any sort is actually useful or whether it becomes a ritual. Evaluation is only worthwhile if the judgments are subsequently considered in decision making. Usually, the decision making to which evaluative information is most relevant is that aimed at improving performance or product. In nursing, the concern with improvement would be related both to performance by personnel and to the care rendered to a patient or group of patients. For that reason, evaluation judgments must be viewed as inputs for a new cycle of the management of nursing care. Personnel performance evaluation must be communicated to the worker, and group performance data must be analyzed for trends and for needed changes in policy, in management practice, or in staff development. Thus, evaluation of nursing care should provide the basis for activities designed to improve care through direct individual practice and through associated care management activities for groups of patients.

Methods of Evaluating Nursing Care

As a professional nurse, you will be expected to know not only the general steps in each phase of nursing management but also the current specific activities that are used in each phase. This is as true for the evaluation phase as it is for implementation or for any other phase. For this reason, the next several pages are devoted to providing information on techniques used in evaluation of care and in the evaluation of personnel performance, both of which areas are the concern of the professional nurse who is "manager and managed".

Over the past several years the nursing literature has contained increasing numbers of articles on the topic of evaluation of care. The focus of these articles has moved from concern with whether care *could* be evaluated, to increasingly complex *techniques* for doing the evaluation. The reasons for the change in focus are complex. They include: (1) an emerging concern in nursing for accountability for practice; (2) the recognition of the need for evidence of the effect of nursing care; (3) rising concern with the cost of health care; and (4) the mandates of the various agencies for hospital accreditation, including the Joint Commission on Accreditation of Healthcare Organizations and certain federal legislation, particularly PL92-603, which mandated review of care provided to recipients of Medicare and Medicaid.[1] The result of this growing interest in evaluation of nursing along with interest in other aspects of health care is the presence of a potentially (to be described below) confusing array of terms and techniques.

Nursing Care Evaluation and Quality Assurance

The several systems of evaluation that have been developed over the past few years are similar in that the general evaluation process as outlined in this chapter can be identified in each. One major change is that evaluation of nursing care now tends to be viewed as an element in a broader program of evaluation called Quality Assurance. Typically, in hospitals the nursing quality assurance activities are a part of an agency-wide program of quality assurance. This approach is consistent with standards of the JCAHO. Each of these programs is developed to meet the needs of the agency, but all have in common the assumption that the feedback from the quality assurance activities should be the basis for corrections in performance and/or change in procedure and policy designed to assure desirable quality. The methods used to evaluate nursing as part of this process will reflect the general process of evaluation described above. The differences among the approaches result from choices in three major areas; source, specificity, and type of criteria used; timing and methods of data collection; and the manner in which judgements are make. Table 15.1 describes these differences in more detail.

---

[1] Staff of Subcommittee on Health and Environment of the Committee on Interstate and Foreign Commerce of the U.S. House of Representatives, *A Discursive Dictionary of Health Care* (Washington, D.C.: U.S. Government Printing Office, 1976)p.119

TABLE 15.1 Basic Differences in Evaluation Systems

1.*Source, specificity, and type of criteria used.* Some systems focus on general criteria dealing primarily with the structure within which care is delivered and the process or action of the nurses giving care. Other systems combine very specific criteria about patient outcomes related to particular disease conditions with some process criteria about patient outcomes related to particular disease conditions with some process criteria. For the more general criteria, the source is a standard system from the literature augmented by local review and refinement. For the more specific disease-related standards, the source of criteria is the local review group. The standards are generated or collected from published material and are then ratified by the nursing staff whose work is to be evaluated.

2.*Timing and methods of data collection.* Some evaluation methods use a retrospective review of the patient or family record as the only approach to data collection. These reviews are referred to as *audits.* Other evaluation methods use a concurrent combination of review of records and care in progress, whereas still other methods combine a retrospective review with a concurrent chart analysis for problem areas. In each case the data are collected and analyzed, at least in part, by professional nurses who are oriented to the method in order to provide reliable data collection.

3.*The manner in which judgments are made.* In each of the more formalized methods, judgments are made prior to the collection of data. Either numerical scores or totals of appropriate answers are related to decision categories such as "unsatisfactory" or "excellent." Situational judgments are more often used in "homemade" systems of evaluation or in informal unit level activities.

The history of the development of evaluation of nursing care has seen trends moving from the use of retrospective review of patient records to concurrent approaches; from a focus on criteria related to the *process* of care, to the outcomes and structures associated with care. Current methods seem to combine approaches, with the emphasis placed on creating programs of evaluations which are flexible and can result in feedback to the direct care level.

In *A Guide to JCAH Nursing Service Standards*[2], the seven required characteristics of nursing department monitoring and evaluation activities are listed. You will note that these characteristics *do not* outline a single standard program for evaluation, but describe characteristics which a program must have to be acceptable. The are:

- planned, systematic, ongoing activities to provide an organized method to determine if care is acceptable at any given time
- comprehensive
- based on indicators and criteria agreed to by staff
- use routine collection and periodic evaluation of data

2 Pattersen, C., D. Kranz, and B. Brandt *A Guide to JCAH Nursing Services Standards* (Chicago, Illinois: Joint Commission in Accreditation of Hospitals, 1987)p.145.

- result in appropriate corrective action
- are continuous
- are part of the hospital wide QA program

Quality Assurance - Your Role

A typical view of quality assurance activities at the direct care level is that from time to time one will be asked to participate in data collection, to audit records or care in progress in regard to one or more standards of care. For example, the unit's plan may specify that a weekly review of a sample of current records will be conducted in regard to at least two standards of care. On your unit staff nurses rotate the assignment for data collection. The standards chosen for this week's review are "(1) Each patient has an admission assessment documented by the assigned primary nurse within sixteen hours of admission and (2) Each patient who is conscious and able participates in developing the plan of care."

Suppose the requirement of the evaluation plan is that you sample 30 percent of the patients. Thus, you have criteria (the standard) and an initial element of your data collection plan identified. Identifying the patients whose care will be sampled could be by random choice or by some prescribed method. Other choices to be made regarding data collection include what data will be relevant. For example, will only the narrative chart be considered appropriate data for standard 1 or will a flow sheet also be considered? Will the patient be asked a set of standard questions regarding standard 2? What are the possible categories of data based on the evaluator's response? (categories called criteria met, not met, partially met, not applicable, are often used, but some standards can only be met or not with no partial category acceptable.)

As a data collector, you may encounter a major ethical concern. That is, when you are collecting data from patients and identify a problem with care, do you correct it immediately or simply note it? If you correct it, do you identify the unmet criterion or note it as met? The concern for validity and reliability of data collection must be balanced against the immediate concerns for patient well-being.

When the sampling and critical review of care is complete, the results are calculated. The data are compiled for annual statisical purposes and to review for possible trends. The feedback from the specific review is the basis for direct feedback to the unit personnel. The Manager (Head Nurse or other title) is responsible in most Quality Assurance programs for developing and putting in place any needed corrective action as well as for relaying positive feedback for good results.

Another way in which Quality Assurance Programs may vary among health care facilities is the degree of centralization of the QA function and its various activities. In one extremely centralized program, decisions about all program aspects will be made at a central level, with some involvement of nurse managers for input into the decision. In a unit-based system, the central QA staff will serve to guide process and to facilitate data compilation, primarily. This latter approach is consistent with efforts to decentralize decisions about patient care to the delivery level, a strategy consistent with promoting individual professional nurse accountability.

Computerization offers a way to deal efficiently with the mass of data that are collected in the QA evaluation processes. A standard database program can be tailored to compile the data and provide reports that will show change over months or years. With the power available in microcomputers, a personal computer rather than a large mainframe is all that will be required to manage the information. A review of health related software vendors indicates that development of data management programs for quality assurance is an area of current development. This supercedes an interest in centralized evaluation systems designed to manage the evaluation process, such as the Rush-Medicus System.[3]

Given the concern of the public for quality in health care, the increasingly litigation-conscious health care consumer, and the increasing complexity of care, it is to be expected that the emphasis on monitoring quality will continue. As the major accrediting agency, JCAHO will exert a great influence on the type and extent of processes used to perform this monitoring via the commentary of its accreditation teams and its official publications. As a professional nurse, knowledge of current accreditation requirements and of the concept of the process of evaluation will prepare you to understand the methods used in the facility where you work. Your leadership will be an important factor in demonstrating to colleagues that there is value to participating in the evaluation process and using the feedback it provides.

Evaluating Personnel Performance

The general evaluation process described earlier in this chapter is a useful framework for analyzing and understanding methods that are used for personnel performance evaluation. In this section you will look at

3 Richard C. Jelinek et al. *A Methodology for Monitoring Quality of Nursing Care* (Bethesda, Md:U.S. Department of Health, Education, and Welfare, Division of Nursing, 1974).

performance appraisal activities from two perspectives, that of the evaluator as well as that of the recipient of an appraisal.

Purposes of Performance Evaluation

Typically, organized nursing services have a regular schedule for the completion of an evaluation summary for each employee. The schedule will very likely require one or more formal reviews during the first six months of employment, a review at one year, and yearly thereafter. The early reviews frequently coincide with a probationary employment period. The specific terms of the probationary period vary from agency to agency, but the assumption is that for a period of a few months, the new employee is learning to function in a new organization.

A variety of systems, forms, and results are found among the many approaches to personnel performance appraisals. However, there is a good deal of similarity in the purposes for which these systems are developed, although some agencies may identify only a few of these purposes. Table 15.2 lists the most common reasons for the presence of an ongoing personnel appraisal system.

Table 15.2 Purposes for an Ongoing Personnel Appraisal System

1. To provide information to the employee about performance in order for improvement to occur.
2. To provide information that can serve as a reward and positive reinforcement for good performance.
3. To identify personnel for potential development and promotion or additional responsibilities or other positions.
4. To document the performance basis for salary increases.
5. To document the basis for demotion or terminations.
6. To provide data for development of inservice education activities.
7. To formalize communication between supervisor and employee about job expectations and performance.
8. To promote overall high-quality performance within the organization toward its goals.

The purposes accepted for performance review in the agency should be stated since these purposes will determine logical choices of methods for the system. If you find, as one new to the work setting, that these purposes are not stated or that you have not been informed of them, do not hesitate to ask. It is an important question since you are certain to be evaluated and may be responsible for the evaluation of others as well.

The evaluation *should* provide feedback about how well an employee is performing, fitting in with the expectations of the nursing service. At the best, performance evaluation can be very helpful in encouraging and stimulating improved performance. At the worst, it can become a time-consuming ritual. The key to which direction the evaluation system takes is the attitude of the participants. If, as recipient of the evaluation, you accept both positive and negative feedback gracefully, and if you make efforts to use the suggestions you receive, the process will be helpful to you in your professional development. Your willingness to participate in evaluation in this positive manner will also be affected by the way in which your supervisor approaches the activity. If it seems that she gives little thought to the ratings, if all areas are rated the same, if the review is discussed with you in a superficial way, or if you know that there have been no systematic observations of your work, the performance appraisal will be of little value to you. It follows that when you are in a position to evaluate another's performance, your approach could well have the same effect. You can make the evaluation experience of the highly motivated employee very positive, and a positive approach can certainly do no harm even with the minimally motivated worker.

The Criteria

Recall the general evaluation process. You will note that the initial phase in developing any evaluation system (as well as understanding one) is to identify the criteria that serve as standards for the evaluation. The source for performance appraisal criteria must be the job description. This means that the expectation of each position must be identified before a useful appraisal can be developed. This excludes the use of abstract personal traits as elements of the evaluation.

Joann Marshall and Edward Schau described the development of criteria and subsequent creation of a method for evaluating the performance of nursing assistants.[4] The criterion development was focused on carefully analyzing the elements of good job performance and deriving behavioral statements that reflected such performance. Evaluation scales using this process are described as Behaviorally Anchored Rating Scales. A behavioral statement is one that supplies a description of the desired action in explicit terms. In this way, a performance area such as "independent action" is converted to a series of statements that describe typical activities in which

---

4 Joann Marshall and Edward Schau,"An Evaluation Process for Nursing Assistants," in *Quality Control and Performance Appraisal*, Vol. 2 (Wakefield, Mass: Contemporary Publishing, 1976),pp.2-25.

independent action is demonstrated. An example is: "Identifies unassigned work tasks on unit and completes them voluntarily." The resulting statements are then organized by category on a form that can be used to summarize the evaluation.

Another approach to criterion development is one that is consistent with Management by Objectives (MBO). This approach is especially useful when the job being considered is one in which the employee has a relatively high degree of control over work that is not highly structured or routine. The position of head nurse or other administrative positions are examples. With the MBO approach, the employee meets with the immediate supervisor to plan goals and specific criteria for the next evaluation period. These criteria are to reflect the organization's job objectives and must be stated in terms that the employee and supervisor can understand in order to evaluate subsequent performance.

It is common to state these objectives/criteria as descriptions of outcome rather than as processes or activities. The reason for this is that the persons in positions for which the approach is used will generally use a variety of techniques and will work with and through others to accomplish their objectives. This is in contrast to the workers whose functions are generally evaluated by criteria that focus on the processes or manner in which more routine work is accomplished.

The development of these objectives and their approval by the supervisor is intended to be a two-way process, with negotiation being used to arrive at mutually agreeable expectations. In some agencies, an adaptation of this approach is used. This involves requiring that the general job description be used as a guide for developing one or more objectives in each area of job responsibility.

Whatever the specific approach, there are at least *three* primary concerns that must be kept in mind in considering the criteria used for performance evaluation. These are listed in Table 15.3.

TABLE 15.3 Three Primary Concerns for Performance Evaluation

1. The criteria chosen should reflect the purpose of the evaluation activity. These purposes may include improvement of performance, decisions about pay, decisions about promotion, and others.
2. The criteria should be directly related in the job requirements.
3. The criteria must be stated in terms clearly understood by both employee and evaluator *before* the evaluation period.

Methods for Collecting and Using the Data
for Performance Evaluation

The most obvious, valid method of collecting the data that will be compared with performance criteria is direct observation. Certainly, there is no substitute for eyewitness accounts of the process or outcomes of an employee's work. The need for some means of accurately recalling these observations has led to the use of "critical incident reports" or "anecdotal notes." These were described in Chapter 14. Because these notes include a variety of observations, collected over time, it is possible to form impressions about overall performance based on the facts. At the time an observation is made, no evaluation is attached. Rather, the circumstances and observations are recorded as succinctly as possible. The disadvantage of this method of data collection is the amount of time required to make the notes. However, this problem is offset by the quality of information available for developing improved performance. Of course, if the performance observed is obviously substandard or technically incorrect, immediate action must be taken to correct the problem. Without a routine of collecting anecdotal records, all the supervisor has at evaluation time is the written counseling that accompanied a remedial action and a few vague "impressions" of observations.

The person being evaluated can also collect data for the performance appraisal. This method is most useful when the criteria specify outcomes, but it can also be used when processes are the focus of the appraisal. For example, you might collect your own description of ways in which you taught several patients and combine these with chart audit information about those patients. You could then supply this as a part of the data for your own evaluation when teaching activity is a relevant criterion. Some authors recommend having an employee complete an entire copy of her own evaluation form, covering each area of the appraisal. This is based on the idea that the employee can both provide basic information about performance and make judgments about that performance.

Another source of data for performance evaluation is the patient or his family. However, this should not be viewed as a primary data source since many factors can confound the type of information that a patient or family may provide about care received. But this is no reason to overlook this as a source of unsolicited information in the form of both positive and negative input.

The forms used to compile the collected observation and judgments vary widely. Some have little structure, leaving opportunity to create a narrative related to each job performance area. This is compatible with the MBO approach described above. Other forms provide rating scales developed to describe degrees of accomplishment in each criterion area. The various levels of accomplishment may also have numerical values attached, and each separate area may be weighted. The more elaborate the rating and weighting scheme, the greater is the need for proper instruments or tools to establish validity and reliability.

In addition to the need for properly developed rating forms, there is a need to provide training in the use of the specific forms, data collection methods, and all other activities in the evaluation process. Even though many nurses who are responsible for evaluating other personnel will be acquainted with the general process of evaluation, it is important to establish that they understand the specific procedures associated with the forms in the agency. Unless this is assured, both validity and reliablity of the ratings will be questionable.

The most difficult part of using the evaluation method is making a judgment, based on observations, of just what rating will be assigned or what sort of narrative statement will be composed. The main concerns must be objectivity (Is the person being judged fairly, on the same basis as others in the same job?) and accuracy (Do the observations support that there are facts upon which to base the judgement?). It is tempting to simply mark "good" or "above average" on all blanks or to develop an entirely complimentary narrative. Although this may not damage the individual's personnel file, such an evaluation does not give accurate feedback for improvement either. Knowing that objectivity and accuracy are important concerns and acting in accord with them can prompt the evaluator to develop a fair and useful evaluation.

Evaluative Counseling

When the general evaluation process is applied to personnel evaluation, the final phase is when the employee is provided with the evaluation. Just as in evaluation of the quality of care, the evaluation is of little value unless it is communicated to the person or persons who can make changes. From your perspective as a *recipient* of evaluation, you can probably appreciate the anxiety that a counseling discussion can generate. As mentioned earlier, it is important to approach the session with a constructive attitude if you want to gain useful information. Likewise, when you are the person who is communicating the evaluation results, your approach must be positive and constructive. In either position, it is helpful to keep in mind that the performance, not the person, is the focus of the evaluation.

There are some guidelines for counseling activities that can prove helpful in making the session productive. These are presented in Table 15.4. As you read, keep in mind that practice will help prepare you to be the evaluator in such sessions. Role-playing this activity can be very useful in providing that practice. It is not necessary to reserve role-playing for students or for classroom use only. Ask a friend to be your "employee", set the scene, and begin. Be sure to refrain from using the actual employee's name in order to maintain confidentiality. When you are through, each of you can analyze the activity and the feelings of each participant.

TABLE 15.4 Guidelines for Evaluative Counseling Sessions

1.Notify the employee in advance of the time, place, and purpose for the meeting. If you have had an ongoing supervisory relationship with the employee since the last evaluation, you may have invited her to prepare for self-evaluation at this time. The employee needs time to prepare if she is bringing evaluative data. If the employee has not been asked to bring evaluative data, one day's advance notice is the minimum for adequate notification.

2.Choose a time that will permit an unhurried, thorough discussion for both participants. If you schedule a meeting at peak hours, you may notice that the employee is distracted and seems only interested in finishing the conversation, or that you feel pressure to attend to other matters yourself.

3.Schedule the meeting in a private place. Interruptions are common in many patient care areas. If it is at all possible, the meeting should be away from the work area in a private office.

4.Plan the discussion so that you know the main points you intend to mention and the general order in which you will proceed, including a summary at the close of the conference. The summary should include the main points mentioned and any plans that you have for improved performance. You should also plan to get feedback from the employee, which will let you know what she has understood and what plans she has for improving her performance. It takes great restraint to keep from simply asking, "Do you understand?" Or "Do you agree?" However, such yes/no questions give no opportunity to hear the employee state, in her own words, her understanding of the content of the conference.

5.The employee should see the form on which the evaluation is completed. One way to do this is to place the form so that you are both able to see each section as it is discussed. Most evaluation systems require that the employee and supervisor both sign the evaluation form to indicate that the conference has been held. In some cases there is also a requirement for a review of the rating by a person at the next supervisory level. Also, should the employee disagree with the rating, most systems have a plan for an appeal of the rating at the review level. If the disagreement is not to be settled at that level, there is typically a grievance procedure available to the employee.

6.Finally, you should assure that each employee's evaluation is properly confidential. Only those supervisory personnel who have a need to know should have access to the form on which the rating is compiled. Although you may verbally assure the employee that this confidentiality exists, she may doubt it if she is allowed to see others' ratings lying about in full view. Keep your materials in a safe, private place.

Other Feedback from the Evaluation Process

The counseling session provides the most direct feedback from the evaluation process. However, it is not the only kind of feedback that is useful. There are two other kinds of information that can be derived from the personnel evaluation process. The first is information about job-related learning needs. Statements of individual needs for education can be deduced from the individual evaluation summary and can be validated with the employees. Also, when you consider the evaluation of several employees with whom you work, you may note that there are similar needs for learning among the group. If there are indications of educational needs, the person(s) responsible for providing or assisting in developing staff education can be helpful in planning ways to provide the necessary learning activities.

The other kind of useful feedback from personnel evaluation is that directed toward improving the evaluation system itself. As with the evaluation of care, every phase of the evaluation activity should be examined in light of the information the process provides. For example, when you have considered every criterion and have given a rating to an employee, yet "feel" that you have left something out, you need to see if other criteria need to be included. Or if you find that the form used to compile the evaluation is difficult to understand, you should take action. There are several directions that this type of feedback may take. You may speak directly to your supervisor, or you may decide to write your comments and suggestions to your supervisor with copies sent to the personnel department. Perhaps there is a staff nurses' organization in your agency. One way to gain support for a change in the evaluation system is to discuss the matter with this group and move for the group to recommend revision of the evaluation system.

There are many ways to initiate action, depending on the agency. The way you choose should be based on your knowledge of formal organizational channels of communication, the amount of anticipated resistance to the suggestion, your own power base and comfort with the issue, and the importance or urgency you place on the issue. The best source of information for improvement in evaluation procedures is this type of feedback. As either evaluator or recipient of evaluations, it is your responsibility to provide this feedback.

A Current Issue In Performance Evaluation - Peer Review

The personnel evaluation activities described above are appropriate in organizations where a typical hierarchy exists within the nursing department. This means that there is at least one "layer" of persons who are responsible for supervising the performance of others who work there. The number of levels of supervisors and the number and types of personnel will vary depending on the size and type of organization. But, whether the structure is flat or tall, a common factor is that those at one level report to and are supervised by a person at another level. This relationship is widely accepted as being appropriate for assuring coordination among the actions of various workers and for controlling (evaluating) both work and workers.

The tradition of autonomy of professionals is not at all consonant with their functioning in a hierarchical structure. The occupational groups that have been historically recognized as professional, notably law and medicine, have served as the model for definitions of "professional". One distinguishing characteristic of these occupations has been the autonomy of the group as a whole as well as the independent status of the practitioner. The resulting ability to control one's own standards and methods of practice is seen as appropriate since the professional fields require use of a body of knowledge that is not acquired by those outside the field. The traditional method of evaluation of practice in these fields has been self-evaluation and loosely structured peer evaluation through voluntary organization. This method of evaluation, along with a strong focus on internalizing an ethic of primary concern for the well-being of the patient or client and of personal responsibility for the consequences of one's practice, was for many years the only mechanism for internal controls on quality of practice.

Nursing as an occupation has had a different evolution than medicine or law. The exclusivity of a field of knowledge was not a hallmark of early nursing. Nursing was, to begin with, simply an extension of the activities performed by families and others for those who were ill. Over the years, the special knowledge of the field of nursing has grown. Along with this, there has been increasing concern for achieving for nursing the recognition of some of the same aspects of professional practice as are recognized in other professional fields. Among these aspects has been the achievement of professional control of practice, that is, more autonomous practice. The creation of methods for peer review to replace or augment agency or organizational evaluation as described above has been proposed as one way to achieve the desired autonomy. It remains to be seen whether: (1) peer review promotes autonomy, (2) autonomy increases individual accountability, or (3) whether either is compatible with high-quality nursing care. Research on these issues is needed. At the same time, as a practitioner it is important for you to be acquainted with the methods that are typically proposed for nursing peer review. As mentioned in Chapter 13, efforts to promote shared governance are likely to include a peer review system, at least a portion of which will focus on personnel evaluation activities. To function effectively in such a system will require an understanding of the advantages and potential disadvantages of such arrangements.

The main problem faced in developing a peer review system for nursing is the problem encountered when an attempt is made to model the system on the one currently used for medicine. Peer review in medicine is accomplished through the review of the diagnosis and treatment of patients, using the medical record as the source of information. The medical quality assurance program is a formalized version of this technique, now institutionalized in order to meet federal reimbursement requirements.

For some, the nursing quality assurance program is also viewed as a peer review mechanism. This is a legitimate notion when staff- level personnel participate in the process at each step. However, due to the manner in which nursing practice is structured, the nursing quality assurance program is not generally equivalent to a peer review of individual performances. The nature of nursing practice is currently such that groups of nurses care for any particular patient. Under such circumstances, the review of the care given by an individual nurse is difficult to accomplish through the typical review performed in quality assurance system. In circumstances where there is a one nurse-one patient relationship, such as in community health or in agencies where one nurse is a patient's primary nurse, this type of review is more realistic. Another confounding factor is that in many nursing settings, direct care of patients is only a part of the responsibility ascribed to the nurse. She may be expected to provide supervision or coordination for other levels of personnel and to consult with other professional nurses. For this reason, review of care will not constitute review of the total realm of the nurse's responsibility. It is obvious that for peer review to be useful, the activity must be consistent with the purpose for which it is developed and with the mode of practice in the individual setting.

The first concern then must be to understand the purpose for which peer review is chosen. Simply to emulate another professional group is insufficient reason to prompt any activity. If *increased* professional autonomy and accountability are the desired outcome, peer review can then be considered, along with other options, as a possible method for achieving this objective. Strictly speaking, the general evaluation process described earlier in this chapter can serve as a guide for the development of a peer evaluation system just as for any other evaluation. The key element is that if *peer* evaluation is what is being designed, the process will focus on the involvement of peers in the process rather than supervisors. The relationship of the peer review to organizational structure must be carefully thought out, and the system preferably should be pilot-tested before any large-scale adoption is planned.

Assuming that it is demonstrated that there are positive outcomes from peer review techniques either for nursing as a profession or for the nurses practicing in a particular agency it is useful to consider some of the problems that may be anticipated as such a system is developed. One of the first difficulties to be overcome is the lack of practice that nurses have in peer evaluation activities. The educational process in nursing seldom focuses on peer evaluation as a professional requirement, and actual practice in peer evaluation is even less often provided. Therefore, since peer evaluation is unfamiliar, some may hesitate or do a poor job when they participate. A second obstacle is that many individuals are either unwilling or unable to criticize another's performance directly to that person. This prompts a tendency to "downplay" any negative comments. Thus, the evaluation becomes a polite ritual, useless and time-consuming. A third factor that must be dealt with is the fact that peer review, if used as an adjunct to or replacement for a supervisory action may threaten the persons in those supervisory positions and may prompt their resistance.

It is clear that instituting a system of peer review that focuses on individual performance will be more difficult than developing a peer level review of care reflecting a group's efforts. There is growing support for the idea that both are important for the improvement of the professional practice of nursing. Only careful evaluation of pilot projects will provide the answer.

SUMMARY

The evaluation phase of management in nursing involves evaluation of the nursing care rendered as well as evaluation of the performance of personnel who provide care. The first half of the chapter has presented an "all-purpose" process of evaluation, followed by specific discussion of some programs and techniques for the evaluation of care. The second half of the chapter deals with the evaluation of personnel performance from two perspectives, that of the evaluator and that of the recipient of the appraisal.

The general process of evaluation is composed of the following steps: identification of criteria or standards; collection of relevant data; comparison of data with standards; making an evaluative judgment; provision of appropriate input; and uses of feedback, including evaluative counseling; and evaluation and change of the system itself.

Additional Reading

Blanton, Nina E., Mary Jane Bogner, Helen L. Collins, Jo Ann Futrell, Suzanne Lagina and Alice Rolison, "Putting Peer Review Into Practice", *American Journal of Nursing*,85:11 (Nov.,1985)1284-1287.

Council, Jan D. and Roger J. Plachy, "Performance Appraisal is Not Enough", *Journal of Nursing Administration*,80:10 (October,1980)20-26.

Coyne, Christine and Marcia Killien, "A System for Unit-Based Monitors of Quality of Nursing Care",*Journal of Nursing Administration*,17:1 (January,1987)26-32.

Davis, Sallie E., "A Professional Recognition System Using Peer Review", *Journal of Nursing Administration*, 17:11 (November,1987)34-38.

Edmunds, Linda. "A Computer Assisted Quality Assurance Model", *Journal of Nursing Administration*, 13:3 (March,1983)36-43.

Harrington, Patricia and Nancy Koniecki. "Standards and QA - A Common Sense Approach" *Nursing Management* 19:1(January,1988)24-27.

Hastings, Clare E. "Measuring Quality in Ambulatory Care Nursing" *Journal of Nursing Administration*,17:4 (April,1987)12-20.

Hughes, Florence S. Y. "Quality Assurance in Home Care Services" *Nursing Management*, 18:12 (Dec,1987)33- 36.

Lachman, Vicki D. "Increasing Productivity Through Performance Evaluation"*Journal of Nursing Administration*, 14:12 (December,1984)7-14.

Lawler, Theresa G. "The Objectives of Performance Appraisal - or Where Can We Go From Here?",*Nursing Management*, 19:3 (March,1988)82-88.

Nauright, Lynda "Toward a Comprehensive Personnel System: Performance Appraisal - Part IV", *Nursing Management*, 18:8 (August,1987)67-77.

O'Brien, Barbara. "QA: A Commitment to Excellence" *Nursing Management*, 19:11(Nov.,1988)33-40

Pelle, Denise and Leonard Greenhalgh. "Developing the Performance Appraisal System", *Nursing Management*, 18:12 (December,1987)37-44.

Purgatorio - Howard, Kathy, "Improving a Quality Assurance Program" *Nursing Management*, 17:4 (April,1986)38-42.

Smeltzer, Carolyn H.,Barbara Feltman and Karen Rajki. "Nursing Quality Assurance: A Process, Not a Tool" *Journal of Nursing Administration*, 13:1 (January,1983)5-9.

Verran, Joyce. "Patient Classification in Ambulatory Care" *Nursing Economics*, 4:5 (Sept/Oct,1986)247-251.

Wright, Dominique "An Introduction to the Evaluation of Nursing Care: A Review of the Literature" *Journal of Advanced Nursing*, 9(1984)457-467.

Chapter 16

Staff development

The words *staff development* have always brought to my mind an image of a group of personnel engaged in calisthenics. My immediate connotation of "development" is one of gaining strength and maturity. In many ways, staff development is similar to the image it inspires since it comprises educational activities directed toward increasing the ability of the staff to function with greater competence and/or to move to new positions or functions within the organization. The term *inservice education* is frequently used interchangeably with staff development. For some people, however, inservice education has come to mean something more circumscribed than staff development, in that inservice is viewed as being conducted only within and by the agency for which one works. By contrast, staff development may use learning activities conducted either in or outside the agency, depending on the learning need that is to be met. In each case, what distinguishes staff development and inservice education from other sorts of educational activities is the *intent*; that is, the purpose of both is to improve the ability of the learner to function on the job.

There are times when you are a student in a basic nursing program when you feel that you will never want to learn another thing. All you want is to be finished with school and to practice as a "real nurse". But the first job and each position thereafter make each of us a learner once again. There is a need to learn about the employing agency and its policies, organization, and procedures, and even the floor plan and the fire drill activities. As a new technique or new equipment is available, new skills must be learned. As one set of functions is mastered, you may wish to move to another set in order to expand your ability or to maintain your interest. Staff development can help by providing the learning activity for each of these learning needs.

Educational Activities After the Basics

Just as inservice eduction and staff development are members of the same class, so is the term *continuing education*. However, it is a term with a much broader meaning than the other two. The idea of continuing education grew from the adult education field. The idea that the adult needs access to a variety of learning experiences, even though formal schooling is completed, is the basis for the concept of continuing education. The topics of adult education cover every conceivable subject. It is intended that these "lifelong learning" experiences should provide skills and knowledge for better living, making it possible for a person to keep pace in a rapidly changing world. The same principle is the basis for continuing education in nursing, a specialized form of adult education. The field of nursing changes so rapidly that much of one's knowledge can become obsolete in five years or less.

Figure 16.1 depicts the relationship among continuing education in nursing, inservice education, and staff development. Notice that staff development encompasses inservice activities and makes use of external continuing education opportunities to provide for the staff member's increased knowledge.

Because nursing is a human service occupation, its practitioners have accepted the responsibility of providing this service at the highest level of excellence. For this reason, schools of nursing, the professional organizations, and in many states the legal agencies regulating nursing (state boards) all emphasize the need for continuing one's education as a necessary part of the professional life of a nurse. Because of public concern for quality of health care practice, some state boards regulating nursing practice have statutes or rules requiring continuing education for relicensure.

This continuing education can be conducted in the work agency as inservice education, or it can be generated to meet the needs of an audience wider than the employees of one agency. Continuing education can be provided as short-term workshops, semester- length courses, independent study, or programmed instruction, to mention a few methods. Some continuing education efforts in nursing are exploring the use of problem-oriented consultation as a method of offering continuing education. Due to the large interest in continuing education among nurses, it is likely that other new forms of continuing education delivery will be developed. The array of offerings is becoming more and more extensive, with professional journal companies sponsoring national workshops, private companies developing "packages" of seminars, professional organizations sponsoring special-focus programs, and colleges and universities attempting to serve their constituencies.

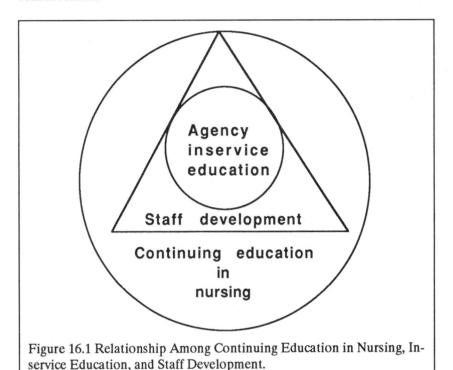

Figure 16.1 Relationship Among Continuing Education in Nursing, In-service Education, and Staff Development.

The need for continuing education in nursing has been accepted more as a result of belief in education generally than from consistent research evidence that it causes changes in practice. One investigator noted that even though the nurses in her study showed gains in knowledge, there was no significant change in the behavior described in the "practice" objective of the experimental course.[1]. Her explanation is that for practice behavior to change, knowledge is necessary but not sufficient and that the key lies in the reward structure of the practice environment. In this study, nurses demonstrated on tests that they knew more about medication following a course and that they were better able to question medication orders than was true

[1] Dorothy del Bueno, "Continuing Education, Spinach, and Other Good Things," *Journal of Nursing Administration*, 7 (April 1977),32-24

before the course; yet these same nurses showed no change in actually giving medication information to patients, the desired practice change.

You, as the consumer of continuing education, can make careful use of the variety of opportunities to build a very useful professional experience. To do so, you will need to have learned how to be a self-directed learner. Since staff-development is a particular position-focused sort of continuing education, the following paragraphs describe how you can participate in staff development in this self-directed fashion. This behavior can serve as a model for your whole continuing education program. The information should also acquaint you with what you might expect from staff development in your agency.

Staff Development Organization and Purpose

The staff development function in health care agencies can be organized in several ways. In some large hospitals, there is a separate department that provides educational experiences for all personnel, including nursing services. This same hospital-wide approach may be used when staff development is a function of the personnel department. The staff development function for nursing may also be placed in the nursing department. Some nursing departments may define the staff development personnel as consultative, with head nurses or clinical specialists deemed responsible for developing the actual staff development activities. Others have a large complement of staff development personnel who develop, implement, and evaluate the educational offerings. As with other questions of organization, there is no single correct answer. The decisions about how to structure the staff development function should be made with the following factors in mind:

1. The philosophy and objectives of the nursing service should be complemented by the structure.
2. The staff development function should be accomplished as efficiently, economically, and effectively as possible.
3. Nurses should be participants in the planning, implementation, and evaluation of the offerings for nursing personnel.

As an employee, new to an agency, it is to your benefit to identify the structure through which staff development is provided. This information is basic to your becoming an active self-directed participant. And when you are responsible for the work of others, you will need to assist with identifying needs for learning indicated by their performance or interest. Therefore you will need to have knowledge about the structure and services available to help these learners as well.

As mentioned earlier, staff development is a specialized form of continuing education in nursing. As such, it is a special form of adult education. This field has been improved in recent decades by research on the nature of adult learning and related education techniques. Some of the elements that distinguish the adult learner and his education from the young student and his schooling have been described by Malcolm Knowles in his book *The Modern Practice of Adult Education.*[2] His assumptions about the behavior of an adult learner are listed in Table 16.1.

TABLE 16.1 Assumptions about Behavior of an Adult Learner

1.As a person matures, self-concept moves from one of being dependent toward one of being a self-directed human being.

2.He accumulates a growing reservoir of experience that becomes an increasing resource for learning.

3.His readiness to learn becomes oriented increasingly to the development tasks of his social roles.

4.His time perspective changes from one of postponed application to immediate application.

From Malcolm Knowles, *The Modern Practice of Adult Education* (Chicago: Association Press, 1980)p.43-45.

On the assumption that the adult has certain learning characteristics, such as shown in Table 16.1, educators have proposed specific approaches to teaching adults. These methods are designed to capitalize on the readiness that springs from a problem-centered or self-perceived learning need. This suggests that the learner should be a participant in planning the educational experience. Other "adult-ed" methods include extensive use of discussion techniques, group activities, and problem-solving sessions. Lecture presentations, when used, should be thoroughly laced with real-life examples or descriptions of the potential application of the material. In each case, the key is involvement of the learner in activities that he can see as relevant to his present life. The assumptions in Table 16.1 about adult learners seem plausible enough; yet it is probably inaccurate to view any of them as "all or none" conditions. Rather, it is more likely that at any particular time a person can be viewed as more or less self- directed, more or less in possession of a reservoir of experience, somewhere on a continuum

[2] Malcolm Knowles, *The Modern Practice of Adult Education* (Chicago: Association Press, 1980)p.43-45.

of concern with one or more tasks of social development, and varying in willingness to postpone application of learning. This view of the adult as functioning somewhere along a continuum as the "model" adult learner offers insight about how to proceed as a learner or as one assisting other adults in meeting job-related learning needs. That is, the adult learner model and the techniques that are proposed to fit it will be effective only to the extent that the learners are accustomed to pursuing learning in a self-directed manner.

Many nurses who have just completed their basic nursing program will be unaccustomed to having learning activities presented according to the adult education principles. In many nursing programs there is some discussion of the need for students to develop the ability to be self-directed learners. However, it is relatively seldom that active effort is devoted to systematically aiding students in developing that ability. As a result, you may experience some concern that staff development conducted according to adult education principles is not "real education." However, as a practicing professional, you will find that directing your own continuing education, using staff development, can be the "most real," most meaningful learning you will do. Since self-direction in learning is a key to making the best use of staff development and other continuing education in nursing, the next section will focus on that approach to learning.

Self-Direction in Learning-A Key to Making Staff Development Work for You

Before going farther, a definition of self-direction in learning should be stated, to clarify its use in this text. *Self- directed learning* is defined as an approach to learning in which the learner chooses what, how, when, where, and to what extent he will learn. The degree to which a learner functions in this manner may depend on personal attributes and motivation, his physical ability to perceive, his cognitive ability to gain and process information, and factors determined by the teacher and/or school if the learner is in a school setting or the environment in general if the learner is not in a formally designed learning situation. The *prime element* in self-directed learning is that the student retains choice or control (to some degree) over what is studied as well as when and how.

Individualized learning and *individualized instruction* are terms that are frequently related to self- direction. Individualization refers to attempts to tailor content and methods to learning needs and to the learning style of the individual learner. There is, however, no necessity in this approach that the student be "in charge" of the learning process. In fact, much of the literature in this area speaks to the teacher's role as one of diagnosing learning needs and prescribing appropriate activities, followed by evaluating the learner's performance. Therefore, although individualization is an important concern in educational efforts, it is not the same as self-directed learning.

Given this contrast, the image of self-directed learning is sharpened. It is clearly imperative that for learning to be self- directed, the learner must be "in charge" of at least some portion of one or more of the elements of learning-the what, when, how, and how much of learning. The greater the learner's control, the more self-directed the learning is. What is not clear from the definition and contrast with individualization is whether there is some particular type of learner behavior that comprises *effective* self-directed learning. Surely, anyone can choose to perceive herself as "in charge" of her own learning. But what sort of actions by the learner are likely to result in satisfying, effective gains in knowledge and skill? Since the primary element in self-direction is decision making, it seems that gaining the ability to be self-directed would require three factors: (1) skill in decision making, (2) a knowledge of a systematic process for acquiring learning, and (3) a continually growing store of information about available resources for learning.

This least commonly considered of these factors-a systematic process for learning-will be discussed here, along with a warning. The warning comes first. As you learn to be more self-directed in learning, it is tempting to prescribe that behavior and the underlying attitude of personal responsibility are the desired state for *everyone*. Yet you must recall that the desire, willingness, or ability to function in this fashion depend on a number of factors. To expect everyone to function at the same level of self-direction is to deny that individual differences exist. This attitude is just as rigid as the one that expects that adult learners should behave like child learners. Enough for the warning. There are probably numerous ways to be systematic in your efforts at learning. The sequence of steps shown in Table 16.2 presents one such way.

TABLE 16.2 Sequence of Steps for Acquiring Learning

1. Define desired knowledge or skill.
2. Identify present level of knowledge or skill.
3. Compare step 1 with step 2: If step 2 is less than 1 = learning need.
4. Identify possible learning resources.
5. Plan for use of learning resources.
6. Use resources-implement plan.
7. Evaluate-compare present level of knowledge or skill with desired level.

Determining Learning Needs

If you were approaching your own staff development in the systematic manner shown in Table 16.2, how might you proceed? Let's assume that there is to be a change in the patient population of your unit. You have, until now, had only orthopedic patients. The census has been low, and as a result several beds have been assigned for neurological patients. None will be craniotomy patients, but some will have had laminectomies, and others may have been admitted for neurological diagnostic tests. The first step, defining the desired knowledge or skill, will necessarily be imprecise. You may only know *generally* the topic areas you need to explore. This is a first point at which the staff development service may be of use to you. Consultation with someone from that department or possibly with other nurses who have worked in neurological units may help you define the desired knowledge and skill more clearly.

It may well be that the staff development personnel have been given information about the change on your unit and, doing their job, are already developing a description of the knowledge needed for the nursing care of the new patients.

When you have identified what type of knowledge is needed to give care, you can identify what you know and do not know. The *discrepancy* between what is desired knowledge and what is already known can be called the *learning need*. Perhaps staff development personnel can give you a test to help with a more precise identification of what the learning need is. Kate Lorig described several methods of needs assessment that a staff development department might use.[3]

1. *Checklists*-The respondent simply indicates *yes* or *no* to learning needs she perceives, skills she possesses, or topics in which she is interested.

[3] Kate Lorig, "An Overview of Needs Assessment Tools for Continuing Education," *Nurse Educator* (March/April,1977),p.12.]

2.*Reiterated checklists-*An expanded or refined "second time around" for a checklist. This is designed to get more specificity and, in some cases, a rank order of preferred topics.

3.*Delphi II-*This is a rather involved technique in which respondents begin by answering some rather broad questions about their jobs and the skills required and subsequently respond to feedback about the responses of the total group and to more specific definitions of need. When done by mail, for a widely scattered group, this method may take several weeks. When used in a group, 4 to 6 hours may be needed.

4.*Asking-*This is the simplest method. Each learner is *asked* to state what she needs to learn.

5.*Matrix-*The results of "asking" are placed in a matrix. Then each person may agree or disagree that each cell represents a personal learning need. There is also space for additional items to be added by the respondent.

6.*Pyramid-*This technique gives groups of increasing size (2, then 4, then 8) a time limit to produce lists of learning needs on which the group agrees.

The techniques in the above list all assume, to some extent that the educator will be dealing with a *group* of learners in providing the needed information. For this reason, such methods *do not* always suggest that the learner be told of the outcome of the assessment. Therefore, as a self-directed learner seeking your own "diagnosis," you and your request for the results of your self-assessment test may be a surprise to the staff educator. It is likely that identifying your learning need by using the discrepancy model described, along with expert consultation, will provide the information you want most directly.

Developing Objectives

The next level of refinement about the learning needs is that of developing objectives. As in general planning, objectives for learning are statements of specific intent. As indicated in Chapter 12, the most useful objective is one stated so that the condition, the desired behavior, and the standard or criterion level for accomplishment are stated. It is probably easy to understand why it is important to state very explicit learning objectives when you plan to teach someone else. The objectives will help you focus your teaching efforts on those pieces of information, activities, and situations that will prompt the needed learning. Otherwise you might find that you have used up your teaching time and have omitted some important aspects. When you are a learner, it may seem unnecessary to take the time to carefully identify your objectives. However, the development of objectives helps you to clarify the level and types of learning necessary to meet your learning needs. That knowledge then helps you to choose appropriate learning experiences. Finally, as with other planning, having objectives makes precise evaluation possible.

Making Use of Taxonomies of Objectives

Moving from objectives for general plans to objectives for learning requires that you be able to identify just what level and type of learning you want to accomplish. A body of literature has developed in education that focuses on the various types or domains of learning. Different authors have developed taxonomies, or classification systems, for each of these domains. These taxonomies define levels of learning within each domain. Since the levels are hierarchical, each succeeding level includes the previous lower level as a part of or prerequisite for its accomplishment. The descriptions of learning outcomes at each level are stated in terms of the behavior of the learner. In your case, as a self-directed continuing learner, the decisions you will make about what to learn and at what level will be reflected in statements you choose to describe your own learning outcomes.

The taxonomies mentioned, and the original work in which they are found should help to clarify just how each system can be useful to you. The three taxonomies, the *cognitive*, the *affective*, and the *psychomotor*, should be viewed as guidelines. As educational research and development continue, these organizing schemes may be revised and/or be elaborated upon. Certainly some complex forms of behavior (learning outcomes) may combine elements of two or more taxonomies. Yet even in light of this stage of development, the concept of domains and levels of learning outcomes is very useful to you as either teacher or learner. The usefulness is in the fact that such a notion can help you to move from generality to specificity in defining the intended learning outcomes. It is only with such specificity that the choice of learning activity can become efficient and evaluation can address accomplishment.

The taxonomy of the cognitive domain. The handbook by Benjamin Bloom that details the cognitive domain has become a classic since its publication in 1956.[4] This work deals with learning outcomes that are intellectual, such as knowledge and thinking skills. The cognitive domain is composed of six categories. The are (1) *knowledge*: recall of previously

---

[4] Benjamin Bloom, ed., *Taxonomy of Educational Objectives, The Classification of Educational Goals, Handbook 1: Cognitive Domain* (New York: D. McKay, 1956).

learned material; (2) *comprehension*: grasping the meaning of material; (3) *application*: using material in new situations; (4) *analysis*: breaking material into underlying structural units; (5) *synthesis*: putting parts together to form a new whole; and (6) *evaluation*: judging material according to criteria.

As you can see, it is relatively easy to agree that knowledge is basic to the other categories. Therefore, the next step after gaining new information is comprehending it (category 2). From that base you may then decide just what other types of learning may be needed. Typically, objectives arising from needs defined through work interest or experiences will require application- level objectives (category 3), since your interest has been prompted by a need to use (apply) the information you gain. In such cases, the collection of facts will not be a sufficient learning experience. In order for you to practice application of knowledge, the learning activity must furnish something more than facts. For example, there could be a written presentation of a case study demonstrating the use of the information about changes in level of consciousness. An audiovisual presentation may have a series of questions to which you respond, requiring use of knowledge. Another possibility is that a series of readings, discussion, and a movie might be complemented with a guided experience in nursing the type of patient you want to learn to care for.

The abilities of analysis, synthesis, and evaluation are important in that they represent abilities to think critically, to produce new information, and to judge the value of material or activity. Can you think of occasions when your purpose in learning might involve one of those levels?

The taxonomy of the affective domain. The next taxonomy, the affective, deals with learning outcomes that focus on emotions, interests, attitudes, and other elements of the ways in which individuals react to and adjust to facets of the world about them. The categories of the affective taxonomy are arranged in ascending order as were the cognitive group. The assumption is that each higher category incorporates behavior in all lower categories. The types of behavior include the following. (1) *Receiving*: attending to a stimulus; (2) *responding*: reacting in some way to a stimulus; (3) *valuing*: attaching some worth to a stimulus object, behavior, or idea; (4) *organization*: putting values together, and resolving conflicts between them: (5)*characterization by a value or value complex*: values affect behavior and become part of the way of life.[5].

Media presentations, interactive experiences such as seminars, "thought questions," and reading, plus many other techniques, are used to

5 D. R. Krathwohl, B. S. Bloom, and B. Masia, *Taxonomy of Educational Objectives: The Classification of Educational Goals, Handbook 2: Affective Domain* (New York: D. McKay,1956)

develop interests and to prompt consideration of personal values and attitudes. For example, the value of the worth of every client or patient is one aspect that receives emphasis in most schools of nursing in this country. More recently a concern with the awareness of different cultural pracitices has been added to the nursing curricula. In any case, the learning experiences, if directed to the highest level of that affective taxonomy, will need to be provided over a period of time.

Less is known about precisely how planned learning experiences influence values and attitudes than about the effect of learning experiences in producing cognitive outcomes. As a self-directed learner, you may find less stimulus to seek experiences specifically aimed *only* at the affect; but many learning activities seek to influence attitudes while providing information. Therefore it is worthwhile to understand this taxonomy so that your choice of learning can be made with more complete information.

The taxonomy of the psychomotor domain. The taxonomy for classifying movement behavior was developed primarily as a result of concern for creating appropriate learning experiences (movement activities) for childern.

The levels of Anita Harrow's version of a psychomotor domain taxonomy are as follows.[6]. (1) *Reflex movements:* require no conscious effort; (2) *basic fundamental movements:* combination of reflex movements which are inherent such as walking; (3) *perceptual abilities:* interpreting stimuli from environment; (4) *physical abilities:* characteristics of vigor, stamina, and flexibility needed for coordinated skilled motion; (5) *skilled movements:* intricate patterns based on fundamental movements; and (6) *non-discursive communication:* conveying meaning through body movements.

As you can see, there are levels of this taxonomy that are also relevant for specifying the teaching and learning purposes related to certain nursing techniques. For example, using a stethoscope to auscultate bowel sounds involves both perceptual abilities and some skilled movements. Making use of the sounds perceived requires some cognitive learning also. This is one example of how the learning related to the various taxonomies is interrelated, although the three domains (cognitive, affective and psychomotor) are arbitrarily separated for purposes of analysis.

Suppose that part of your concern about the learning needs as related to your neurological patients involves assisting with the measurement of spinal fluid pressures. This would involve the manipulation of certain types of equipment and accuracy in visual perception, both of which functions are

---

[6] Anita Harrow, *A taxonomy of the Psychomotor Domain* (New York: D. McKay, 1972),pp.104-6

characterized by levels in this taxonomy. Can you identify which levels from the descriptions given?

Identifying Learning Resources

When objectives are identified to a level that is clear enough for you to know what you want to accomplish and to guide you in evaluating what you learn, you are ready to move on to another phase in you own self-directed learning.

Identifying learning resources is the next phase in this systematic process of directing your own learning. The categories listed in Table 16.3 should all be considered as you make decisions about how you will pursue learning.

The lists in Table 16.3 are not exhaustive, but they do suggest the

TABLE 16.3 Categories of Learning Resources/Activities

---

1. Activities you pursue alone -- some examples
    (a) Reading from textbooks and journals
    (b) Using audio or videotapes or slide programs
    (c) Using programmed instruction
    (d) Practice of skills,using simulated patient situations
    (e) Using other individuals or individual-machine interactive learning activities

2. Activities in which you participate with others
    (a) Direct consultation with a "knowledgeable other"
    (b) Small group discussion
    (c) Planned classes, using lecture
    (d) Planned classes, using methods including participation by learners in discussion, problem-solving activities, and return demonstration
    (e) One-to-one interaction with a teacher in a tutorial session

3. Series of activities combining two or more of the approaches listed above

---

variety of possibilities available to you. Although most of the items listed are self-explanatory, a few may require explanation. For example, in the first list, "programmed instruction" is mentioned. Perhaps you will use materials such as those published occasionally in some nursing journals. These programmed units have been well received and generally do a good job of providing factual and basic conceptual information.

Your agency may also be affiliated with a school of nursing that has a learning center with simulated patient care activities, or there may be practice areas available in the agencies. If staff development provides opportunities of this sort, it is likely to be based on an assessment that a group of learners will have a similar need. If you are the only one needing such practice, plan to seek the learning opportunity wherever it exists. If the staff development department is attempting to provide individualized education, your indicating a recognized need for such an experience will prompt them to help you get such practice.

Numerous audiovisual and/or computer systems have also been developed that provide an opportunity for the learner to provide responses and receive feedback. These systems can provide instruction on a variety of topics, and for some these are more stimulating than reading or workbook-form programmed instruction. Again, if such teaching systems are available in your agency, staff development personnel can acquaint you with the hardware necessary to operate them and with the topics and the level of content.

Consultation with a colleague is not often thought of when learning resources are identified. Yet if you are specific about the information you seek and genuinely view the colleague as an expert, it is unlikely your request for information will be refused. Consultation will be most useful if you reserve this resource for gaining *other* than basic facts that can be found in texts. The consultation can best be used for information about problems, questions of judgment, or recent research or special techniques based on his or her experience. This kind of interaction is less formal than the one-to-one tutorial approach. In this latter interaction, the tutorial, there is a contract, either explicit or implied, that one is the teacher, the other the learner.

Classes of various sorts are the most common learning activity provided by staff development departments. When several learners are likely to have similar learning needs, group instruction may be an efficient method. For some learners, the formal lecture is a comfortable activity. It provides predigested material on a topic without the necessity of seeking out other sources. For those who have begun to function in a self-directed fashion, a lecture alone is seldom sufficient for complete learning, although a good lecture on a topic of interest may meet a specific learning need.

For the choice of learning activity to be made on a rational basis, those who plan classes should indicate, as "advertising," what one can expect to learn from attending and any preparation of prerequisite knowledge that is expected of the learner. An indication of the topic is not enough. In order to make a decision about participating in a particular learning activity, you will need to know the depth or level of ability a learner is expected to reach by using the learning activity. There is a vast difference between being able to describe the surgical procedures used for a laminectomy and being able to individualize the care of a laminectomy patient. It is also obvious that there is a difference between being able to identify the pieces of equipment necessary to perform a lumbar puncture and being able to assemble the various pieces of equipment for use quickly and correctly.

If you have specified your objectives at the level necessary to meet your learning needs, these objectives can now be used to help choose learning activities. For example, suppose one of your objectives is to be able to properly perform an assessment of gross neurological function. This objective involves knowledge, performing some tests (dexterity and manipulative skills required), and perceptual ability coupled with the ability to evaluate responses against some preexisting criteria (normal or expected reponses). To accomplish this objective, you may choose reading, observation of a demonstration by a skilled nurse, practice and return demonstrations (you show me, I'll show you in return), and either a group discussion or one-to-one consultation about case studies. This process demonstrates how the objective you define and subsequently refine as you identify your learning needs can guide your choice of activities.

Making a choice of learning resources to use must, of course, take into account what is available. The choice must also reflect an understanding of your own preferences and performance with each of the possible resources. If you are put to sleep by lectures in a room full of people, no matter what the subject, then the lecture is probably a poor choice of activity for you; whereas the fact that you find programmed instruction fun to use means that this is a good method for you. It is worth your time to consider carefully which methods work best for you.

Other factors that should be considered in your decision about how to learn are the costs in both money and time. Perhaps the ideal way, from your viewpoint, to prepare for the neurological patient responsibilities would be to go to a unit where such patients are presently cared for. At this other hospital, perhaps in another city, you would plan a combination of work with a skilled nurse, consultation, and reading. This process would take approximately one to two weeks. Would it be necessary or possible to replace you in your absence? If staff development could arrange such an experience, could your agency afford the monetary cost? Could the agency afford to set the precedent of such an expensive experience? If the hospital could pay for your salary and replacement but not your travel, would you be willing (or able) to pay that cost? If the costs are too great for you and/or your employer, what are your options? This discussion demonstrates that choices can only be made in light of resources, both human and financial, and that in some cases you cannot make your choices of learning activities without information and/or approval from others.

Planning and Implementing of Learning Activities

The choice of learning activities is followed by, or perhaps is actually simultaneous with, planning for their use. As with any sort of planning, the purpose is to determine which activities, in what sequence, and over what period of time will accomplish your purposes. Here again, it is important to consider your typical pattern. Do you read rapidly? Do you work best for long periods or for short intermittent periods? What information or skill is prerequisite to what? Your sequence of activity should be detailed enough to assure that, for example, you have reviewed the anatomy and physiology of the neurological system before you attempt to learn the techniques of neurological assessment that will be required for your new patients' care.

A working professional nurse has to fit learning activities in with the other demands of her life. If you have a full-time job and a life full of friends, family, and other interests, you may have to schedule your learning activities in relation to both the time available at work and the multitude of other activities in which you are involved. It is at this point that you will determine what priority you place on the continued learning. Although much staff development is conducted on site at the work place, the professional nurse is unlikely to satisfy her learning needs without many outside learning activities. The primary difference between planning for your learning and simply soaking up what is available is the fact that the planned sequence of experiences is designed to accomplish some specific purpose. The incidental or nonplanned activity is certainly not a bad thing. In fact, much serendipitous creativity can result from encountering an unexpected idea. But when *only* happenstance, such as which journal arrives, what program is scheduled when you are on duty, or which nurse you will happen to consult with over coffee, predicts your learning activity, the result is likely to be less than high quality.

Planning might be approached by focusing primarily on the learning need topic. Suppose, using the neurological unit example, you develop a plan for meeting that need, assembling your learning activities and identifying your sequence. In one approach, the period of time over which you will accomplish the plan will be predicted by the need and the activities. Another approach is to identify a time period, say one year, and develop a plan to meet one or more learning needs within that period. The latter approach assumes that you may use the discrepancy approach or some method of learning needs identification to develop the basis for one or more series of activities that can be completed during the period of time. The only real difference in approaches is whether the time requirement defines or is defined by the rest of the planning activity.

The result of your planning process is, of course, a plan. A written plan can serve as a contract with yourself. If you need the encouragement of knowing that others are interested in and are aware of your plan, a staff development person might be an appropriate colleague with whom to share your plan. In fact, such "contracting", initiated by a staff development person, a head nurse, or others might be the beginning of some nurses' developing self-directed learning behavior.

The plan you have developed should be flexible in that it allows for necessary adjustment as you begin implementation. If you find that one book leads you to pursue another you had not planned to read, you might add the second as an additional activity. When a conference in nursing techniques to use in dealing with pain is cancelled, you will choose other methods to meet the same objective. Perhaps you will even revise the objectives you have set. As you learn about caring for your new patients, you may come across information on therapeutic touch as a nursing measure. Your interest may be piqued so that you will develop a portion of your plan to give you greater depth on this topic. Such flexibility is critical if you are to make *planning* a useful part of the way you go about your learning. Your plan should also be realistic in that it does not define unreachable goals or list overly extensive activities for the time period. After all, learning of this sort will continue throughout you professional life. It is not necessary to make drudgery or frustration of what can be a delightful and challenging aspect of being a professional nurse.

Evaluating Learning Activities

Evaluating your own self-directed learning is an important way of identifying what you have accomplished. The simplest way to do this is by asking yourself, "Did I learn what I intended to?" Or you may say, "Can I demonstrate the outcomes indicated by my objective?" *Testing* is one way to find the answer to your question. Many learning experiences have exams as a planned part of the experience. For example, the learning units contained in some professional journals are followed by a professionally developed test. Some staff development teachers may provide tests as a method for giving feedback to learners and for evaluating the effect of classes they have offered in the agency. These are "ready-made" ways to assess your learning, assuming you seek specific feedback rather than simply a score.

When no written test is available, there are other ways to evaluate your learning. For example, you can serve as your own sternest critic. With your objectives as a reference you can assign yourself to *prove* what you have learned. Perhaps you will need to present the information orally to a colleague, who can tell you when your explanations are clear. A coworker may also be helpful by providing peer review of your care. This could be especially useful when the learning you intended to do involved techniques of care. In any case, as a self-directed learner, you should be the final judge of your learning. You will ask yourself if a "very good" from your staff development instructor means you have gone far enough or if you feel that you need more depth. You will be the one to determine whether a colleague's indication that care was given satisfactorily is a signal you have done enough. The key is that you should evaluate rather than assume that because you read, or watched a film, or practiced a skill, you learned.

Besides evaluating your achievement, the *outcomes*, it is also important to evaluate the *process* of the learning. Stop a bit and think back to the original choice of topic, the decision about objectives, the plan for and use of learning experiences. Were these decisions well made, efficient, and effective? Above all, was the experience satisfying to you?

Staff Development for Those with Whom You Work

The previous pages focused on you as the target of staff development, the person in charge of continuing your own education. It is possible that some nursing personnel with whom you work, for whose work you are responsible, will have a different perspective on learning. You may encounter wide variations in motivation and in skills. Therefore you may find it is important to be able to help in identifying learning needs, in developing learning experiences, and in giving feedback in staff development for others. As a professional, you should accept the responsibility for such functions if your agency defines this as part of your position. A job description is one good source of information about this expectation. If there is no clear definition of this responsibility, it is to your patients' benefit as well as that of the staff for you to clarify just how you can best aid in improving the work performance of the nursing staff with whom you work.

The process for staff development for others is analogous to that for directing your own learning. The first step is defining the needs for learning. However, caution is needed to prevent viewing every deficit in performance as a clue to a need for learning. Robert Mager and P. Pipe point out in their book *Analyzing Performance Problems, You Really Oughta Wanna* that there are other blocks to performance besides lack of knowledge.[7] One such block is produced when the person feels that performing is punishing. For example, a nurse may *know* procedures for caring for patients who have had a stroke. However, she may have a strong emotional reaction against performing, based on her own father's recent illness. In this case, the nurse's difficulty in performing has nothing to do with a learning need. Rather, performing as required produces discomfort. It is "punishing" in that sense. Another performance problem is produced when the employee finds that doing the job, although not punishing, is not rewarding. This is a fine distinction, obviously based on the individual's reaction. But the final effect of this is a lack of motivation to perform. Here again, the inference that a learning need exists is incorrect. A third block to function is lack of proper tools or other resources or other actual physical restraints to the performance. When these are ruled out as possible causes of nonperformance or inadequate performance, then a learning need may be present.

After defining the need for learning, one proceeds through the steps of choosing objectives, choosing learning activities, and evaluating the learning, all of which involves the same kinds of decision making as when dealing with your own learning. The staff development personnel can function in a consultative/supportive role by helping to identify learning resources and to plan programs for groups and generally assisting you as the supervisor to work with your employee(s). An alternate role for the staff developer is to work directly with the employee(s) once a learning need is identified until the providing reward for subsequent use of the new knowledge. The appropriate role in your agency should be clear from your job description. No one arrangement of functions is "right." Any system can be effective as long as there is clearly a responsibility for the provision and support of the educational development of staff.

SUMMARY

As manager and as professional you are doubly concerned with the learning needs of yourself and of the staff with whom you work. This chapter presented a systematic process of self-directed learning as a model for guiding your own learning and as a prototype for staff development activi-

---

[7] Robert F. Mager and P. Pipe, *Analyzing Performance Programs, You Really Oughta Wanna* (Belmont, Calif.: Fearon, 1970).

ties. Different types and levels of objectives for learning were described as were several types of learning activities.

Additional Reading

Benner, P. *From Novice to Expert* Menlo Park, Ca:Addison Wesley Publishing Co.,1984

Bodnar, B. and J. Lavery, "Journal Reports - A Unit Event", *Journal Of Continuing Education in Nursing*,19:3 (May/June,1988)p.109-112.

Farley, J. and P. Fay., "A System for Assessing Learning Needs of Registered Nurses", *Journal of Continuing Education in Nursing*,19:1 (January - February,1988)p.13-16.

Knowles, Malcolm, *The Adult Learner:A Neglected Species*,3rd ed., Houston:Gulf Publishing Co. 1984.

Tobin, Helen M., Pat S. Yoder Wise, and Peggy K. Hull, *The Process of Staff Development: Components for Change*, 2nd ed. St. Louis, Mo.: C.V. Mosby,1979.

Chapter 17

Processes of planned change

Ever-present, distressing, challenging-these and many other adjectives at either extreme come to mind when the topic is "change." A huge variety of alterations and innovations comprise the almost continuous changes potentially confronting you as a professional nurse. The unit of change may be the individual, the health care agency or some of its operating units, some element of the environment, or some combination of these.

Changes in organization can be described in a variety of ways. One convenient set of descriptions classifies change as developmental, innovative, reactive, or planned. Change may occur as a part of the developmental process of the target. The concepts of human development are well-known to you since they serve as a framework for understanding much of human behavior that is basic to nursing. Certainly the individual human developmental changes that nursing personnel encounter will affect their interaction with coworkers. However, these individual changes are probably not as influential in the work setting as the developmental phase of the small work group or of the organization as a whole.

Some authors have presented the idea that both small groups and organizations as a whole experience developmental phases. Robert Chin describes the use by social scientists of developmental models for understanding an organization's "condition" as a use of this approach.[1] According to Chin, there are five terms that are common to developmental models: *directions, states, forces, form of progression,* and *potentiality.* Direction refers to the idea that development proceeds toward some end state. In human development, physical development proceeds in a cephalocaudal direction, and there are considerable data from which to estimate typical milestones

---

[1] Robert Chin, "The Utility of System Models and Developmental Models for Practitioners," in *The Planning of Change,*3rd ed.,Warren Bennis,Kenneth Benne, and Robert Chin,eds.(New York: Holt,Rinehart & Winston,1976),pp.90- 115.

of development by age. These are referred to as *stages* or *phases*. However, there is far less evidence accumulated about the milestones anticipated for various types of groups and organizations. For this reason, the direction of organizational development is generally thought to be toward mature, efficient accomplishment of goals.

Change is also experienced as an expression of creativity or innovation. There may be no real problem requiring the introduction of an alteration in the time and type of conferences held on the unit where you work. The work group may simply be interested in doing "something new." Such changes are spontaneously generated and are tentative in nature. The attitude is frequently, "Oh, that's an interesting idea, let's try it for awhile." For an innovation to be accepted as quickly as just described, agreement among all significant members of the work group is likely to be present, along with a low degree of threat or anticipated disruption of already satisfying circumstances.

Reaction to circumstances or to changes in other elements of the same agency or in the other elements of the environment may also be the basis for change. It is possible that such change will be planned and systematic, but reaction more often prompts random responses rather than systematic planned change. Suppose that your community health agency is responsible for operating a health station in a low-income area. At a meeting of the residents' advisory committee, there is angry discussion of the presence of nursing students at the station. The message is, "We are poor but we have our rights. We will not be 'guinea pigs' for those students to practice on." The next day, the medical director orders that no more nursing students will be a part of activities at the facility. The schools of nursing are quite distressed at the loss of clinical facilities. At the same time, agency personnel agree that the director's reaction is proper, a necessity to keep good community relations. Further, they agree that the change will not really alter the amount and kind of service they can give since they did not depend on students for service.

Three different types of change have been mentioned- *developmental*, *innovative*, and *reactive*, although many aspects of these changes may be similar no matter what the stimulus. Furthermore, all three types may also have some similarities with elements of *planned change*. Planned change is change that is usually prompted by attempts to solve problems or to improve function or output. It is systematic alteration with a specific goal. The rest of this chapter is devoted to considering planned change from your perspectives as manager and managed, sometimes instigator, and frequently as the target of change.

Planned Change-
A Social Phenomenon

The health care industry is a field of rapid growth and technical improvement. As the various groups involved in providing health care evolve, their techniques prompt the recognition of new problems. Growing awareness by the public of the possibilities and the problems in health care forces continuing consideration of the emerging problems and creates new problems as well. For these reasons, nurses are frequently confronted with the need to develop changes in procedures, in practice roles, and in organizational relationships. To understand fully the ways in which change can be accomplished efficiently and effectively, a general view of change as a social phenomenon is useful.

A body of literature on change has been developed in the social sciences and in the applied field of management and administration in the past several years. The fact that change is sometimes difficult to produce effectively and to experience gracefully has created a market for consultants in organizational development. The specific tools and techniques used by these consultants and as described in the literature may vary, but the theoretical orientation is generally one that relies on a *systems view* of organization or on Kurt Lewin's approach called *force field analysis*.[2] Both of these approaches recognize the many variables and the several levels of interaction present in any social setting and relate this to the analysis and prediction of the effects and responses to change.

A Systems Theory View

The view of organizations or units of an organization such as a health care agency as social *systems* allows concepts from general systems theory to be used as tools for the description and analysis of activities that occur when change is attempted. This view is consistent with systems approaches used by individuals in a variety of fields from biology to engineering. The degree of precision and of quantification of the concepts varies from rather imprecise to highly exact. For example, a simple, not too precise diagram of a system might serve nicely to demonstrate the relative interdependence of the parts of the whole system, whereas this same degree of precision would be inadequate to serve the computer scientist.

---

[2] Kurt Lewin, "Frontiers in Group Dynamics: Concepts, Methods and Reality in Social Science," *Human Relations* Vol. 1(1947),pp.5-42.

Even with the wide differences in function and detail among systems, there are some generally used terms and some basic concepts that are common to all. These are useful as you begin to take a systems view of the work situation as a site of planned change. The following paragraphs detail some of these important concepts.

System is the first term requiring definition. It is a whole combined of interdependent parts or subunits. One major precept is that the whole (system) is greater than the sum of the parts. This implies that because there is an essential dynamic interaction among the parts, they together become something more than simply a collection of separate parts. The automobile is an example. All of the parts for a sports car can be stored in a loose collection in a corner of a garage. When these same parts are connected in a unique and interdependent way, they become a system greater than the total number of separate parts. In the same way, a group of nurses together in a space becomes a care-giving system when their actions function for a common purpose and when they are tied together, however loosely, by elements of interdependence.

Any particular system is also a part of one or more larger systems. However, in order to focus on a single system for purposes on analysis, it is necessary to identify what is and is not a part of the system under consideration. Determining the *boundary* of the system may be as simple as pointing out a physical limit or edge. For example, the body of an individual defines the boundary of that person's physical system. The boundary may likewise be abstract or imaginary. All the nurses providing maternal and child services in a visiting nurse service may constitute such a system. The limiting boundary here is abstract, imaginary.

The surrounding variables (again physical or abstract) about a system form its *environment*. The *open system* is one that is thought of as having the ability to receive and respond to information or stimuli from the environment, across its boundaries. Living systems of all sorts are open systems. Logically, then, a *closed system* is one that lacks this quality of interchange with the environment.

The open system concept that there is an exchange of energy with the environment is not intended to imply that the exchange is always equal. This is because the system uses energy in certain ways. In other words, energy may be used to create an output, and may be used efficiently. In addition, the system may apply some of the input energy to *evolution*, growing toward a higher level of organizaiton, increasing in complexity. On the opposite extreme is the possibility of dissipation of energy or waste, which leads to draining of the system. This tendency to dissipation is called *entropy*, in systems terms. Another relevant notion when considering the energy of a system is that of *feedback*. This is a mechanism where a portion of the *output* (transformed energy) is directed back into the system to allow for self-correction in the process of creating the output.

There are some other concepts of systems theory that are useful when considering change in work organizations. One such concept states that *a change in any element of a system will produce changes in other elements of the system*. This is true because of a tendency for a system to seek an equilibrium or balance among the forces of its elements. If the system's tendency is to return to a particular point, *equilibrium* is the proper term. Suppose there is a fire drill (the change) that prompts removal of all patients and nurses from a hospital unit to a place of safety. When the drill is over, all the elements return to their previous places and relationships, and the system begins as before, in equilibrium. On the other hand, when the system retains relative balance among elements with no fixed point to which the system returns, the balance is called a *steady state*. In the fire drill example, if everyone returned to the same unit but to different places and if some exchanged functions but with the same eventual effect, the balance would be a steady state. In either case, changing one element or function in a system creates an imbalance or disequilibrium in the system. The other elements then act to compensate, to return the system's balance.

Another important concept is that *all systems change with time*. That is, in a way, similar to the developmental view. However, in systems theory the notion is broader. As Arlene Putt states, "Most real systems change with time, either decaying or growing toward a higher level of organization. With increasing complexity comes increasing centralization."[3]

When these concepts of systems analysis are applied to the analysis of a work setting where planned change may occur, the picture created is of a dynamic situation with numerous interdependent elements and one or more functions that will, at least to some extent, respond predictably to a stimulus for change. Later in this chapter, these ideas are applied to examining a planned change. However, before that, it is useful to add some other tools, as discussed below.

---

[3] Arlene M. Putt, *General Systems Theory Applied to Nursing* (Boston: Little, Brown, 1978), p.3.

Force Field Analysis and a Process of Planned Change

As mentioned above, planned change is systematic alteration typically directed to solving some problem or producing improvement in function or output. As we consider the nature of these changes as they occur in nursing settings, we can identify that they constitute alteration in environment, in purpose, in goals, in structure of relationships, or in procedures. Thinking back to the systems concept, it will be evident that any one of these types of changes may create changes of one or more of the other types as well. For example, a change in goals in a mental hospital might produce a new concern with family involvement in the care of patients. As a result, changes in staff relationships and in procedures may be required to meet the new goal.

As long ago as 1947, Kurt Lewin described a rather simple model of stages of change that is still a useful tool today.[4] This model indicates that there are three phases to a social change: (1) unfreezing, (2) moving to a new level, and (3) refreezing or stabilizing. The unfreezing phase is the point at which the status quo is questioned, stimuli for change are created, and some discomfort or dissatisfaction with the present situation is induced. It is during this phase that the change agent can usefully apply the force field analysis technique for clarifying the nature of the situation. (At this point, assume that the term *change agent* applies to the person or group responsible for instigating a change. This term is explained more fully later in this chapter.)

The force field analysis is a way of identifying the elements in a situation that are responsible for creating the status quo or the current equilibrium. If you think of the present situation (status quo) as being represented by a vertical line, you can then conceive of a series of opposing forces as the elements that keep the line perpendicular and stationary. The driving forces are those that push toward a new or changed position, and the restraining forces are those that militate against that change by maintaining the status quo.

Status quo

Driving	Restraining
Forces	Forces

FIGURE 17.1 Force Field Model

---

4 Lewin,"Frontiers in Group Dynamics,"pp.5-42.

In general, comfort with routine or habit is a major restraining force in any existing social situation such as is present in a work setting. Personal satisfaction produced by valued interpersonal relationships, by a feeling of competence gained from mastering a job or elements of it, or by positive comments received from patients and their families are examples of restraining forces that may be present in some nursing situations and that act to preserve the status quo. Therefore, in some situations, an anticipated change may produce major concern about the loss of such satisfaction, and the resulting fear can itself be a restraining force.

Driving forces may be positive, in the form of anticipated rewards and satisfaction, or they may be essentially negative, as in the case of threatened loss of rewards. In either case, the driving forces cause motion toward a change.

The initial use of this model is to serve as a set of categories for identifying the major forces operating in any situation. As the forces are identified and sorted, the relative strength of each can be estimated. For example, if a group whose procedures are to be changed is a relatively newly created and loose-knit group, disruption of interpersonal relationships may be a relatively weak restraining force. In the same situation, if each group member is considerably rewarded by the feeling of mastery over the task he or she currently performs, this may be a major restraining element when new unmastered tasks are part of the change.

The principle inherent in the model of "what is" is that in order to produce change, either restraining forces must be weakened or driving forces must be added or strengthened. The task then is to develop strategies for change that will accomplish this alteration in the balance between restraining and driving forces.

Strategies for Change

The use of the term *strategy* implies that there are identifiable clusters of actions that represent differing approaches to accomplishing a given intent. The intent, in this case, is change. The categories of strategies presented here are probably not so clearly defined that there is no overlap among them. But they do serve to identify the several typical approaches to change, for purposes of analysis. The framework that they provide can also be helpful in actually plannig a change. The descriptions are those developed by Robert Chin and Kenneth Benne.[5] In their work, these ideas are directed to an audience primarily of social scientists who function as practitioners of change, "change agents," a role that is discussed in more detail later in this chapter.

Rational-Empirical Strategies

The first cluster of strategies is the *rational-empirical* strategies. These strategies are based on the assumption that individuals are rational, that they always act in a reasoned fashion toward what they perceive to be their own self-interest. Some strategies mentioned by Chin and Benne in this group are basic research and dissemination of knowledge through general education.[6] This approach is directed to building the base of available knowledge and making that knowledge a part of what is generally available. This is a long- term strategy, primarily applicable to large groups such as a whole segment of society. The incorporation of health-related information in public school curriculum is one such strategy since it is assumed (hoped) that when individuals know how to maintain their health, seeing that good health is in their best self-interest, they will choose to use the information, and a general change in health practice will emerge in society.

The widespread public information campaign conducted on the topic of cigarette smoking and health is another more specific example. This information is based on research collected by the U.S. Department of Health and Human Services , Office of the Surgeon General. The information is being disseminated with the expectation that individuals will understand that smoking is *not* in their self-interest and will, as a result, cease or reduce smoking. Even so, with all the available information, you will note that there are cigarettes consumed all around you each day. Therefore it is logical to conclude that this strategy is only partially effective.

Other approaches among the rational-empirical strategies include the use of systems analysis, and the development of applied research projects and associated linkage systems for the diffusion of research results. These approaches are not discussed in detail here because they apply mainly at the societal level rather than at the organizational or organizational subunit

---

[5] Robert Chin and Kenneth D. Benne, "General Strategies for Effecting Change in Human Systems," in *The Planning of Change*,4th ed., Warren Bennis, Kenneth Benne, and Robert Chin, eds. (New York: Holt, Rinehart & Winston,1985),p.22- 45.

[6] Ibid,pp.24-31.

level. If you wish to pursue the topic of change in greater depth, the bibliography at the end of the chapter furnishes a useful starting point.

Normative-Reeducative Strategies

The second cluster of change strategies listed by Chin and Benne are the *normative-reeducative* strategies.[7] The assumption behind this series of approaches differs from those upon which the rational-empirical group are built. Rather than viewing humans as consistently rational, this approach assumes that individuals are a part of a continuing transaction with the environment and are constantly attempting to satisfy needs.

Men are guided in their actions by socially funded and communicated meanings, norms, and institutions, in brief by a normative culture. At the personal level, men are guided by internalized meanings, habits, and values. Changes in patterns of action or practice are, therefore, changes, not alone in the rational information equipment of men, but at the personal level, in habits and values as well and, at the sociocultural level, changes are alterations in normative structures and in institutionalized roles and relationships, as well as in cognitive and perceptual orientation.[8]

The strategies in this group have certain common elements, although they differ in specifics. In common, they all stress the importance of involvement of the target system (individual, group, or organization) in the development of the program for change.

Another common point is that there is *no* assumption that simply providing better, more complete information will be the basis for prompting a solution to the target system's problems. This is in direct contrast to the rational-empirical strategies. Other elements common to the group of normative-reeducative strategies have to do with the approach of the change agent and the process by which that agent works with the client system. First, there is an emphasis on a mutual, collaborative relationship between change agent and client. Second, there is a recognition of the value of the use of methods and ideas from the behavioral sciences as tools in change, along with the specific focus on bringing to a conscious level the nonconscious elements that may affect the change process.

One of the strategies in this group is focused on efforts to improve the problem-solving capabilities of a system. The intent is to design and institutionalize techniques that include: (1) the collection of information that can serve as feedback about process and output of the system, (2) analysis and problem identification based on the feedback, and (3) generation of

---

7 Robert Chin and Kenneth D. Benne, "General Strategies,"pp.31-39.

8 Ibid.,p.31.

solutions to the problems identified. Much of the current literature on the topic of "organizational development" is an elaboration of techniques that implement this strategy.

In a health care agency this strategy might be implemented at any of several levels. For example, a consultant might work with persons in key administrative positions as a group, to help create a group that will be able to recognize and solve organizational problems. Activities of the group, initiated by the consultant, might include: (1) exercises designed to analyze current problems of the organization, (2) development of interpersonal communication skills, (3) discussion of typical patterns of dealing with problems of interpersonal and intergroup conflict in the organization, and (4) examination of the roles and functions of individuals in the organization in order to identify how newly learned skills and approaches can become a part of the usual operation of the organization.

On a smaller scale, this normative reeducative approach of focusing on developing the problem-solving capabilities of a system could be applied at the unit level in a hospital. Perhaps there is a concern that the care given to families of cancer patients on the unit is not adequate. The change agent, in this case the new clinical specialist, could institute group and individual problem-solving sessions. These meetings would have two purposes. One would be to solve the problem at hand. The other would be to improve the problem-solving skills of the group and its individual members.

Closely related to the strategy of focusing on problem solving, is a second strategy-that of promoting personal growth in the individuals who are the target system. This strategy aims to prompt personal growth through individual and/or group experiences designed to help persons become better able to function effectively in life. Since the individual is ultimately the basic unit of any social change, it is reasoned that persons who are more capable of mature functioning will be inclined to create better social situations, that is, to create needed change. The techniques used include laboratory training in self- confrontation and interpersonal interaction, individual counseling, group therapy, and other related activities.

In both strategies-the problem-solving and general growth strategies-the emphasis in the overall change effort is toward helping individuals learn new general ways of behaving. This is intended to promote both improved function and satisfaction as well as a desire to change toward optimum function in all endeavors.

Power-Coercive Strategies

The third cluster of strategies for producing change is called by Benne and Chin the *power-coercive* approaches.[9] These authors note that power, in the sense of the use of efforts to influence behavior, is a component of any change strategy. In this group of strategies, the emphasis is on the coercive and non-reciprocal aspects of situations that are created to promote change. Coercive situations can be characterized as those in which the responsive behavior change is directed to "reducing-pain" rather than gaining pleasure. Or stated another way, coercive means are effective when the targets of change are caused to recognize that some negative sanctions can result or that some positive sanctions will be lost if change does not occur. Although this may appear to be a very negative and possibly unethical approach to producing change, in fact, many of the socially legitimized institution in our culture are designed to function in this fashion. For example, administrative authority in many large organizations is based on the potential to provide or withhold economic rewards for performance. Another example is the U.S. Army, which relies on the legitimacy of command and its associated coercive ability to assure compliance with its orders. The list of examples could be extensive.

The primary elements that distinguish the power-coercive strategies from the rational-empirical is that the power-coercive set tends to rely on economic and political forms of sanctions, although clearly this set of strategies agrees with the assumption that individuals behave in their own self-interest. The rational-empirical, however, depends on self-interest as defined by the individual or the determinant of behavior, whereas the power-coercive assumes that economic and/or political forces will be common denominators of self-interest.

One example of power-coercive strategies is nonviolent activities. These include picketing, parades, sit-ins, and other public demonstrations as well as peaceful civil disobedience. These activities are typically employed by groups that lack the power of position and direct economic sanction, and the activities are therefore essentially directed "upward" as a means of influencing those who are in a dominant position (in possession of the usual means of control).

Labor strikes are an example of nonviolent coercive means to prompt change. As with any attempt to use coercion, there are risks inherent in the use of this tactic. In the case of the strike, as well as other nonviolent means directed against a person or group possessing power, there is the risk of

9 Ibid.,pp.39-45

retaliation. Perhaps strikers will be fired, or demonstrators may be arrested. The strategy recognizes these risks. Those who favor nonviolent methods contend that even the retaliation can benefit the change effort by provoking moral outrage in the general population against the change target. The idea is that the general public will side with the "underdog" when the situation is exposed. Do you suppose that this holds true when, for example, nurses strike for better working conditions through contract demands that include a greater role in decision making? The fact that public sentiment may not be favorable if health care is interrupted points up the degree to which well-planned mass communication efforts are necessary for these means to actually effect change. The message-that the strike is related to patient care conditions-is a fine distinction, since wages are the typical concern of negotiations, but a necessary one if any public sympathy is to be aroused.

Another power-coercive technique is the use of political institutions to produce change. This strategy characterizes the actual effect of all the elements of our political system-the legislative, judicial, and executive branches of government at federal, state, and local levels-all have the power to effect changes within their jurisdiction. Individuals and groups are able to influence changes prompted by these systems to the extent that they are able to influence the persons holding positions within the various branches. Theoretically, at least, the voters control these political institutions through choice of representatives and through referendum. For this reason, groups such as the state nurses associations will ask the candidate's position on specific health-related issues during his campaign, will contact the representative as votes on critical bills are called, and will review the records of service by these persons as they seek reelection.

If such political activity seems remote and not strongly tied to the care you are able to give as a nurse, perhaps an example will be helpful. Assume that you are working in a county hospital, the budget for which is approved each year by the county commission, an elected body. During the past two years, the acuity of illness of patients in this hospital has risen steadily. Very few of the patients are admitted for elective surgery or diagnostic workups. The typical patient is in need of extensive medical and nursing care. The staffing pattern for nursing has been revised to account for this increased need for care, with a resulting request for 23 new positions in the nursing department. When the budget hearing is held, several of the commissioners question the request in a year when the total budget must be held to minimal increases. Although a strong case is presented by the hospital administrator and nurse executive, the commissioners eliminate the new positions for the budget. The result is that several units will work at a severe disadvantage for the next year, with fewer staff than needed. In order to change this situation, the commisssioners must be the target of change. More correctly, it is the decisions made by the commissioners that must be changed. The political process can effect this change. New commissioners or the old commissioners with new understanding are the answers.

There are seldom "pure-type" uses of these strategies. Typically, those planning a change will choose combinations of strategies, based on their past experience in producing change. The value of considering these approaches as separate types lies in the possibility of making better choice of strategies related to the analysis of the force field present in the target situation.

The Change Agent

Understanding strategies for producing change is important, just as is using a model such as Lewin's for analyzing the target situation.[10] However, simply grasping this information about change will not necessarily cause you to produce successful changes. Another important ingredient, at least when your perspective is that of the manager, is an understanding of the role of change agent. The idea of a special role for someone who is responsible for facilitating planned change was originally defined as "change agent" by the social scientists who first began to deal with planned change as a field to study. Numerous allusions to this role have been made in nursing literature. In fact, you may have been told that a major responsibility of the professional nurse is to be a change agent. It is useful then, to consider just what this role might entail.

The prescription for the role of change agent usually focuses on two elements: (1) the personal characteristics of the change agent and (2) the process used by the person to bring about change. The ideal change agent is characterized as having excellent skills in communication and in knowledge of group process. Thinking back to the various change strategies, you will notice that these skills would be most important when either normative-re-educative or rational-empirical approaches are used. It is these approaches that are typically used by consultants who consider themselves professional change agents. These are the practitioners of social science who work as consultants to organizations desiring change. The literature on "change agentry" is largely the result of their experience.

[10] See Fig. 17.1.

You might wonder if a person within an organization, a regular employee, can function as a change agent. Experience has shown that this can be the case. But when the individual is within the organization, the advantage afforded the outsider of functioning from a base of *expert* power combined with implied support from legitimate authorities in the organization is lost. Instead, the potential for successful change agent function will be related to the extent to which those two power bases exist *and* the extent to which the individual is *not* viewed as developing undue *personal* gains from the change at the expense of the group or organization.

Previously existing trust of the change agent can be a positive factor. The internal person who is acknowledged as having expert ability may, in fact, have an advantage in facilitating a change, especially if the change is clearly related to the scope of that knowledge. As you consider the attributes useful for a change agent, you can see that it would be rather difficult for a nurse who is a recent graduate and is new to an agency to have either the full benefit of the expert power base, the trust of the group, or the sanction from legitimate administrative authority. Herein lies an explanation for the all too common frustration experienced by recent graduates who attempt to promote major changes in their work setting early in their careers. Further, if the choice of change strategy is power-coercive, it is not likely that the "new nurse" would command sufficient resources to have a base of power that would make this a realistic strategy.

Planning a Change

Besides the personal characteristics attributed to the individual promoting change, another key element in change in an organization is the process by which the change is brought about. Keep in mind that these following statements are not so much descriptive as normative. That is, they reflect a view of how change ideally *should* be accomplished rather than how it *is* accomplished. This is in contrast to the earlier comments on strategies for change. Those comments were descriptive, indicating a typology of change as viewed by the authors cited.

There are a number of ways to describe the series of steps involved in creating a change. One of the more common ways is to describe a problem-solving process and to imply that the problem solution results in the change. Surely, when change is directed to solving a problem, this is true. On the other hand, the activities might be a bit different if the change involved were primarily an innovation rather than a problem solution. In either case, the change itself should be carefully planned. If the change were directed to problem solving, the planning would begin at the solution planning stage after other solutions had been ruled out. In the situation where change is simply for the sake of "doing something new", the process would essentially reflect only the planned change process.

In any event, the overall planning would require at least the following phases:

- Assessing and analyzing.
- Identifying and choosing strategies.
- Developing an activity plan.

Following the planning phase, the change would enter the implementation phase, including the following:

- Implementing the activity plan.
- Adjusting the plan as needed.

This is followed by a final phase which must be planned at the outset:

- Evaluating and stabilizing the change.

These phases combine Lewin's concepts of force field analysis and the three-phase change process (unfreezing, moving, refreezing) with a systematic planning process. If the change agent views the best approach to most changes as at least partially normative-reeducative in nature, this will determine who is involved in each of these phases. This change agent would have as a basic orientation the notion that the best change is created when those who will be implementing the change participate in its development and planning. This is the premise that is often implicit in much of the literature on change.

The initial assessment and analysis by the change agent should include a force field analysis. This will clarify what are the restraining and driving forces related to this change. If the target group is sufficiently skilled, this may be the initial point of their involvement in the change. One warning is important in making the decision to involve the target group. There is nothing quite so detrimental to group morale and to the status afforded the change agent as the irritation that can be produced by "pseudo-involvement." This happens when the indication is given that the group has the option to make choices, to give direction, to use its own way to solve a problem, only to learn later that the decisions have already been made. If, in fact, some decisions have already been made or some options are not open to the group, that should be made clear at the outset.

The assessment and analysis phase should result in an understanding of who is involved in the change, what precisely will be necessary to produce the change (resources, approval time, etc.), and what forces are producing the present situation, as well as what forces may be increased or reduced in order to produce movements. Using systems theory terms, the change agent should gain an understanding of the critical elements of the target system, the relationships among its subsystems, its major inputs, function and outputs, and the relationship of this system to its relevant environment.

Also, an effort should be made to estimate the impact of the desired change on the target system and on its subsystems and environment. This latter piece of the analysis is important in order to know if complementary changes in other functions, subsystems, or the environment will be necessary in order to produce the desired change.

This phase of planning should be given plenty of time. If you are the change agent, even though you may be working with and through the target group, you may find that the enthusiasm you feel for the change can cause you to rush past critical details or overlook significant restraining forces. One major restraining force may be that identified as potential losses for any of the individuals affected by the change. Considering the change from a variety of perspectives, are there potential personal losses in resources or status for any who will be affected?

One of the surest ways to check for the hazard of "too quick" an analysis is to consult with a disinterested person. The key question to ask is, "Why won't this work?" As long as you ask this question and continue to get new answers, you can usefully spend more time in analysis and assessment.

Following the analysis is the choice of strategy or combination of strategies. This choice should reflect an understanding of the nature of the resources available to the change agent. What is the power base? What money, time, and personnel are available? What strategy or combination of strategies have worked before in similar situations? Also important is the change agent's personal philosophy. Some persons will find that the normative-reeducative approach is more compatible than any other strategy with their personal view of desirable interaction. Others may consider a variety of strategies on the assumption that no one strategy is philosophically or ethically better than another.

When the decision about strategy has been made, the next step is to make a specific activity plan. The development of this plan would be just as described in Chapter 12. There is at least one special consideration in developing the activity plan for change; that is determining with whom or at what point in the target system the change will begin. Edgar Schein describes one key factor in that decision as identifying "linkages"[11] This means the manner and degree to which a portion of a system (a person or group) is connected to other parts of the system. In an organization, it is obvious that the administrative hierarchy has more linkage than any other element of the system. Conversely, a small group on a hospital specialty unit is very likely to be rather weakly linked with all other elements of the hospital, for purposes of diffusion of a change targeted at the whole hospital. So the best choice for a place in a system to begin change must be as highly linked as possible to other relevant elements of the target system.

Also, the choice must reckon with whether the highly linked person or group is *willing* to be changed and to aid in the subsequent efforts to spread the change. For example, if a head nurse is unwilling to be the "entry point" for a change, even though she is the best linked person on the target unit, it may be wiser to begin initially with an enthusiastic assistant head nurse. This assumes that the head nurse would not attempt to block the change but is simply not interested in helping. If she were sufficiently negative toward the change, she might be considered a restraining force. If she were sufficiently powerful, it might be futile to begin a change on her unit at all, and so it would be better to seek to begin at a step above her in the organization.

After a starting place has been identified, other elements of the planning should produce a list of activities and time lines as well as milestones or objectives that can serve as the basis for continuing evaluation and readjustment of the plan as needed. This is a phase in which many change agents will choose to involve members of the target change group. This involvement can serve a purpose if the intent is to produce competence to accomplish future change and/or if the intent is to produce a sense of ownership of the activities, and as a result, a commitment to the change. The matter of a commitment to change is delicately balanced against the possible sense of frustration resulting if members of the target group are led to believe that their choice is *whether* to change rather than *how*. This issue must be clear from the outset. If the "whether" is a possible option for the group they should legitimately be involved from the beginning analysis and assessment phase rather than only at the activity planning phase. If there is no such choice intended, for such reasons as receiving mandates from organizational superiors or the need to institute procedures to meet governmental regulations, then the members of the target group need to have that information from the onset.

[11] Edgar Schein,*Professional Education* (New York: McGraw- Hill,1972),p.91.

Implementation follows, accompanied by readjustment of the plan as needed. Perhaps time estimates were overly optimistic. Possibly the strategy itself does not seem to be accomplishing the objectives. Perhaps new restraining forces have emerged. In each case if there are points included in the activity plan at which adjustment can occur, crises and/or failure may be obviated. It is sometimes difficult in the glow of enthusiasm for a change you "know" is right to step back and view things coldly and objectively enough to inject an adjustment in the plan, especially if you are the prime mover in that plan.

Evaluating the change serves two purposes. First, it can confirm the extent to which the change has been effected and the degree to which the results expected from the change are being achieved. A systematic evaluation would require the series of actions described as needed in any evaluation (Chapter 15). The criteria chosen would relate certainly to the intended outcomes of the change and possible to the process by which it has been achieved. Appropriately, data collection may involve both objective and subjective data gathered from a variety of sources.

The second purpose of evaluation is to begin the final phase of change, the refreezing or stabilization. This process can be aided by involving members of the target group in the evaluation. As the evaluation results emerge, the recognition of this change as a real part of the system becomes firm. The change begins to be transformed from something new (possibly temporary) to something completed and accepted.

Reactions to Change

Think back to when you were 14 years old. What would have been your reaction if your parents had told you that the family was going to move to another city in two weeks? Many people's responses would be extremely negative. The possibility of leaving friends, familiar surroundings, pleasant activities, and school could be quite anxiety producing. Such a reaction to change is not limited to moves from city to city nor to teenagers. On the other hand, some teenagers may be eager for new faces and new experiences and quite ready for a change. So also may others respond at least neutrally if not very favorably to the prospect of some changes. Therefore, it is not safe to assume that all people resist any and every change. Perhaps the reason that the topic of reaction to change usually brings thoughts of resistance is that resistance is the only reaction that can become a restraining force, potentially blocking the change. It would seem useful, though, to give consideration to favorable reactions as well, since enthusiasm could serve as a driving force in a change process.

A logical question is what prompts the reaction to change? Depending on the basic theoretical orientation, a variety of explanations can be given. A behavioral approach might explain that the present relatively constant situation produces reinforcing stimuli that prompt the individual to repeat learned behavior in pursuit of continuing rewards. Disrupting the reinforcing situation prompts random and nonfunctional behavior in pursuit of renewed reinforcement. This same theoretical approach would imply that to produce a change in people's behavior, one manipulates the reinforcers and moves in successive steps toward the new and desired behavior. If this approach is used, the result should be no major disruptions. This technique seems rather mechanistic, does it not? Somehow, it is easier to accept when rats are the target of change rather than human beings.

Another theoretical approach that could supply an explanation for reactions to change is consistent with humanistic psychology. This would explain that an individual carries certain perceptions about himself that influence his view of life situation. For that person, his perceptions are reality. The needs of the individual include a need to achieve self-esteem, to gain some sense of mastery or competence in some life activities, and to have satisfying interpersonal relationships. If the current situation or pattern of behavior is seen to contribute to meeting those needs, "making me feel good," then changes could prove to be distressing in that they are a potential threat to meeting those needs. Alternately, if the change can be perceived as having greater potential for meeting those needs, then it may be welcomed.

Social exchange theory offers the idea basic to the use of power-coercive strategies of change. That is, an individual will act in what he believes to be his own self-interest. Resistance or favorable response, from this theoretical view, will have less to do with the substance of the change than with the perceived net value of the change to the individual. Again, this theory implies that neither favorable nor unfavorable response to change is standard.

A specific application of role theory has been developed to explain the behavior of some individuals who consistently resist almost any change in a situation of which they are a part. The particular role behavior was labeled by one author as the "defender role".[12] His notion is that in some groups,

12 Donald Klein, "Some Notes on the Dynamics of Resistance to Change: The Defender Role," in *The Planning of Change*, 4th ed., Warren Bennis, Kenneth Benne, and Robert Chin, eds. (New York: Holt, Rinehart & Winston, 1985),p.98.

that role serves to maintain the integrity of the target system by helping to focus on the maintenance of the core values of the system. The role is viewed as an important social, group-related (rather than individual, psychological) force, which is created by the group and is embodied in one individual. Of course, returning to the psychological view, one might wonder why some individuals are apt for the role and others are not. In any case, this concept does emphasize that although change is occasionally necessary in any system and is frequently necessary in many systems, stability also deserves attention, and many groups cultivate it by nurturing the defender role.

The range of possible reactions to change is wide. The best prescription for the planner of change is to remain as accepting and objective as possible in the face of either favorable or nonfavorable responses, placing no labels on the individual or the behavior involved. Rather, an attempt shoud be made to continually incorporate the reactions into making decisions about adjustments in the plan for change.

Your Part in Planned Change

As a member of a health care agency, you will have many occasions to be a part of a target group for change and some opportunities to be a change agent. The fact that you understand something about planned change can make you a valuable asset to a change. But it does not in any way prevent your feeling anxiety if a particular change is threatening to you, or responding enthusiastically if you are challenged by it. Being a professional nurse does not in any way define you as *always* favorable toward change.

Your education and experience will probably produce the expectation by others that you are capable of managing a change. Hopefully, you will not avoid that responsibility if you are in a situation where you are sufficiently powerful and competent to do the job. Equally hopefully, you *will* avoid acting out the tendency so common in new graduates to want to produce change in practically everything almost immediately.

SUMMARY

Change in health care agencies is an example of social change, a topic of literature, and a matter for consultation in a number of organizational settings. This chapter has described a systematic approach to the development of planned change, the functions of the change agent, and some human reactions to change.

Additional Reading

Bennis, Warren, K. Benne, and R. Chin (Eds) *The Planning of Change*, 4th ed.,New York: Holt, Rinehart and Winston,1985.

Blend, Deborah, "Change: Are You a Resistor or Creator?"*Journal of Post-Anesthesia Nursing*,1 No.2(May,1986)92-96.

Brooten, Dorothy, L. Hayman, and M. Naylor, *Leadership for Change*,2nd Ed.,Philadelphia: J.B. Lippincott Co.,1988.

Goren, Suzanne and Richard Ottaway, "Why Healthcare Teams Don't Change: Chronicity and Collusion"*Journal of Nursing Administration*,15:7/8(July/August,1985)9-16.

Haffer, A.,"Facilitating Change: Choosing the Appropriate Strategy", *Journal of Nursing Administration*,16 No.4 (April,1986)18-22.

Lawrence, Paul, "How to Deal With Resistance to Change", in *People: Managing Your Most Important Asset*,Boston, Ma: Harvard Business Review,1987,36-44.

Pinkerton, SuEllen and P. Schroeder, *Commitment to Excellence*, Rockville, Maryland: Aspen Publishers, 1988.

Rosenman, H. and M. Jenkins, "A Nursing Staff Designs Its Own System" *Nursing Management* ,17 No.2,(February,1986)32-34.

PART III

A Final Note:
You-A Reintegrated
Professional Nurse
and
Your First Position

This final chapter is meant for only some of the readers of this textbook. Some have already made the step from student to graduate and have use only for the earlier portions of the book, the sections designed to help increase their ability to manage the care of patients. This last chapter is primarily for those who are beginning their practice as professional nurses. It is guidance on developing a reintegrated professional nursing role and advice on seeking a position. Also, it offers suggestions for dealing with the reactions you may experience as a new graduate.

Chapter 18

Your first position

Your First Position as A Reintegrated Professional Nurse

Chapter One mentions the concept of the role of the Reintegrated Professional Nurse. This text has focused on the managerial aspects which are often a part of a professional nurse's clinical position. In contrast, this chapter emphasizes a view of the basic elements of one's professional role, a reintegrated role which returns the elements of clinical practice, educative function, scholarly activity, and community service to the basic definition of any professional nurse role. This reintegrated role definition is seen as the basis for planning one's career path, for selecting a first position, and for fitting together personal and professional life.

The concept of reintegration of professional nursing was first described by Langford, et al, as it guided development in the Texas Tech University Health Sciences Center School of Nursing.[1]

> Reintegration is a term chosen to reflect our belief about how professional nursing must proceed at this point in tis development. Re-, means "again" and implies that at some previous time the situation/act/concept was complete. *Integrate* means to " bring together parts of a whole" These are the basic elements of the word *reintegrate*. The action this describes is what we believe professional nursing requires, a bringing back together of what was and should be a whole, nursing. Reintegration, then is a verb form that functions as a noun, and can describe both the process and product of efforts to bring about this return to wholeness for our profession. As we view reintegration of nursing, it is the process of creating a whole, professional nursing, by the synthesis of clinical practice, educative function, scholarly activity, and community and institutional

[1] Teddy Langford,et al. "Past Unification to Reintegration: One School's Effort to Emphasize Wholeness in Professional Nursing" *Journal of Professional Nursing, 13,No.6, (Nov./Dec.,1987)362-371.*

service. We view these elements as being present in the "whole" of professional nursing in varying amounts, depending on one's choice of professional employment role. Thus, a reintegrated professional role might be carried out in one way if a person practices in a hospital and in another way if one is a member of a faculty. But, in each case, the role's definition would encompass all elements of the professional role, not only the parts emphasized if one takes a "job" view of professional function.[2]

The parts of the whole of professional nursing have become increasingly differentiated, seeming at times almost to have disparate purposes. Therefore, efforts at integration are required. *Reintegration* describes this effort best because it emphasizes a pre-existing wholeness, rather than a creation of a completely new entity. After all, each of the elements of nursing that we preface with the word "nursing" were once historically connected or integrated.[3]

With reintegration as a guiding concept, one might be tempted to see it as a prescription for life. Not so. For good health and personal development, each of us must establish a balance between the personal and professional aspects of our lives. Certainly there will be areas of overlap among role aspects. Yet when one sees only friends and colleagues who share the same profession or job site, when one's only social outings are aimed toward improving professional opportunities, when accepting frequent overtime at work means no time for family activities and insufficient rest, this balance is disturbed. In the same way, when the professional role shrinks from the full reintegrated set to only the clinical aspects, the professional view has been eliminated, what is left is a job. (See Figure 18.1.)

Value of Reintegration as a Guiding Concept

Planning professional goals is one especially beneficial use of the idea of reintegration of professional nursing. Beyond annual goals, using the planning guide can help clarify desirable career goals for extended periods of time. Of course, as with any other plan, career planning should be flexible, so that one's opportunities are not inappropriately limited. (See Fig. 18.2)

2 Ibid. p.362
3 Ibid p.363

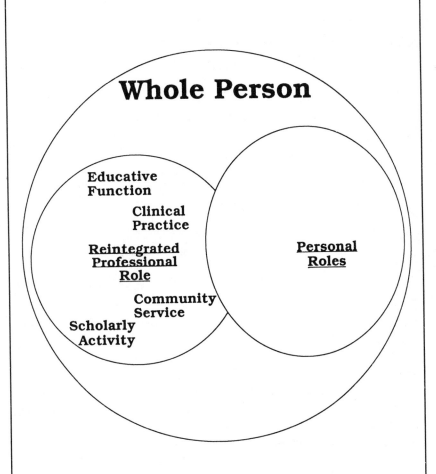

Figure 18.1 Relating Reintegrated Professional and Personal Roles

ROLE AREA/PROFESSIONAL	GOALS
CLINICAL	
EDUCATIVE	
SCHOLARLY/SYSTEMATIC INQUIRY	
COMMUNITY SERVICE	
OTHER JOB RELATED ROLE AREA	
CREATING THE WHOLE (DESCRIBE HOW ACTIVITIES FOR VARIOUS GOALS CAN HELP MEET OTHER GOALS, HOW GOALS ARE COMPLE-MENTARY, AND HOW)	

Figure 18.2 Planning for Reintegration

Consider each role area and speculate about goals/activities in each area that interest you or to which you aspire. What would you like to be doing in 5 years? After considering each of the four areas, ask yourself these questions:

- Have I considered the priority of goals in my personal life to see if the personal and professional are compatible?
- Will the goals and interests I have listed work together so that my energies are conserved as I pursue my goals?
- Are the goals realistic in combination, in conjunction with my personal level of stamina?
- Are the goals consistent with my education?
- Will my experience and opportunities in the position(s) I have or seek help meet these goals?

Answers to these questions will help you refine your career goals. The concept of a reintegrated professional role can give guidance and a high priority on balancing personal and professional life will help maintain human wholeness.

Beyond these values, a view of oneself as practicing a reintegrated role can reduce your sense of dependence on a single job. The very idea that you are a member of a profession, of a community of colleagues, encourages you to know that you are in charge of deciding to be in your job, that you are not trapped, that you do have choices. With this goes a sense of professional identity that returns quality to your efforts in each aspect of your reintegrated professional nurse role. Consider this perspective as you read the following paragraphs.

Finding Your Job

The business of finding and securing a position can be a challenging task, especially if you set out to find the best job for you rather than simply taking the first one offered. Careful thought is necessary to decide what sort of position to pursue and how to go about presenting yourself to the nursing service there. The type of position you set out to get should be chosen as a result of your interest and your abilities. A plan that includes some estimate of what you would like to be doing at the end of one year or at the end of two years will help you clarify directions. For example if you have to be ready in two years to enter graduate school, you may consider general medical-surgical practice in a hospital a good first step toward deciding what specialty to pursue in graduate school. If more education is not in your near future plans, perhaps you would want to enter a practice area that you did well in as a student, so that you can do well and advance quickly in your position, especially if you plan to stay in one geographic area for a long time. Table 18.1 lists a series of questions that you may ask yourself in regard to your job-seeking decision.

Suppose that after you consider all of these questions, you have narrowed the possiblities of positions to seek down to one geographic area, one type of health care agency, and one or two types of positions. Now, you can begin to be more specific. Are there other factors that are absolutes that would limit your choices? For example, will you only consider a 3-11 shift, since that is when you seem to be at your best? Or will you only look for jobs that are near to or offer child care? List any *real limitations, but be certain that your reason is firm before a concern becomes an absolute limitation.*

TABLE 18.1 Questions to Answer Before Seeking a Job

Where (geographically) would I like to live? (If I have made a location choice already, where will I live?

What am I most comfortable with in nursing; what do I do well?

What do I want to prepare for doing two to five years from now? What other interests will I want to maintain, and how will certain positions affect these?

Do I want to do something new, try a new type of life-style now? If so, what type of position or location is most conducive?

Do I have responsibilities that my job will influence, such as child care needs?

Do I want to work full-time or part-time?

Which of these items takes priority in affecting may choice of positions? Now you are ready to seek information about available positions. Consult all of the following sources (see Table 18.2). The first three items in Table 18.2 are the typical sources most nurse applicants consult. The "possibles" list developed from these sources is real, indicating presently available jobs. However, other vacant positions may exist and may be quite attractive. For example, a hospital with relatively low turnover rates may not find it necessary to begin to advertise since person-to-person information may result in a sufficient pool of applicants. Positions may also be listed with state and/or city employment services. These services do not charge a fee and are usually notified quickly about state or city personnel system positions.

Although there are some positions that are listed with commercial (private) employment services, other sources such as classified advertisements and city or state agencies probably furnish all necessary information and will save you the fee charged by the private agencies. The main types of positions for which commercial (private) services are really very helpful in nursing, either for nurses or employers, are the top-level administrative positions when a national search is required.

The telephone book can be a guide to potential places of employment. You can call the nursing service or personnel department of any agencies that appeal to you to find whether vacancies exist. This technique will result in a list of places to begin your job seeking, if you are in a city.

TABLE 18.2 Typical Sources of Information Regarding Nursing Positions

---

Individual Personal Contacts - Your Colleague Network

Professional journals.

State and district nurses association newsletters.

City telephone books.

City or state employment services.

Other employment service or nurse service agencies.

If, however, you are interested in practice in a rural area, you may need to identify general geographic areas of interest and then plan to consider the health care facilities in several small towns in those areas. Some facilities may be actively advertising, but others may have had so little response in the past as to discourage them from doing so.

Other possible positions exist in the armed forces, government volunteer agencies such as the Peace Corp, and religious orders; but these will not be considered here because the selection and recruiting process for these depends primarily on some initial decisions to make a long-term life-style commitment, a very individual consideration.

The information that follows regarding presenting yourself and seeking information about the organization will be useful for those who have made this type of long term decision, as well as for those who are simply seeking a good first position as a graduate professional nurse.

Resumé or Not

The list of possible positions that you have now assembled is the begining of your search activities. The next step is the application. Depending on time and distance, call or write the agencies to which you want to apply to request information and application material. If you do telephone, make notes of date and request as well the name of the person with whom you spoke. You can then confirm your request in writing if you do not receive the materials immediately.

Some individuals prefer to send a personal resumé along with the request for information and application. Although there is nothing against this, it seems more useful to save the resumé until you receive application materials since, for entry-level positions, no applicants would be (1) ruled out on the basis of a resumé and/or (2) considered without complete agency application forms. Therefore, the resumé has no real purpose. This situation changes as you become eligible for more specialized positions. At that point, if you seek a new position, a resumé can be a quick way to let a health care facility see if there is a possible match between your qualifications and its need.

Even as you look for entry-level jobs, a prepared resumé can be a useful guide in completing the agency application forms. If your resumé contains all the pertinent facts, you will not need to stop and try to recall your last supervisor's name or the statement about professional goals that you wrote. If you cultivate the habit of keeping a resumé and updating it periodically, it will save time and effort and result in a thorough and complete presentation of your qualification whenever needed. The guide below (see Table 18.3) indicates the types of information usually included in a professional resumé.

TABLE 18.3 Resumé Content

Personal Information

Name
Date of birth
Present address
Nursing license number and state in which licensed.
Social Security number

Professional Experience

Position title, name, and location of agency, brief description of functions and responsibilities. If you were promoted or responsibility was increased, state that.
Name of direct supervisor may also be included here.
If this is your first nursing position, you can list previous jobs held, if any.
As you gain experience in nursing, you can separate nursing from nonnursing positions and drop the nonnursing after two or more years of experience in nursing.

Educational Background

Schools, Date of completion, degrees or certificate.
Additional special educational activities (such as continuing education activities).

Special Achievements

List any major honors or awards you have received or any special projects.

Professional Organizations

List membership in professional organizations and indicate any offices held.

Community Service/Institutional Service

Memberships
Committee responsibilities

Scholarly Interests

Describe succinctly your area(s) of interest in application or conduct of research, professional inquiry.

Personal interests

This can be a brief statement indicating you major avocational interests.

Professional Goals

This should indicate what you plan for your professional future, especially as the position currently sought may relate to it.

There is no single right way to prepare a resumé, so evaluate your materials with the perspective of the agency in mind. Certainly you should have the document typewritten on good quality paper. Conservative presentation is better than "cute". Also, it is acceptable to add an additional page to an agency application to provide information that is not requested but that you may want to furnish, such as your goals statement or description of a major project you were responsible for in your last position.

The Interview

After you have submitted your application, or perhaps even as you receive the materials, you will set a time for an interview. If you have not heard from an agency within a maximum of two weeks after submitting your application, call to clarify the status of you application. Be certain that there is an answer to whether (1) the application has been received; (2) it is being considered, you will hear about an interview no later than --; (3) it is no longer being considered, no interview scheduled; or (4) the agency wants to schedule an interview now.

If you find that the application has been rejected, you might benefit from any feedback you could gain by asking if there is a specific reason for the decision and why you had not been notified. Although any agency may have selected other applicants due to a variety of good reasons, there is little reason to justify failure to notify applicants that they are no longer being considered. It is worthwhile to ask, when applications are submitted, if there is a negative reporting system, meaning that if you do not hear something in a specified period to time, you may correctly assume that the position has been filled. Sheer volume of applications make this rather impersonal system necessary in some agencies, so it is to your benefit to know if this is the method in use.

The initial interview may be conducted by someone from the personnel department or an interviewer from the nursing department, or both, depending on the agency. The concern from you perspective should be whether you can gain the information you need in the interview, as well as presenting yourself for consideration. Do not hesitate to ask for other sources if you lack the answers you need as the interview nears an end.

Punctuality is important for the interview. Since you may be unfamiliar with the agency's location, be certain to allow plenty of time for travel. If you arrive early, it will give you time to get a sense of the atmosphere of the agency as you wait. In some agencies, you may be requested to complete other application forms or material when you are on site; so plan to take your license, social security number, and other such basic information along for reference.

Of course, appropriate attire is a factor in making a good impression on interviews. There are no "glove and hat, or suit and tie" rules today as there once were, but good judgment about what is too casual or too dressy should be your guides in selecting what you will wear to your interview. Again, consider the interviewer's perspective as someone who does not know you, in making your choices of what to wear.

During the interview, you should attempt to answer questions completely but without excessive rambling, and make an effort to focus on the interviewer in order to reduce anxiety you may feel. Make the assumption that the interviewer is positive toward you.

Take a small note pad so that you can take notes on any facts you want to retain for comparison. The same pad can be useful for holding brief reminders of questions you want to be certain to ask. Remember that this interview is for your benefit as well as the agency's, so do not hesitate to ask questions as the opportunity presents itself. The position should be clear to you, its responsibilities stated, and the lines of responsibility specified by the time the interview is complete. You should know all the specific details about the job such as shift rotation, type of assignments, benefits, salary range, and potential for advancement as well as when you will be notified about the position.

In addition, you should be sure that you have had an opportunity to describe your strong points, your previous experience, and any other special personal abilities or special concerns such as the time by which a job decision will be made. It is helpful, if the interviewer does not take the initiative to do so, to summarize the major points before the interview is concluded. Simply say, "Before I leave, I would like to check briefly to see if I have correct information." Then state briefly the major points of the interview. Follow that with, "Are there any other questions that you might want to ask me? I have enjoyed the opportunity to talk with you. Thank you."

You may be thinking, "I couldn't possibly do that." Perhaps that's because you have not practiced this sort of behavior. But you have interviewed patients, have conducted teaching conferences, and have met with teachers many times. The big difference is the newness of the situation. You have the skills to handle it, but you may not have used them in this type of situation before. One good way to prepare is to role-play the interview. Another nursing student can be your partner, or perhaps you know someone who has interviewed through the campus placement service with corporation representatives who would be willing to role-play the situation. Ask for feedback on your performance and analyze your own reactions to the situation, in order to be well prepared.

As you go through the interviews, you will begin to compare agency with agency and job with job. Try to withhold a final judgment until you have finished all of your interviews and can make a careful decision among the job offers you will receive based on the concerns you identified before you began seeking a job. An impulsive "yes" to a dramatic looking job in the burn unit may not be wise for the person who really functions best in a slower-paced atmosphere. The fact that an agency may press you for an answer is flattering but should not prompt you to be less than judicious since your reaction to positions early in your career can color your reaction to all of nursing.

Adjusting and Enjoying

The previous chapters have provided information on theories, principles, and processes useful in managing and being managed as a professional nurse. As you move from student to a beginning nurse practicing a reintegrated professional role, you may find that you are at times surprised by the differences between being a student and being a professional and by your reactions to those differences. Perhaps you have been employed in nursing while you were a student. Even so, you may find that the two sorts of employment prompt different reactions from you. Because such reactions are not uncommon, this final note contains some advice regarding adjustment to your new function as a professional nurse.

Why These Reactions?

There are probably a number of individual personal reasons why you find yourself reacting to your new role. Some of the several possibilities are the following: expectations, multiple life changes, concerns about competence, and the burden of responsibility and accountability.

In the book *Reality Shock* and several subsequent publications, Dr. Marlene Kramer described the reaction of many new nurse graduates entering practice.[4] These individuals have a preconceived notion of the role they will enact and are frequently influenced by strong idealism and high hopes

4 Marlene Kramer, *Reality Shock* (St. Louis,Mo.: C. V. Mosby,1974).

for personal success and satisfaction. When they enter practice, their expectations, which may in some cases be unrealistically high, are often not met. They find that some of the people they work with seem uncaring and uninterested in their work. They encounter poor nursing care and some questionable medical practice. Their supervisor may maintain an attitude toward accomplishment of treatment and routine that seems incompatible with individualized care. Thus, the new graduates may go for weeks at a time without a definite plan for the care of any patient and seldom feel satisfied with the day's accomplishments. Their expectations about work and their roles do not match the reality they encounter.

Kramer described the result of this situation as "role deprivation" and noted that some experience it to a much greater degree than others.[5] The responses to this reaction vary, but for many it means leaving nursing, or less drastic but perhaps more eventually problematic, they return to graduate school to become teachers of nursing. These responses are usually the long-term ones, taking from six months to several years after graduation.

The more immediate responses include anger, depression and/or stress-related somatic problems like fatigue, inability to concentrate, irritablity, and sleep disturbances. Kramer's solution is to present the students with opportunities to deal with the conflicting demands of work reality and with the resulting asault on their professional ideals *before* they actually enter the professional world. She describes this as a sort of inoculation against reality shock, a way to help the new nurse find integrative solutions to conflicting role demands.[6]

Another source of reaction may not relate to the position at all. Rather, it may relate to the series of major like changes surrounding the move from student to graduate and subsequently to the new job. This series of changes may involve any or all of the following: new geographic location, new living quarters, change in roommates/housemate/spouse, changes in friendship interaction, change in amount of time available for leisure activity, need to reorganize/reorder priorities, and change from casual to more professional type of interaction. There is the potential that although any one or all of these factors may not produce stress effects for some individuals, they may for others. If the stress is greater than the individual can adapt to readily, several stress-related responses can occur, including anxiety, irritability, fatigue, and even a wide range of physical symptoms.

A third source of reaction to beginning to function as a professional is the major difference in scope and degree of responsibliity for self and

5 Ibid.
6 Ibid.

others (both staff and patients), between the student status and your new situation. Athough you have expected and been eager to merit the responsiblity, you may find that you spend a good deal of energy coping with this new weight that you carry. You are confronted with the fact that work cannot be "cut" like class could be without affecting the lives of others. Those affected include both coworkers and patients. Even if you are working only part-time or for a supplemental service agency where you go on different assignments each day, someone is expecting you to be there when you have said you will.

Dealing With Your Reactions

The physical and mental results of the reactions you are experiencing can be frustrating, even frightening, if you do not realize their relation to your experiences. One important factor in dealing with this period of reaction is regular rest and adequate diet and exercise. As trite as that may sound, a careful analysis may lead to your recognizing that you have been missing lunch five days out of seven and that your new schedule has changed your hours of sleep. Perhaps you have missed your game of tennis for three weeks and no longer bicycle each day. The advice you would give your patients is good for you also. That is, make a plan to take care of your health through a routine of good diet, exercise, and rest. Although this plan may not cure your aggravation or your feelings of anger if you are disappointed with reality, it can help reduce the negative effect that excessive stress can have.

Dealing with the reasons for negative reaction may be more complex than the "good health" efforts. It will require that you consider carefully, *before* you take a position, what your expectations are and, in addition, examine whether they are realistic. Can you really expect to have the shift, the specialty, the type of assignment, the pay rate, the environment, and the type or orientation you would like, all within walking distance of an apartment you love? Or can you list in priority order the factors that are most important to you? After that, can you specify for yourself just *why* a certain item is high on your priority list? Why, for example, is it important to you that primary nursing be the assignment method used? Is it because that is the only way patients can receive good care, because that is what your instructor told you, or because you have carefully examined each other assignment method and found them inadequate? When you have a clear notion about your "must have" items, you are then in a better position to make decisions about jobs. You can ask questions that will be sufficiently specific to tell you about what you will find as actual practice, not simply what the stated philosophy of the nursing service is. You can explain what you want in a job and ask if you are likely to be able to find it at the agency with which you are interviewing. You can attempt to evaluate the fit between you and the job you are offered.

The reactions caused by the stress of several simultaneous life changes is best amenable to careful planning. Can you make your new house move a bit later, so that it does not coincide exactly with both the new job and the beginning of a new diet? A key to knowing just how much you might handle gracefully is whether you continue to feel that you are in charge of what you are doing. The feeling of being disorganized, pushed, out of control, or "done to" are signals that too many things are acting as stressors at one time. Adjustment of plans and, again, the regular exercise, rest, and good diet are all helpful in making such difficult times less so.

And After the Newness Wears Off

One day, without realizing it is happening, you will no longer consider yourself a new graduate. Rather, you will think of yourself as a nurse. More than that, if you are enjoying yourself, you will think of yourself as a nurse, a reintegrated professional nurse. More than that, if you are enjoying yourself, you will think of yourself as a *person* who is a nurse. In hopes that that will happen, one last bit of advice is offered here. Do not allow the rest of your person to be overshadowed by the professional concerns you may have. The energy you can devote to helping others can only come from a whole and healthy person who has a strong sense of interest in life and a reverence for its value. Cultivate that by allowing your own full development as a person. Have hobbies, avocational pursuits, friends, and fun. Build a support system for yourself that does not depend at all upon your being a nurse but rather upon your being you. Enjoy!

Additional Reading

McDonagh, Kathryn J. and Mary Ann Sorensen. "Restructuring Nursing Salaries: A Mandate for the Future" *Nursing Management*, 19:2(February,1988)39-41.

Langford, Teddy, N. Ridenour, K. Dadich, P. Wise, H. Cox, S. Axton, B. Harsanyi, and S. Cooke, "Past Unification to Reintegration : One School's Effort to Emphasize Wholeness in Professional Nursing" *Journal of Professional Nursing*, 3 No.6(Nov/Dec,1987)362-371.

Index

A

B

C

D

E

F